WP 870 RAY

Medical Therapy of Breast Cancer

There have been very significant advances across many areas of the study, investigation and treatment of breast cancer. This new publication brings these developments fully up to date and surveys how scientific advances have influenced, improved and extended modern therapeutic options. The volume spans prevention, screening, genetics and treatment of preinvasive breast cancer, before focusing in depth on modern management of established breast cancer. This includes chapters on the various therapeutic options available and their role in treating breast cancer from the very earliest stage through to advanced and metastatic breast cancer. In addition, the text looks forward at the potential for emerging experimental strategies to become adopted into medical management in the future. The volume concludes with a chapter on palliative care.

This wide-ranging modern account will be essential for breast cancer specialists, trainees in oncology and clinical research scientists.

Zenon Rayter is Consultant Surgeon at Bristol Royal Infirmary and Honorary Senior Lecturer at the University of Bristol. He is Director of the Bristol Breast Unit and Vice President of the Surgical Section of the Royal Society of Medicine.

Janine Mansi is Consultant Medical Oncologist and Honorary Senior Lecturer at St George's Hospital Medical School, and also Lead Clinician for Cancer Services for the Trust, and an executive member of the Association of Cancer Physicians.

This book is due for return on or before the last date shown below.

Medical Therapy of Breast Cancer

Edited by

Zenon Rayter

Bristol Royal Infirmary, Bristol

and

Janine Mansi

St George's Hospital, London

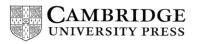

CAMBRIDGE
UNIVERSITY PRESS

PUBLISHED BY THE PRESS SYNDICATE OF THE UNIVERSITY OF CAMBRIDGE
The Pitt Building, Trumpington Street, Cambridge, United Kingdom

CAMBRIDGE UNIVERSITY PRESS
The Edinburgh Building, Cambridge CB2 2RU, UK
40 West 20th Street, New York NY 10011-4211, USA
477 Williamstown Road, Port Melbourne, VIC 3207, Australia
Ruiz de Alarcón 13, 28014 Madrid, Spain
Dock House, The Waterfront, Cape Town 8001, South Africa

http://www.cambridge.org

First published 2003

Printed in the United Kingdom at the University Press, Cambridge

Typeface Minion 10.5/14pt   *System* Poltype® [V N]

A catalogue record for this book is available from the British Library

Library of Congress Cataloguing in Publication data

Medical therapy of breast cancer/edited by Zenon Rayter and Janine Mansi.
      p.   cm.
Includes bibliographical references and index.
ISBN 0 521 49632 2
1. Breast – Cancer – Treatment.   I. Rayter, Zenon, 1951–   II. Mansi, Janine, 1955–
RC280.B8 M42 2002
616.99′44906 – dc21   2001043947

ISBN 0 521 49632 2 hardback

Contents

6   The management of in situ breast cancer   126

Zenon Rayter

9   Predictors of response and resistance to medical therapy   209

9a   Cell kinetic parameters and response to therapy   210
R. S. Camplejohn

10   Primary medical therapy in breast cancer   264

Janine L. Mansi

11   Medical therapy of advanced disease   283

Alison Jones and Karen McAdam

Contributors

R. S. Camplejohn
Senior Lecturer
Richard Dimbleby Department of Cancer
Research
Guy's, King's and St Thomas' School of
Medicine
St Thomas' Hospital
London, UK

John Crown
Consultant Medical Oncologist
St Vincent's University Hospital
Elm Park
Dublin, Ireland

A. G. Dalgleish
Professor of Oncology and Visiting
Professor
Institute of Cancer Research
Department of Oncology
St George's Hospital Medical School
Cranmer Terrace
London, UK

T. R. J. Evans
Senior Lecturer and Honorary Consultant
in Medical Oncology
CRC Department of Medical Oncology
University of Glasgow, UK

Rosalind Given-Wilson
Consultant Radiologist
Duchess of Kent Breast Screening Unit
Blackshaw Road
London, UK

H. Gogas
Clinical Research Fellow in Medical
Oncology
St George's Hospital
Blackshaw Road
London, UK

Janet Hardy
Department of Palliative Medicine
The Royal Marsden Hospital
Downs Road
Sutton
Surrey, UK

Tamas Hickish
Consultant Medical Oncologist
Poole General Hospital
Longfleet Road
Poole
Dorset, UK

Stephen R. D. Johnston
Senior Lecturer and Honorary Consultant
The Royal Marsden Hospital
Fulham Road
London, UK

Alison Jones
Consultant Medical Oncologist
Royal Free Hospital
Pond Street
London, UK

David Landau
Clinical Research Fellow
The Royal Marsden Hospital
London, UK

R. C. F. Leonard
Professor of Cancer Studies
University of Wales
Swansea, UK

Janine L. Mansi
Consultant Medical Oncologist
Department of Medical Oncology
St George's Hospital
Blackshaw Road
London, UK

J. Marsden
Clinical Research Fellow
The Royal Marsden and St George's
Hospital Trusts
London, UK

Karen McAdam
Macmillan Consultant Medical Oncologist
Peterborough District Hospital
Thorpe Road
Peterborough, UK

V. Murday
Consultant Clinical Geneticist
St George's Hospital
London, UK

A. H. G. Paterson
Tom Baker Cancer Centre and
University of Calgary
Canada

Zenon Rayter
Consultant Surgeon
Bristol Royal Infirmary
Bristol, UK

Gillian Ross
Senior Lecturer in Clinical Oncology
Institute of Cancer Research
London, UK

N. P. M. Sacks
Consultant Surgeon and Head of Breast
Unit
The Royal Marsden and St George's
Hospital Trusts
London, UK

Andrew Tutt
Clinical Research Fellow
Institute for Cancer Research
London, UK

History of breast cancer therapy

Zenon Rayter

Bristol Royal Infirmary, Bristol, UK

History of surgery for breast cancer

Introduction

Breast cancer is an ancient disease and was described by the Egyptians 3000 years before Christ. Subsequently various articles about breast cancer and its treatment were written by Greek and Roman physicians. Surgery is the oldest method of treating breast cancer with different operations described which sometimes reflected beliefs held about its causes and natural history. However, a variety of 'medical' therapies have also been described, especially in the Middle Ages, which to the modern observer were more akin to witchcraft than the application of scientific knowledge to the treatment of the disease. Changing fashions in the treatment of breast cancer have reflected not only changes in beliefs regarding its pathogenesis but also a growth in knowledge about the disease as well as advances in science and technology. Thus four periods can be discerned in the evolution of treatment over the centuries. The first period could be described as the Empiric era of the pre-Galen period. Subsequently, breast cancer was regarded as a systemic disease and this characterized the Pessimistic period. By the eighteenth century, breast cancer was thought to be a local disease leading to the Optimistic era in which it was believed that larger operations than performed previously could eradicate the disease. By the twentieth century, knowledge about the biology of breast cancer had started to grow which led to a realization that breast cancer was a more complex disease than previously had been supposed and led to the establishment of the Realistic era in which we now find ourselves. The twentieth century also saw the introduction of radiotherapy in the treatment of breast cancer, and medical therapy began to emerge from its primitive treatment concepts of the Dark Ages to emerge as a major new therapeutic tool. Philosophically, the emergence of medical therapy was conceptually different to that of surgery (apart from surgical endocrine manipulation) in that it was a systemic therapy as opposed to a local therapy. The emergence of these non-surgical modes of treatment has been pivotal to the way that surgery has changed in the management of breast cancer over the last 50 years.

The empiric period

The earliest record of breast cancer comes from the Edwin Smith surgical papyrus which dates from Egyptian times (3000–2500 BC) and describes eight cases of tumours or ulcers of the breast, the writer admitting that there was no treatment, although one case was treated by cauterization with a fire stick. Writings dating from 2000 BC on cuneiform tablets from Assyria only mention the occurrence of breast cancer, but those from India mention the treatment of breast cancers with surgical excision, cautery and arsenic compounds. The first recorded 'cure' is credited by Herodotus (484–425 BC) to Democedes, a Persian physician living in Greece who treated the wife of King Darius. The most famous of Greek physicians, Hippocrates (460–370 BC) mentioned breast cancer only twice and advised no treatment. The early Romans performed extensive surgery for cancer of the breast, including removal of the pectoral muscles, although the Roman scholar Aulus Cornelius Celsus (42 BC–37 AD) advised against surgery, caustic medicines and cautery.

The pessimistic period

Galen (131–203 AD), the legendary Greek physician who worked among the Romans refined Hippocrates' theory that breast cancer was caused 'by the particular humor that prevails in the body'. Galen attributed cancer to an excess of black bile in the body. This systemic concept must have accorded well with the prospects of cure for women with breast cancer. Despite this, Galen excised those tumours that were removable, recommending excision through surrounding healthy tissue. The control of haemorrhage was by the use of pressure on surrounding veins as ligatures were thought to cause local recurrence of breast cancer. Leonidus (180 AD) was more concerned about haemorrhage and he used the knife and cautery alternately as he proceeded around the tumour until the breast had been amputated. This method of amputation as well as the avoidance of ligatures persisted for more than 1000 years and must have been a totally horrific experience without anaesthesia.

Little progress was made during the Dark Ages and surgery was discouraged by the Church, cautery and caustics remaining the mainstay of treatment. In France, Ambrose Paré (1510–90) excised small breast tumours but substituted sulphuric acid for hot cautery. Large tumours were treated with milk, ointment and vinegar. A variety of other topical treatments in this era included goat's dung, frogs, laying on of (preferably royal) hands and compression of the tumour with lead plates. Towards the end of the sixteenth century, new techniques were introduced to surgery, Vesalius (1514–64) used ligatures instead of hot cautery when excising breast cancers. Guillemeau (1550–1601) advocated removal of the pectoralis muscle along with the breast. Severinus (1580–1659) advocated removal of axillary lymph nodes along with the breast and both he and Paré were among the first to appreciate that axillary lymph nodes were part of the malignant process. During the seventeenth century, various instruments began to be developed which allowed very rapid amputation of the breast, perhaps in as little as 2 or 3 seconds. The majority of these techniques involved using metal rings or forks to transfix the breast and distract it from the chest wall, thereby allowing rapid amputation with either a knife or a hinged scythe. The large wounds thus created took months to heal and therefore these were gradually abandoned. During this period cancer remained conceptually a systemic disease. After the discovery of the lymphatic system, Descartes (1596–1650) proposed a lymph theory of the origin of breast cancer that was perpetuated by John Hunter (1728–93), who taught that breast cancer arose when defective lymph coagulated. This was conceptually little better than Galen's black bile theory, but it may have been a stimulus for encouraging surgeons to remove obviously affected axillary lymph nodes.

The optimistic period

In 1757, a French surgeon, Henry LeDran, advanced the theory that cancer began in its earliest stages as a local disease (LeDran, 1757), spread first to the lymph nodes and subsequently entered the circulation. This theory offered the hope that surgery might cure the disease if performed sufficiently early. Other surgeons embraced this pivotal concept during the nineteenth century and it gradually replaced the humoral theory of breast cancer, although, almost a century later, Henry Arnott still felt obliged to reiterate the local origin of breast cancer (Arnott, 1871). With the acceptance of the local origin of cancer, the principles of curative surgery were to perform wide *en bloc* operations at the earliest moment. As early as 1773, Bernard Peyrilhe advised an operation that removed the cancerous breast with the axillary contents and the pectoralis muscle, the same operation introduced by William Halsted 100 years later. Lorensius Heister (1683–1758) removed ribs as well if necessary, an operation still occasionally performed today for stable local disease.

During the nineteenth century great advances were made in science and medicine that included the introduction of general anaesthesia in 1846, antisepsis in 1867 and microscopic pathology. By the end of the nineteenth century, Beatson had demonstrated that breast cancer was hormonally dependent in at least a proportion of patients (Beatson, 1896) and X-rays and radium had been discovered. The results of surgery for cancer of the breast at this time were still poor, partly because of a high operative mortality (up to 20%) due to overwhelming infection. Even those patients who survived rarely lived longer than 2 years. Sir James Paget (the eminent surgeon from Guy's Hospital, London) confessed to never having seen a cure. However, the two forces that pushed radical surgery forward were the theory of local origin and the need to eliminate local recurrence, and these reinforced each other.

In 1867, Charles Moore at the Middlesex Hospital in London renewed the case for the local origin of breast cancer when he published a paper in which he observed that recurrences after limited operations for breast cancer were generally near the scar and that their pattern suggested centrifugal spread from the original site (Moore, 1867). His principles of surgical cure were to remove the whole breast (including as much skin as was felt to be 'unsound'), avoiding cutting into the tumour, and removal of diseased axillary glands as advocated by Peyrihle nearly 100 years earlier. The importance of Moore's paper lies in the fact that it produced evidence for the local origin of breast cancer and the routine removal of the breast is clearly traceable to Moore. Routine removal of the axillary glands is also believed to be due to Moore's influence as although he originally advocated the routine removal of 'diseased' glands, he subsequently became aware of the difficulty in knowing whether the glands were involved or not and stated that they can never be assumed to be normal (Power, 1934–35). Banks in Liverpool subsequently continued to argue for routine axillary surgery and in a paper presented in 1882, he reported 46 cases in whom he had routinely removed axillary nodes (Banks, 1902). Küster in Berlin had also advocated routine axillary dissection with mastectomy as early as 1871 (Küster, 1883) with the effect of drastically reducing axillary recurrence to 1% (Schmid, 1887). The next structure to receive attention was the pectoralis fascia. With the advent of the microscope and developments in pathological anatomy, it was discovered that the pectoralis fascia was occasionally microscopically involved with tumour not obvious to the naked eye. Von Volkman in Germany was one of the first to supplement removal of the breast and axillary contents with routine removal of the pectoralis fascia (Halsted, 1894–95). A view that went further was proposed by Heidenhain, after microscopically examining Küster's cases, who suggested removal of the entire pectoralis muscle if the cancer was infiltrating part of the fascia or muscle (Heidenhain, 1889).

William Halsted, professor of surgery at Johns Hopkins Hospital in Baltimore, USA was aware of developments in Germany and also advocated removal of the entire pectoralis major muscle save occasionally for its clavicular portion. Halsted's operation employed a tear-drop incision, removing so much skin that grafting was subsequently required, removing the whole breast, pectoralis major and the axillary contents after dividing pectoralis minor. In 1894 he published the results of 50 patients so treated with a dramatic fall in local recurrence to 6%

compared with the 56–81% reported in Europe (Halsted, 1894–95). By the current definition of local recurrence this would actually represent 18% over a relatively short follow-up. Nevertheless, after 37 years, this had only risen to 31.5% in this group of patients (Lewis & Rienhoff, 1932). The radical mastectomy was an operation whose time had arrived. Professor Willie Meyer of the New York Postgraduate Medical School reported a similar operation in 1894 (Meyer, 1894). The differences in details of the operative technique were that Meyer used a diagonal incision, dissected the axillary contents first and excised pectoralis minor, a modification which Halsted subsequently adopted. The radical mastectomy operation was supported conceptually by the centrifugal permeation theory proposed by William Sampson Handley of London, who stated that cancers originated at one focus and spread from it exclusively through lymphatics. This lymphatic spread was by growth in continuity (permeation) rather than embolic spread and occurred equally in all directions. Regional lymph nodes halted the progress of permeation only temporarily, but thereafter growth through the lymph nodes allowed haematogenous embolization (Handley & Thackray, 1969). Such was Halsted's reputation as a teacher and surgeon, the radical mastectomy soon became the standard operation for breast cancer worldwide. However, the main achievement of this operation was the reduction of local recurrence rates compared with lesser operations and it became clear subsequently that little had been achieved in terms of overall survival. This may in part have been due to the fact that many patients who underwent radical mastectomy had relatively advanced disease. The contraindications to radical mastectomy were subsequently defined by Haagensen with improved results in terms of local recurrence and overall survival in line with better case selection and earlier diagnosis (Haagensen, 1971).

It soon became apparent that radical mastectomy did not cure patients with breast cancer and Halsted extended his operation by removing supraclavicular lymph nodes after dividing the clavicle. He also occasionally removed internal mammary lymph nodes and this procedure was lent support by the work of William Sampson Handley who advocated treatment of involved internal mammary nodes with interstitial radium (Handley, 1922). This line of study was extended by his son, Richard S. Handley, who routinely biopsied internal mammary lymph nodes during the performance of a radical mastectomy in a series of 119 patients and found metastases in 34% of patients. The radical mastectomy was subsequently extended by a number of surgeons to include removal of internal mammary lymph nodes (Sugarbaker, 1953; Urban, 1964). This 'extended' radical mastectomy was extended even further to include removal of the supraclavicular lymph nodes at the time of mastectomy (Dahl-Iverson & Tobiassen, 1969). Some surgeons even went as far as amputating the upper arm *en bloc* with the mastectomy specimen in an attempt to cure relatively advanced local disease (Prudente, 1949). This increasingly radical progression culminated with the 'super-radical' mastectomy in which the radical mastectomy was combined with excision of supraclavicular, internal mammary and mediastinal lymph nodes, first in two stages and later in one stage (Wangensteen et al., 1956). This procedure was later abandoned because of its high operative mortality of 12.5% and the lack of any improvement in long-term survival.

The realistic period

By the mid twentieth century, surgery for breast cancer had reached its limits. Surgeons began to critically reevaluate the efficacy of radical operations for several reasons. First, it became apparent that radical surgery was unable to cure breast cancer in over a third of patients. A greater awareness of postoperative morbidity such as deformity of the chest, lymphoedema of the arm and occasional irradiation-induced sarcomas led to some surgeons becoming increasingly critical of radical surgery and led to a reevaluation of less radical surgery for breast cancer. Secondly, there had been an enormous explosion of knowledge about the biology of breast cancer, killing off old theories of cancer spread and redefining the indications for surgery. Thirdly, the development of medical oncology added to the therapeutic armamentarium which was available to the extent that adjuvant hormonal therapy and chemotherapy was beginning to lead to statistically significant improvements in survival in patients at high risk of relapse (Chapter 3). Fourthly, earlier diagnosis, advocated for centuries by physicians, had become a reality with the development of high-quality mammography and the introduction of mass screening programmes to detect asymptomatic breast cancer in a number of countries including Sweden, Great Britain and the United States of America. Finally, the possibility of preventing breast cancer in high-risk probands is currently the subject of a number of studies using a variety of agents of which tamoxifen is the best-known example.

The rise and fall of endocrine surgery for metastatic disease

A final legacy of the nineteenth century was the discovery that breast cancer was a hormone dependent tumour, at least in some patients. It had been observed in the nineteenth century that the growth of breast cancer in patients sometimes fluctuated with the menstrual cycle and that the disease grew more slowly in postmenopausal women. However, the landmark observation was that by Thomas Beatson who observed temporary regression of metastatic breast cancer in two patients treated by surgical oophorectomy (Beatson, 1896). For the first time, a systemic treatment for breast cancer became available and its hormone dependence demonstrated. The importance of the hormonal milieu was subsequently confirmed by the use of adrenalectomy (Huggins & Bergenstal, 1951) and hypophysectomy (Luft & Olivecrona, 1953). In the one-third of patients who benefited, the mechanism by which this occurred was thought to be oestrogen deprivation and the scientific foundation for this was confirmed by the discovery of the oestrogen receptor (ER) in breast tumours (Jensen et al., 1967). Ablative endocrine surgery has now largely been superseded by the development of medical endocrine therapies. Thus, the oestrogen antagonist tamoxifen has mostly replaced surgical oophorectomy, the aromatase inhibitors (which block peripheral synthesis of oestrogens) have replaced adrenalectomy and the luteinizing hormone releasing hormone (LHRH) agonists have replaced hypophysectomy in the management of patients with metastatic breast cancer.

Introduction of radiation therapy for breast cancer

History

By the beginning of the twentieth century radiotherapy had been shown to be effective in treating breast cancer. Keynes, a surgeon at St Bartholomew's Hospital in London, described the results of conservative treatment of breast cancer using implanted radium needles (Keynes, 1937). Originally used in 50 patients with inoperable breast cancer in whom good local control was achieved, it was extended to 85 patients with stage I disease and 91 patients with stage II disease. Tumour was excised and radium needles were inserted throughout the breast, axilla, supraclavicular fossa and the upper three intercostal spaces. Five-year survival was 71% in patients with stage I disease and 29% in patients with stage II disease. These results appeared to be as good as those achieved by radical mastectomy, but despite this the technique was not widely used due to the limited availability of radium, handling problems and postradiation fibrosis.

In 1932, Pfahler from the United States reported the use of radiotherapy in 1022 patients with breast cancer, of whom 53 had early disease and who had refused or were too frail for surgery (Pfahler, 1932). The 5-year survival of patients with early disease was 80% and even patients with stage II disease fared better than historical controls. In Great Britain, Robert McWhirter of Edinburgh was the foremost proponent of radiotherapy in the mid-twentieth century and he reported the results of simple mastectomy followed by radiotherapy to the supraclavicular, internal mammary and axillary lymph nodes in 759 patients (McWhirter, 1948). The 5-year survival rate of 62% was comparable to that achieved by standard radical mastectomy, implying that radiotherapy was effective in treating nodal disease.

A logical extension of these observations was to investigate whether radiotherapy could be used to treat the primary breast tumour. Much of the pioneering work in this area was done at the Institut Curie in Paris. Thus Baclesse (1965) demonstrated that even relatively large cancers could be successfully treated by giving 66–70 Gy fractionated over a three-month period. Another technique which involved a combination of external beam radiotherapy and an iridium implant extended the role of radiotherapy further (Pierquin et al., 1980). The introduction of iridium implants in the USA (Hellman et al., 1980) popularized conservative surgery for breast cancer and in part was the stimulus to the randomized controlled trials of conservative surgery and radiotherapy subsequently described. Further efforts in this direction confirmed comparable survival to surgically treated patients with operable breast cancer but at the expense of high local morbidity (Hochman & Robinson, 1960). Higher energy sources developed in the 1950s reduced cutaneous morbidity and early survival results indicated that irradiation could be a possible alternative to mastectomy although the issues of long-term morbidity and local tumour control still needed to be addressed (Harris et al., 1983). The realization that long-term side-effects of adjuvant radiotherapy could be serious came with the publication of studies which demonstrated an increased mortality from myocardial infarction after radiotherapy for left-sided breast cancer (Cuzick et al., 1987, 1994).

The first randomized controlled trial of conservative surgery and radiotherapy versus radical mastectomy was performed at Guy's Hospital in London (Atkins et al., 1972). The conservative surgery group underwent only a wide local excision of their tumour and no axillary surgery and received 35–38 Gy to the breast and only 25–27 Gy to the supraclavicular fossa, internal mammary chain and the axilla, whereas the radical mastectomy group underwent an axillary clearance and the same dose of radiation to the gland fields as the conservative surgery group of patients. It was therefore not surprizing that there were significantly more loco-regional recurrences (notably in the axilla) in the wide local excision group (25%) than in the radical mastectomy group (7%). Overall 10-year survival was similar in patients with stage I disease (80%), but patients with stage II disease had a significantly worse survival in the wide local excision group (30%) compared with the radical mastectomy group (60%). This was an extremely important finding for two reasons. First, it probably delayed the more widespread adoption of conservative surgery for breast cancer and, secondly, it contradicted the popular belief at that time that local control did not influence survival.

Influence of radiotherapy on local control and survival

There is general agreement that the majority of patients undergoing conservative surgery for breast cancer should have radiotherapy. The indications for radiotherapy after mastectomy are less certain. In patients with good pathological prognostic factors (node negativity, absent lymphovascular invasion, tumour size <2 cm and clear margins) there is general agreement that postoperative radiotherapy is not required. In patients with one or more adverse prognostic factors (presence of lymphovascular invasion, >4 involved lymph nodes, tumour size >4 cm), most clinical oncologists would advise postoperative radiotherapy. It is in the group of patients who may only have one to three nodes involved or only one other adverse prognostic factor that the question of radiotherapy is more controversial. The importance of local control and its effect on survival has recently been highlighted again by the results of three recently published studies.

In the Danish study of high-risk premenopausal women (Overgaard et al., 1997) a total of 1708 women who had undergone mastectomy were randomized to have eight cycles of CMF (cyclophosphamide, methotrexate and 5-fluorouracil) plus radiotherapy to the chest wall or nine cycles of CMF alone. High risk was defined as axillary node involvement, tumour size >5 cm and invasion of skin or pectoral fascia. The median length of follow-up was 114 months. The frequency of locoregional recurrence alone or with distant metastases was 9% in the CMF + radiotherapy group compared with 32% in the CMF alone group. The probability of disease-free survival (DFS) was 48% in the CMF + radiotherapy group and only 34% in the CMF alone group. This translated to an absolute overall survival (OS) difference of 9% (54% for CMF + radiotherapy *versus* 45% for CMF alone). All these differences were highly statistically significant.

In the Canadian study (Ragaz et al., 1997) 318 high-risk premenopausal women undergoing modified radical mastectomy were randomized to receive CMF + radiotherapy or CMF alone. High risk in this study was defined as any pathological lymph node involvement. After 15 years of follow-up, the women assigned to CMF + radiotherapy had a 33% reduction in the rate of recurrence and a 29% reduction in mortality compared with the women randomized to CMF alone.

In the third study, this question was addressed in high-risk postmenopausal women (Overgaard et al., 1999). In this Danish study, 689 women were randomized to adjuvant tamoxifen and radiotherapy and 686 women to tamoxifen alone at a dose of 30 mg daily for one year. Median follow-up was 123 months. Locoregional recurrence occurred in 8% of the women who received radiotherapy plus tamoxifen and in 35% of those who received tamoxifen alone. DFS and OS was also much higher in the group who received adjuvant radiotherapy (36% vs. 24% for DFS; 45% vs. 36% for OS) at 10 years. One criticism of this study was that the duration of treatment with tamoxifen was much shorter than currently practised.

These studies have highlighted the importance of local control on survival and suggest that micrometastases in locoregional lymphatics are a potent source of systemic metastases. They also suggest that eradication of locoregional metastases improves survival. These studies potentially may increase the use of adjuvant radiotherapy in those patients who have undergone mastectomy and who have any adverse prognostic risk factors. These and other studies and their significance are further discussed in Chapter 4.

Timing of radiotherapy

The majority of patients undergoing breast conserving surgery will be treated with radiotherapy and, as we have seen, there has been a resurgence of interest in the use of radiotherapy after mastectomy. Until recently, the majority of patients who were node negative may not have been offered systemic therapy, but with the increasing use of adjuvant chemotherapy in this group of patients as well as those who are node positive, the question of sequencing these two treatments has become a topic of great interest. Recently, it has been observed that the order in which radiotherapy and chemotherapy are given may have a bearing on outcome. In a retrospective study of patients who had undergone breast-conserving surgery, it was observed that the actuarial rate of local failure in the breast at 5 years was 4% in patients who received radiotherapy followed by chemotherapy, but rose to 41% in patients who had the reversed order (or sequence) of treatments (Recht et al., 1991). This prompted the introduction of a randomized sequencing trial which has recently been published. The increased risk of local recurrence was again noted in the patients randomized to receive all their adjuvant chemotherapy prior to radiotherapy but this group were observed to benefit in terms of DFS as well as OS. The reverse was seen in patients who received radiotherapy immediately after surgery followed by systemic therapy (Recht et al., 1996).

Combined treatment would seem to be the answer to this controversy but carries with it problems regarding the effects of combined treatment on cosmesis and tolerability. There is a suggestion that concurrent treatment with radiotherapy and chemotherapy produces a worse cosmetic outcome in the preserved breast than sequential treatment (Gore et al., 1987) due to an increase in breast fibrosis. This observation has since been noted by some workers (Taylor et al., 1995), but not by others if methotrexate or doxorubicin is omitted at the time that the radiotherapy is given (Wazer et al., 1992). Combined treatment with radiotherapy and chemotherapy has also been found to increase damage to normal tissues such as bone marrow, skin, lungs, ribs and brachial plexus (McCormick, 1997). These issues and attempts to resolve them are further discussed in Chapter 4.

Theoretical considerations in the spread of breast cancer

The permeation theory of breast cancer spread was the stimulus to the development of increasingly radical surgery. This theory was the first casualty of a greater understanding of the biology of breast cancer. In 1931 Gray demonstrated that the lymphatics around a primary breast tumour were neither obliterated nor filled with cancer cells, even when axillary nodes were involved by tumour (Gray, 1938–39). This weakened the *en bloc* principle of radical surgery and contributed to the rationale for the less disfiguring modified radical mastectomy in which the breast is removed together with the axillary contents, whilst preserving the pectoralis major muscle. The great proponents of this operation in the 1930s were Patey in England and subsequently Auchincloss and Madden in the United States (Patey & Dyson, 1948; Madden, 1965; Patey, 1967; Auchincloss, 1970). In 1955, Engell demonstrated venous dissemination of breast cancer cells from early operable tumours. This also dealt a blow to the permeation theory which stated that haemotogenous spread of tumours occurred only very late in the pathophysiology of breast cancer (Engell, 1955). Subsequently, Fisher and Fisher's work demonstrated that lymph nodes were poor barriers to the spread of cancer cells. In a classic series of experiments in rabbits, they demonstrated that tumour cells could pass easily through lymph nodes into efferent lymphatics and also into veins through lymphaticovenous communications (Fisher & Fisher, 1966, 1967).

The above observations helped to foster a new attitude towards the theory of breast cancer spread which in turn led to a new era in the surgery of breast cancer. It became apparent that radical surgery had reached its anatomical limits without contributing to a reduction in mortality from breast cancer. This was because the concept of local origin provides a basis for cure only if the diagnosis can be made before dissemination has taken place. The stage at which an occult or even symptomatic neoplasm disseminates is extremely variable and is dependent on many factors. One factor long thought to enhance tumour cell dissemination is the effect of handling the tumour during surgery. Trauma to tumours increases both cell shedding and metastasis in animal models (Tyzzer, 1913; Liotta et al., 1976). Early studies of tumour cell shedding in humans were beset by problems with sampling and cell identification and this led to a decline in interest in the subject. Recently, there has been renewed interest in this proposed mechanism of tumour cell dissemination. This is because of an enhanced ability to detect more reliably small numbers of carcinoma cells among large numbers of haematopoietic cells using monoclonal antibodies against epithelial-restricted epitopes (Leather et al., 1993; Pantel et al., 1993) or using quantitative polymerase chain reaction (Smith et al., 2000). A recent study using very sensitive immunohistochemical techniques on selective venous samples before, during and after breast cancer surgery has demonstrated increased shedding of breast cancer cells into the circulation during surgery (Choy & McCulloch, 1996). Furthermore, the likelihood of cell shedding was directly related to tumour angiogenesis as measured by vascular density of the tumour (McCulloch et al., 1995).

However, tumour angiogenesis is probably not the only mechanism involved in the ability of a tumour to metastasize. Transformed cells also require a reduction in adhesiveness to detach themselves and enter the circulation (Nigam & Pignatelli, 1993). Thus, for migration to occur, the affinity between cancer cells and endothelium or lymphatic channels needs to change. For a cancer cell to attach to a particular target organ, further changes in expression of adhesion receptors in the invading cell and the target tissue are necessary. A prerequisite for these cells to form a metastasis is an increase in re-expression of intercellular adhesion receptors coupled with a capacity to grow independently (Aznavoorian et al., 1990; Liotta & Stetler-Stevenson, 1991). Two types of receptors mediate cellular adhesion: those that play a part in intercellular interaction and those that regulate interactions between cells and their surrounding extracellular matrix (a scaffold of glycoproteins and collagens supporting the cells). The main receptors responsible are integrins, cadherins, selectins and members of the superglobulin family (Hynes, 1992). Integrins are the prime mediators of cell-matrix interactions and cadherins of intercellular interactions. Recently a variety of integrin receptors have been demonstrated to be expressed in some breast cancer cell lines and have been shown to have some relationship to the invasive potential of these cell lines in vivo (Gui et al., 1995). Likewise, the cell adhesion molecule E-cadherin has been shown to be important in the process of invasion (Marcel et al., 1994) and the E-cadherin/catenin complex can be upregulated by the antioestrogen tamoxifen, thus inhibiting invasion in vitro (Bracke et al., 1993).

Another mechanism by which the invasive ability of a cancer cell may be enhanced is by the production of enzymes which can degrade the basement membrane. Thus, tumour expression of the proteolytic enzymes cathepsin D (Joensuu et al., 1995) and plasminogen activator (Janicke et al., 1991) has been demonstrated to be related to poorer prognosis, especially in patients with node-negative disease. The role of the nonmetastasizing protein nm23 (Royds et al., 1993) is still poorly understood.

This increasing understanding of tumour biology may lead to new strategies in our ability to moderate the metastatic potential of cancer cells in the near future. It also partially explains why ever-increasing local surgery has failed to impact on the long-term survival of patients with breast cancer. The development of high-quality mammography, which can now detect tumours of only a few millimetres in diameter, has increased the proportion of patients suitable for conservative surgery. Finally, the introduction of the concept of the randomized prospective trial as a scientific tool has demonstrated the efficacy of conservative surgery when combined with radiotherapy compared with radical surgery. All these factors have contributed to the evolution and acceptance of conservative surgery for operable breast cancer.

Evolution of conservative surgery for breast cancer

Surgery of the breast

The last 20 years has seen a change in the management of the tumour within the breast from mastectomy to breast-conserving surgery (Harris et al., 1987). This trend has been based on the results of a number of retrospective studies (Levene et al., 1977; Peters, 1977; Calle et al., 1978; Hellman et al., 1980; Durand et al., 1984; Rayter et al., 1990) and prospective randomized clinical trials (Veronesi et al., 1981; Sarrazin et al., 1984; Fisher et al., 1985a, 1989). These retrospective studies suggested that breast-conserving surgery produced similar results in terms of local control and survival compared with historical and contemporary controls treated by mastectomy and this was confirmed by the results of the prospective randomized controlled trials.

The acceptability of breast-conserving therapy has increased to the level of accepted practice for early breast cancer and this has been due to the results of prospective randomized clinical trials (Fisher et al., 1989; Sarrazin et al., 1989; Veronesi et al., 1990a; Blichert-Toft et al., 1992). The six studies cited all have follow-up of between 6 and 13 years and conclusively demonstrate similar loco-regional recurrence rates and survival in patients treated by breast-conserving therapy compared with patients treated by mastectomy for stage I and II breast cancer (Table 1.1). The only exception occurred in an early trial conducted in London which suggested that breast-conserving therapy had an adverse effect on survival compared with mastectomy (Hayward & Caleffi, 1987), but this study has since been criticized for using a combination of treatments which today would be considered inadequate.

These studies have established breast-conserving therapy for the treatment of stage I and II (early) breast cancer. However, not all patients with early breast cancer are suitable for breast-conserving techniques, and other factors which need to be taken into account when considering the type of surgery as the initial treatment are the size of the tumour in relation to the size of the breast and the location of the tumour in relation to the nipple-areolar complex. Therefore, it may be entirely appropriate to perform a mastectomy for a stage II tumour (T2, 2–5 cm diameter) if the affected breast is small, or for any tumour located immediately behind the nipple-areolar complex as breast-conserving surgery in these circumstances will produce a poor cosmetic result at best, or achieve inadequate tumour clearance at worst, a situation known to predispose to local recurrence within the breast (Dixon, 1995).

The use of breast-conserving techniques has been a stimulus to research into the extent of tumour within the breast and to how this might influence the extent of a local excision. Foci of tumour in addition to but separate from the main tumour

Table 1.1. Randomized trials comparing conservative surgery with and without radiotherapy and radical surgery

Authors	Treatment	No. of patients	Follow-up (yr)	Local relapse (%)	Survival
Hayward & Caleffi, 1987	RM + RT	186	10	14	60
	LE + RT	190	10	68	28
Veronesi et al., 1990a	RM	349	13	2	69
	QUART	352	13	3	71
Fisher et al., 1989	MRM	590	8	8	71
	LE + AD	636	8	16	71
	LE + AD + RT	629	8	6	76
Sarrazin et al., 1989	MRM	91	10	10	80
	LE + AD + RT	88	10	6	79
Lichter et al., 1992	MRM	116	5	10	85
	LE + AD + RT	121	5	17	89
Blichert-Toft et al., 1992	MRM	306	2	4	76
	LE + AD + RT	313	2	2	80

MRM modifed radical mastectomy; QUART Quadrantectomy; LE local excision; AD, axillary dissection; RT radiotherapy.

mass can be detected in the majority of resected breast cancers (Holland et al., 1985). However, it is important to distinguish between foci of cancer in direct relation to the main tumour mass (multifocality) and independent foci of tumour elsewhere in the breast (multicentricity). Multifocal involvement of the breast is common, may be extensive and may consist of microscopic foci of the invasive cancer, emboli of cancer in lymphatics or vascular spaces, or most often, intraductal cancer which can occur at a distance of more than 2 cm away from the site of the primary tumour in up to 10% of cases (Holland et al., 1991). In most cases the associated intraductal involvement has a segmental distribution in the breast; that is, along anatomical boundaries within one of the breast lobes. These studies have implications regarding the extent of local excision when combined with radiotherapy and the feasibility of breast-conserving surgery if irradiation to the preserved breast is to be withheld postoperatively.

The above observations naturally lead on to the unresolved questions regarding the optimal implementation of breast-conserving techniques. One such issue is the extent of breast resection required in patients also receiving postoperative irradiation. Gross excision of the tumour is obviously necessary but the extent of resection of 'normal' surrounding breast tissue is still a matter of debate. Some data regarding this issue can be gleaned from the results of the randomized trials of breast-conserving therapy even though they did not specifically address this issue. The National Surgical Adjuvant Breast Project trial (NSABP B06, Fisher et al., 1989) employed a limited gross excision of the tumour (referred to as 'lumpectomy') whereas the Milan trial (Veronesi et al., 1990a) employed an operation which removed a larger area of breast tissue (referred to as 'quadrantectomy'). Local recurrence in the conserved breast was less frequent after 'quadrantectomy' than after 'lumpectomy' (3% vs. 8%). This comparison is made difficult by the fact that tumours in the NSABP study were larger (up to 4 cm, a factor likely to increase local recurrence) than in the Milan trial which only included patients with tumours less than 2 cm and length of follow-up was different in the two trials (NSABP, 8 yr; Milan, 13 yr).

It is customary for patients undergoing breast-conserving surgery for breast cancer to receive postoperative irradiation. In the NSABP study, one group of patients were randomized to undergo 'lumpectomy' without the addition of postoperative irradiation, and in these patients local recurrence within the treated breast reached 39% at 8 years compared with 10% in the patients who underwent 'lumpectomy' and postoperative irradiation (Fisher et al., 1989). A more recent study from Milan has specifically addressed the question of the necessity for postoperative irradiation in the preserved breast (Veronesi et al., 1993) in patients with small breast cancers (<2.5 cm diameter) whose primary surgery consisted of quadrantectomy and axillary clearance. This study randomized 567 women between surgery alone and surgery with postoperative irradiation. Patients who had positive axillary nodes also received adjuvant systemic medical therapy. After a median length of follow-up of 39 months, only 0.3% of patients undergoing surgery and postoperative irradiation developed a local recurrence compared with 8.8% of patients undergoing surgery alone. An analysis of the major factors contributing to a high rate of local recurrence in patients undergoing surgery alone were younger age (<45 years, local recurrence rate 17.5%) and the presence of an extensive intraduct component. Patients undergoing surgery alone over the age of 55 had a low incidence of local recurrence (3.8%) and it may be that older women with a small completely excised tumour may be treated by surgery without the addition of postoperative irradiation to the breast. There is not sufficient information available on whether patients with tumours exhibiting histologically favourable features may be spared postoperative irradiation after primary surgery. The current British Association of Surgical Oncology (BASO) II study for patients who have had small well-differentiated or special-type cancers seeks to randomize atients in a 2 × 2 design to either observation, tamoxifen, radiotherapy to the breast or to the combination of tamoxifen and radiotherapy.

Axillary surgery

Since breast cancer commonly metastasizes to the axilla, no discussion about local treatment is complete without a discussion on the role of axillary surgery. The likelihood of axillary node involvement is related to the size of the primary tumour. The presence or absence of axillary node metastases is still the best prognostic factor (Cancer Research Campaign Working Party, 1980; Fisher et al., 1985b). Knowledge of axillary node status also provides a rational basis for selection of patients for adjuvant systemic therapies, especially in those patients who have a higher number (>4) of involved lymph nodes, where more aggressive adjuvant chemotherapy regimens would be advised.

The goal of axillary surgery has therefore evolved from increasing the likelihood of cure to, more simply, preventing locoregional recurrence in the axilla and obtaining the best prognostic information. A variety of early trials focused on the treatment of regional nodes. These trials consisted of the following important studies:

- comparison of radical mastectomy plus postoperative irradiation with simple mastectomy plus postoperative irradiation (Brinkley & Haybittle, 1966; Bergdahl, 1978);
- comparison of radical mastectomy with radical mastectomy plus postoperative radiation (Paterson & Russell, 1959);
- comparison of simple mastectomy plus postoperative irradiation with radical mastectomy (Bruce, 1971);
- comparison of simple mastectomy plus postoperative irradiation with mastectomy extended to the supraclavicular and internal mammary nodes (Kaae & Johansen, 1969);
- comparison of simple mastectomy with simple mastectomy plus postoperative irradiation (Murray et al., 1977);
- comparison of radical mastectomy with radical mastectomy plus internal mammary node dissection (Lacour et al., 1976; Veronesi & Valagussa, 1981);
- comparison of simple mastectomy with radical mastectomy (Fisher et al., 1977).

The results of these studies suggested that the stage of the disease was the most important predictor of survival (especially node status) and variations in treatment did not affect overall survival. However, postoperative irradiation was effective in improving local control of breast cancer even though this was not translated into improved survival. The same was true for surgical removal of internal mammary and axillary lymph nodes. Finally, it was apparent that the incidence and severity of lymphoedema caused by surgery was increased with the addition of postoperative radiotherapy.

Despite these studies, axillary surgery is an area in which controversy continues to exist, especially the debate over the type of axillary surgery which should be performed. Recently, some authorities have favoured axillary clearance rather than the more conservative surgical procedure of axillary sampling (Fentiman & Mansel, 1991). The rationale of surgery to the axilla is that it provides the best prognostic indicator available (in terms of the number of involved lymph nodes) and thereby provides a rational basis on which to select patients for adjuvant systemic medical therapy. If axillary surgery is performed, what is the best procedure? Proponents for axillary clearance and axillary sampling have recently debated this issue in the literature (Davidson, 1995; Greenall, 1995). The arguments in favour of axillary clearance are that it achieves the best local control of axillary disease, provides the best prognostic information, spares the axilla from postoperative irradiation and therefore avoids the increased morbidity associated with surgery combined with irradiation which can lead to disabling lymphoedema of the arm in up to 40% of patients, compared with 6% in patients undergoing axillary surgery alone (Davidson, 1995). The arguments in favour of a properly performed axillary sampling procedure (removing at least four lymph nodes) are that it also provides excellent prognostic information, is associated with low morbidity, avoids extensive axillary surgery in patients with node-negative disease and has been demonstrated to be just as efficacious in achieving a low rate of axillary recurrence when combined with postoperative irradiation in node-positive disease, as does axillary clearance (Greenall, 1995).

Another controversy regarding axillary surgery is whether it needs to be performed at all. It is nearly 50 years since McWhirter suggested that irradiation was a credible alternative to surgery in the management of axillary metastases (McWhirter, 1948) but it is only recently that the case for the routine use of axillary surgery has again been questioned. It has been argued that the heterogeneity of breast cancer dictates that individual patients should be treated on their merits. It is now generally accepted that patients with ductal carcinoma in situ (DCIS) should not undergo axillary surgery (Chapter 2) because theoretically there should be no spread to the axillary lymph nodes. An exception to this is in patients with extensive DCIS (>5 cm diameter) which is associated with microinvasion and a significant risk of axillary node involvement. Another group of patients who can reasonably be spared axillary surgery are the elderly (age >70 years) who may be adequately managed by wide excision of the tumour and adjuvant tamoxifen. It has also been argued that those patients in whom adjuvant endocrine therapy would be advized on the basis of parameters derived from the primary tumour (for example, tumour size >2 cm and positive oestrogen receptor status) could also be spared axillary surgery (Harris et al., 1992). With the introduction of breast screening programmes in the United Kingdom and elsewhere, an increasingly greater number of small, good prognosis breast cancers are being detected. In the past, patients with these small tumours have undergone axillary surgery to pathologically stage the disease but it has become increasingly obvious that patients with screen-detected cancers have a relatively low (25%) rate of lymph node metastases. In a recent large series of patients the incidence of positive axillary lymph nodes was documented according to the size of the invasive component of the primary tumour (Silverstein et al., 1994). Thus, T1 tumours (<2 cm) were subdivided further according to size (T1a <5 mm, T1b 6–10 mm, T1c 11–20 mm) and the incidence of axillary lymph node metastases recorded within each size category. The incidence of positive axillary lymph nodes for T1a tumours was only 3% but increased markedly for tumours larger than 5 mm (T1b 17%, T1c 32%). However, even for patients with T1b and T1c tumours, up to half the patients with positive axillary nodes will only have micrometastases or only one or two lymph nodes involved. Only 2%, 6% and 9% of all T1a, T1b and T1c invasive cancers respectively have more than three positive lymph nodes (Cady, 1994). It has been argued therefore that patients with T1a tumours should not undergo axillary surgery at all. Other situations in which axillary surgery could probably be avoided are in patients with mammographically detected cancers less than 1 cm in diameter with favourable histological features and in patients with small tumours of special type such as tubular, papillary and colloid cancers in which the incidence of positive axillary nodes is very small (Cady, 1994). The best way of substantiating these opinions is by means of a randomized controlled trial to determine whether axillary surgery confers any survival advantage, although this would require the recruitment of very large numbers of patients requiring prolonged follow-up.

Sentinel node biopsy in the management of the axilla

There has been much interest recently in the concept of the sentinel node in the management of the axilla in breast cancer. Oliver Cope referred to the 'Delphian node' in 1963 as the lymph node that will 'foretell the nature of a disease process' affecting a nearby organ. Therefore, the first lymph node to receive lymphatic drainage from the site of a tumour should be the first site of lymphatic spread. The corollary of this theory is that a tumour-free sentinel lymph node implies the absence of lymph node metastases in the whole of the lymphatic basin to which that organ drains. This concept was introduced into clinical practice in the management of penile carcinoma (Cabanes, 1977) and was based on the anatomical location of the lymph nodes around the superficial epigastric vein. However, the technique employed then (lymphangiography) was relatively crude and the significance of the concept was not appreciated at that time.

This concept was subsequently investigated in the management of cutaneous malignant melanoma by Morton and colleagues. To localize the sentinel lymph node, they developed intraoperative mapping using intradermal vital blue dye to stain the lymphatics, followed by careful surgical exploration of the regional lymphatic basin (Morton et al., 1992). In this series of 237 patients, a sentinel node or nodes was identified in 82% of cases. In all, 72% of patients had a single sentinel node, 20% had two sentinel nodes and 8% had three sentinel nodes. Of the 194 patients who had a sentinel node identified, 40 (21%) had lymph node metastases and only two patients had metastatic deposits in nonsentinel nodes in the absence of tumour in the sentinel lymph node; the false negative rate was therefore only 1%. Of importance was the observation that of the 40 lymph nodes with deposits of tumour, only 23 were diagnosed using haematoxylin and eosin (H & E) staining, the remainder being identified by immunohistochemistry.

The use of vital blue dyes has some drawbacks, notably difficulty in vizualizing the blue-stained lymphatics and the passage of dye to nonsentinel lymph nodes. Shortly after Morton's report, radiolabelled colloids were introduced which allowed the identification of radioactive sentinel lymph nodes preoperatively by scintigrams and peroperatively by means of a hand-held gamma probe (Alex & Krag, 1993; van der Veen et al., 1994). A further study has combined the use of vital blue dye and a gamma probe in a larger group of patients and has shown that all the nodes stained blue also contained radioactive colloid (Krag et al., 1995).

Identification of the sentinel lymph node has recently been extended to patients with breast cancer. Studies which have employed peritumoral injection of a blue dye alone have had success rates which vary from 50% to 100% in terms of the ability to detect the sentinel nodes (Folscher et al., 1997, Giuliano et al., 1994). This variability is probably due to the type of blue dye used and the learning curve involved in using a new surgical technique. If the false negative rate is taken as the proportion of sentinel nodes which are negative for tumour in patients subsequently found to be axillary node positive on more formal axillary staging, then false negative rates vary from 0% to 17% (Table 1.2). For routine use, sentinel lymph node biopsy would need to be more reliable.

Another method of localizing the sentinel lymph node is by the use of a radionuclide and a number of studies using this technique have now been reported (Table 1.2). Essentially, the technique involves a peritumoral injection of a technetium-99-labelled carrier (human serum albumin, sulphur colloid and antimony sulphate have been used) preoperatively. A scintigram may be taken at various times after injection preoperatively and this may make siting of the axillary incision more precise in relation to the sentinel lymph node. Surgery is then performed 2–24 hours after injection of the radioactive colloid and a gamma probe is then used to identify the lymph node peroperatively. In the largest study which has compared preoperative lymphoscintigraphy with intraoperative localization of the sentinel node using a gamma probe (Veronesi et al., 1997), 163 patients underwent a subdermal injection above the tumour site with

Table 1.2. Studies of sentinel lymph node biopsy in breast cancer

Author/Year	Technique	No. of patients	Detection rate (%)	False −ve rate (%)	Predictive rate (%)	Node +ve rate (%)
Giuliano et al., 1994	Blue dye	174	66	12	96	36
Folscher et al., 1997	Blue dye	79	40	12	85	51
Flett et al., 1998	Blue dye	68	82	17	95	31
Offodile et al., 1998	Gamma probe	41	98	0	100	45
Veronesi et al., 1997	Scintigraphy + gamma probe	163	98	5	98	53
Pijpers et al., 1997	Scintigraphy + gamma probe	37	92	0	100	34
Borgstein et al., 1998	Scintigraphy + gamma probe	130	94	2	98	42
Roumen et al., 1997	Scintigraphy + gamma probe	83	69	4	96	40
Albertini et al., 1996	Scintigraphy + blue dye	62	92	0	100	32
Cox et al., 1998	Gamma probe + blue dye	466	94	1	100	23
O'Hea et al., 1998	Scintigraphy + gamma probe + blue dye	59	93	15	95	36

5–10 MBq technetium-99-labelled human serum albumin the day before surgery. Scintigraphic images were taken of the breast and axilla at 10, 30 and 180 minutes and the skin was marked over the first lymph node that became radioactive. The hand-held gamma probe was used to localize the sentinel lymph node(s) which was then excised successfully in 98% of patients. This node accurately predicted the status of the remainder of the axilla in 98% of cases with a false negative rate of 5%. False negative rates in other (albeit smaller) studies vary from 0% to 4% (Table 1.2). Some studies have also been performed using the gamma probe alone, without the use of preoperative lymphoscintigraphy. These have generally been on small numbers of patients, although the authors have achieved similar results as in those studies which have employed preoperative lymphoscintigraphy.

There have been some studies which have used a combination of a blue dye technique and a radionuclide technique, with and without preoperative lymphoscintigraphic scanning, but all using a gamma probe at operation to identify the sentinel lymph node. Although the studies are not strictly comparable in that different blue dyes, different carriers and different doses of technetium-99 were used, all three studies found that the addition of the radionuclide technique to the blue dye technique increased the success rate for identification of the sentinel lymph node from approximately 70% to 93% (Table 1.2). In addition to these variations in the substances and doses of radionuclide, it is worth noting that the time interval between injection of the radionuclide and surgery also varied in all of the studies discussed. Finally, of great importance regarding the timing of surgery after injection of radionuclide is the site of injection within the breast. Thus, subdermal injection near the site of the tumour leads to more rapid migration of the radionuclide to the axillary nodes than peritumoral injection.

These studies suggest that the concept of the sentinel lymph node in breast cancer spread is valid. This is supported by new histopathological studies which confirm that the sentinel lymph node is the axillary node which is most likely to contain a metastasis (Turner et al., 1997). The incidence of skip metastases varies from 1% to 42% (Boova et al., 1982; Forrest et al., 1982; Rosen et al., 1983; Pigott et al., 1984; Veronesi et al., 1990b) but this has traditionally been based on the anatomical level of the lymph node in relation to pectoralis minor in the axilla. Although the variation in the reported incidence of skip metastases may be due to variations in the technique of axillary clearance, individual anatomical variations and failure to identify lower level micrometastases by conventional methods, it seems highly likely that this variation may also be due in part to variations in local lymphatic flow, either due to variations in lymphatic anatomy, or due to plugging of proximal lymphatics by tumour emboli. This is supported by the fact that the sentinel lymph node may be found in level II nodes in 18–23% of cases (Giuliano et al., 1994; Roumen et al., 1997).

Lymphoscintigraphy will also identify 'hot' nodes in the internal mammary chain in 2–20% of patients (Pijpers et al., 1997; Roumen et al., 1997; Uren et al., 1997) although these studies did not confirm metastatic disease in these 'hot' nodes on routine H&E staining. Whilst it is accepted that radical lymph node dissection of the internal mammary chain does not improve survival (Lacour et al., 1976), it does give prognostic information which may influence the decision to give adjuvant medical therapy (Veronesi et al., 1983). This has led to the suggestion that biopsy of an internal mammary node could be carried out via the second or third intercostal space and this suggestion needs to be tested in relation to sentinel lymph node biopsy using lymphoscintigraphy.

It is recognized that routine histological examination of lymph nodes may fail to detect micrometastases. Serial sectioning of lymph nodes and staining of these sections with haematoxylin and eosin allows the detection of additional nodal metastases (Fisher et al., 1978) and the addition of immunocytochemical techniques increases the detection rate (Wells et al., 1984; McGuckin et al., 1996). There is some evidence to suggest that the reverse transcriptase polymerase chain reaction may be even more sensitive in the detection of micrometastases (Noguchi et al., 1996). It was once thought that occult metastases did not influence prognosis in breast cancer but more recent studies do suggest that micrometastases predict for a reduction in long-term survival (Rosen et al., 1991; Cote et al., 1999).

Routine use of methods of detection of micrometastases on all lymph nodes removed following an axillary clearance, such as immunohistochemistry and reverse transcriptase polymerase chain reaction would be impractical and expensive. A possible role of sentinel node biopsy would be to identify one or two nodes on which to perform this more detailed pathological examination. This may allow a faster and cheaper way of obtaining more detailed information than would be available from routine histopathological evaluation of all the lymph nodes retrieved (Giuliano et al., 1995). The implication of this is that if a sentinel node was subjected to this detailed scrutiny for micrometastases then further axillary surgery would not be required if no evidence of micrometastatic disease was found. This hypothesis would need to be validated by a randomized controlled trial, comparing patients in whom the axilla was treated by sentinel lymph node biopsy and no further surgery if no micrometastases are detected, with patients undergoing standard axillary dissection. This will require prolonged follow-up with axillary recurrence and OS as the outcome measures. Such a multinational trial (ALMANAC, Axillary Lymphatic Mapping versus Axillary Clearance), recruiting patients who are clinically node negative, has just started in the United Kingdom.

The work published to date on sentinel node biopsy has confirmed the validity of this concept. However, there remain several problems (reviewed by McIntosh &

Purushotham, 1998). A clear surgical definition of what constitutes a sentinel lymph node needs to be established. Some consensus on what constitutes a 'hot' lymph node scintigraphically needs to be reached and the working definition proposed by Cox et al. (1998) of the ratio of counts per second in the sentinel lymph node being 10 times that of the background, seems to be a good starting point but needs validation. There has also been little consensus on the materials and methods and it has already been demonstrated that type of radiopharmaceutical, type of carrier which is labelled, type of blue dye, site of injection in the breast in relation to the tumour and the time interval between injection and surgery, may all potentially influence the detection of the sentinel lymph node. A further problem with gamma probe localization of radioactive sentinel nodes is the interference with detection of the sentinel lymph node due to the radioactivity at the site of injection in the breast. Thus, the type of gamma probe and whether it is fitted with a collimator to reduce the interference from adjacent radiation also needs to be examined. Finally, almost all series report some patients in whom the sentinel node cannot be identified and it has been suggested that this may be due to plugging of the lymphatics with tumour (Borgstein et al., 1998).

All the above factors are relevant before sentinel lymph node biopsy becomes a standard method of evaluating axillary lymph nodes. In addition to the methodology employed, the strategy regarding the practical management of the patient also needs to be taken into account. Two possible strategies present themselves. First, the patient could undergo sentinel node biopsy at the time of primary surgery for the breast cancer. If pathological analysis confirmed no metastases, then no further axillary surgery would be required and treatment would be based on whether breast-conserving surgery had been performed and the prognostic variables derived from pathological examination of the primary tumour. If micrometastases were detected in the lymph node, then subsequent definitive axillary surgery may be required. Whether this would be acceptable to the majority of patients is unknown. One method of attempting to reduce the need for a second operation to the axilla in lymph node-positive patients is to consider a frozen section examination of the sentinel lymph node at the time of definitive surgery to the breast. However, it is known that frozen section analysis is inaccurate and has been shown to have a sensitivity of only 73% in a recent study (Dixon et al., 1999) and 76% in one sentinel nodes study (Veronesi et al., 1997).

A second strategy which could be employed is to perform a sentinel lymph node biopsy first without removing the primary tumour. When the pathological status of the lymph node is known, definitive surgery for the breast primary is performed together with further axillary surgery if indicated. In order to reduce the reoperation rate to the axilla, careful selection of the patients would be required. An ideal group of patients which could be considered are patients with small or impalpable tumours detected by breast screening, as this group of patients has a low incidence of lymph node metastases and it would be feasible to inject dye or radiocolloid by current methods of radiological localization. However, even in this group of patients, delayed surgery for the primary tumour after sentinel node biopsy would require a second radiological localization and this also may be unacceptable to many patients.

It is clear that the sentinel lymph node concept has validity in breast cancer and that it is possible to identify the sentinel lymph node in the majority of patients. Clearly, a great deal of work still needs to be performed to obtain a consensus on the methodology of the technique. Whichever variations in approach are adopted regarding the strategy of the management of the patient, the validity of whether to perform no further surgery to the axilla when the sentinel node is negative for metastases (whether detected by routine histological methods, immunohistochemistry or the polymerase chain reaction) needs to be confirmed by randomized trials with locoregional recurrence and survival as end points. Finally, the acceptability of this technique to the patient must also be evaluated.

Timing of surgery

It has been appreciated for a long time that in premenopausal women the breast is subject to the normal monthly hormone fluctuations and this has also been observed in breast cancer. In view of these cyclical changes, Ratajzak et al. (1988) postulated that the menstrual cycle may influence the behaviour of breast cancer. His experiments in a mouse model suggested that mice whose tumours were excised in the nearoestrous phase of the cycle fared significantly worse than mice whose tumours were excised in the postoestrous phase. The scientific explanation for this was that tumours were more likely to shed cells during surgery in a hormonal milieu in which there was unopposed oestrogen action. Initial reports of the effect of timing of surgery on survival in premenopausal patients were conflicting until the study published by the Breast Unit at Guy's Hospital (Badwe et al., 1991). In this study of 249 premenopausal women, those operated on between days 3–12 of the menstrual cycle (a period of relatively high unopposed oestrogen), had a 10-year survival of 58% whilst those operated on at other times in the cycle had a 10-year survival of 84%. The major impact was in node-positive women. Similar but less dramatic results were published by the Sloan-Kettering Cancer Centre in New York (Senie et al., 1991) and the group from Milan (Veronesi et al., 1994). Scepticism regarding timing of surgery has persisted despite the results of a meta-analysis which has demonstrated that there was a significant effect of timing of surgery ($p = 0.02$) with a 16% overall reduction in mortality in those patients undergoing surgery during the luteal phase of the cycle (Fentiman et al., 1994). Detractors of these studies emphasize that they are retrospective and currently it is not standard practice to time surgery for the luteal phase of the cycle. It is hoped that the current prospective study organized by the Yorkshire Breast Cancer Group will provide some firmer evidence.

Reconstructive surgery

Despite the increasing use of breast-conserving procedures, many patients still require a mastectomy in order to remove the primary tumour, either because of unsuitability for a breast-conserving procedure or because of local recurrence after such surgery. The option of reconstruction is therefore important as it helps many women adjust to the changes in body image associated with mastectomy (Schain et al., 1984). The purpose of the operation is to reconstruct a breast mound to produce symmetry and this may be performed either at the time of mastectomy ('immediate') or some time afterward ('delayed'). In centres that provide reconstruction as part of the breast service there has been an increase in demand and in the author's experience, more than half the patients offered immediate reconstruction accept. Delayed reconstruction is usually associated with a lower rate of acceptance. There is no evidence that breast reconstruction increases the rate of local or systemic relapse or makes the detection of local recurrence more difficult.

Reconstruction can be carried out by placement of a prosthesis (implant), insertion of a tissue expander or insertion of a flap of skin and muscle (myocutaneous flap) with or without a prosthesis. Tissue expanders and prostheses all have a silicone shell. Prostheses may contain silicone gel (which gives a 'doughy' consistency similar to that of the normal breast), saline (which leads to 'rippling' of the prosthesis which may be visible) or soya bean oil. These are suitable for immediate reconstruction of a small breast in whom adequate skin flaps are present or in delayed reconstruction after tissue expansion has been achieved. Tissue expanders consist of a silicone outer bag and an inner bag which is inflated with saline via a filler port placed subcutaneously. The tissue expander is gradually filled with saline, usually at weekly intervals until the desired volume has been achieved. It is necessary to inflate the tissue expander to a greater volume than the contralateral breast for a period of time to achieve the desired ptosis before reducing to the final desired volume. The tissue expander can then be replaced with a permanent prosthesis or with the more modern expanders, left in situ with removal of just the filler port and its connection to the expander if appropriate.

Silicone gel prostheses have recently been implicated in the development of serious systemic complications in a minority of patients in the form of rare connective tissue disorders. This has led to a great deal of anxiety and legal activity, forcing large compensation payments to be made to claimants by the manufacturers of these devices on the basis of anecdote rather than fact. Recent studies have shown no association with the development of an excess incidence of connective tissue disease in patients with silicone gel prostheses (Sanchez-Guerrero et al., 1995; IRG, 1998) or of breast cancer (Bryant & Brasher, 1995). However, local complications of breast prostheses are well recognized and include capsular contracture (in approximately 10% of patients), infection (in 5% of patients) and implant fatigue and rupture (in 1% of patients).

Myocutaneous flap reconstruction involves moving skin, subcutaneous fat and muscle on a vascular pedicle from a donor site to the chest wall in order to construct the breast mound. The most common myocutaneous flaps are based on either the latissimus dorsi muscle or on the rectus abdominis muscle (transverse rectus abdominis myocutaneous (TRAM) flap). The latissimus dorsi flap usually requires a prosthesis to be placed between the muscle of the flap and the chest wall to achieve a breast mound of sufficient volume. TRAM flaps may be performed either as a pedicled graft based on the superior epigastric vessels or as free flaps employing a microvascular anastomosis between the inferior epigastric and thoracodorsal vessels in the axilla. The TRAM flap is useful for covering large chest wall defects and creating a large breast mound without the need for a prosthesis. Myocutaneous flaps can also be employed for delayed breast reconstruction if the patient has previously received chest wall irradiation. The greatest problem with myocutaneous flaps is postoperative flap necrosis; rare in latissimus dorsi flaps, it may occur in up to 5% of free TRAM flaps and up to 10% of pedicled TRAM flaps.

The final cosmetic result can be enhanced by reconstruction of a nipple on the breast mound and nipple/areola tattooing (Rayter, 1998).

Need for systemic therapy in early breast cancer

The incidence of breast cancer is increasing whilst mortality has recently started to decline. In the United Kingdom alone, approximately 25 000 women develop breast cancer each year and 15 000 die of their disease, despite the fact that the majority of women present without clinical evidence of overt metastatic disease. These facts suggest that the majority of patients with *symptomatic* breast cancer (in contrast to screen-detected breast cancer) have a systemic disease at the time of diagnosis and that the outcome of locoregional therapy is predetermined by the extent of systemic micrometastases present at the time of diagnosis. There is evidence to support this view, as micrometastases in the bone marrow have been detected in patients with breast cancer employing an immunocytochemical technique using an antibody to epithelial membrane antigen (Dearnaley et al., 1981). The presence of these micrometastases has been found to correlate with other factors of poor prognosis such as large tumour size, the presence of positive axillary lymph nodes and vascular invasion in the primary tumour (Berger et al., 1988). Micrometastases detected by this method have been found in 30% of patients with metastases at sites other than bone and in 100% of patients with radiological evidence of bone metastases (Mansi et al., 1989). Long-term results on the significance of micrometastases in patients with primary breast cancer have so far been equivocal with the most mature study (median follow-up 12.5 years) suggesting that the presence of micrometastases is not an independent factor for survival (Mansi et al., 1999), whereas those studies with shorter follow-up (median 36 and 38 months) have shown that it is (Diel et al., 1996; Braun et al., 2000).

The most compelling evidence that some form of effective systemic therapy is required for breast cancer comes from survival data. Thus, patients with 'early' breast cancer as ascertained by clinical staging based on tumour size and clinical lymph node status (stage I & II, T1-2, N0–N1b) have an overall survival of the order of 70% at 10 years. However, overall 10-year survival of all breast cancer patients is only 45.9% and even patients without axillary lymph node involvement (still the best prognostic marker) only have a 10-year survival of 65%. Survival data is often quoted in the context of prognostic factors and their utility has recently been reviewed (Mansour et al., 1994; Miller et al., 1994). The most widely used prognostic factors are pathological tumour size, number of involved axillary lymph nodes and histological grade of tumour. The Nottingham prognostic index (NPI) uses a combination of these three factors (NPI = (0.2 × size) + lymph node stage + grade) to identify cohorts of patients with a good, moderate and poor prognosis. This may be useful in identifying those groups of patients likely to relapse from breast cancer and therefore more likely to gain from adjuvant medical therapy (see Chapter 7).

Conclusion

Over the centuries our understanding of breast cancer has made enormous progress. This has greatly influenced the management of primary operable breast cancer to the extent that breast-preserving surgery has achieved an established place in the surgical management of operable breast cancer. The combination of breast-preserving surgery with postoperative irradiation now achieves similar rates of local control as that of more radical surgical procedures without any detriment to survival (Dixon, 1995). The role of sentinel node biopsy in reducing the morbidity of axillary surgery in node-negative patients is an exciting new development which is in the process of evaluation in randomized controlled clinical trials. A better understanding of the indications for mastectomy has allowed for better selection of patients for ablative surgery and has consigned to history the super-radical procedures described. Reconstructive surgery has done much to alleviate the psychological consequences of mastectomy for those patients in whom it is still required for the treatment of the primary tumour. However, it is apparent that local treatment strategies have failed to cure those women destined to develop metastatic disease which is eventually fatal. The development of effective systemic therapies is crucial so that further therapeutic progress can be made. Surgery which changes the hormonal milieu of the patient in the treatment of metastatic disease has now been superseded by medical therapies. The introduction of adjuvant systemic therapy to treat presumed micrometastases has been a real advance in the management of breast cancer over the last 20 years and the recent introduction of neoadjuvant chemotherapy for operable breast cancer is currently the subject of intense study whose potential requires careful evaluation. Finally, there are still many questions regarding the optimum combinations of chemotherapy and radiotherapy to be answered.

REFERENCES

Albertini, J.J., Lyman, G.H., Cox, C. et al. (1996). Lymphatic mapping and sentinel node biopsy in the patient with breast cancer. *Journal of the American Medical Association*, 276, 1818–22.

Alex, J.C. & Krag, D.N. (1993). Gamma probe-guided localization of lymph nodes. *Surgical Oncology*, 2, 137–43.

Arnott, H. (1871). On the therapeutical importance of recent views of the nature and structure of cancer. *St. Thomas Hospital Reports*, 119, 103–22.

Atkins, H.J.B., Hayward, J.L., Klugman, D.J. & Wayte, A.B. (1972). Treatment of early breast cancer: a report after 10 years of a clinical trial. *British Medical Journal*, ii, 423–9.

Auchincloss, H. (1970). Modified radical mastectomy: why not? *American Journal of Surgery*, 119, 506–9.

Aznavoorian, S., Stracke, M. L., Krutsch, H. et al. (1990). Signal transduction for chemotaxis and haptotaxis by matrix molecules in tumour cells. *Journal of Cell Biology*, 110, 1427–38.

Baclesse, F. (1965). Five year results in 431 breast cancers treated solely by roentgen rays. *Annals of Surgery*, 161, 103–4.

Badwe, R.A., Gregory, W.M., Chaudary, M.A. et al. (1991). Timing of surgery during menstrual cycle and survival of premenopausal women with operable breast cancer. *Lancet*, 337, 1261–4.

Banks, W.M. (1902). A brief history of the operations practiced for cancer of the breast. *British Medical Journal*, 1, 5–10.

Beatson, G.T. (1896). On the treatment of inoperable cases of carcinoma of the mamma: suggestions for a new treatment with illustrative cases. *Lancet*, 2, 104–7.

Bergdahl, L. (1978). Simple and radical mastectomy with postoperative irradiation: a controlled trial. *American Surgeon*, 44, 369–73.

Berger, U., Bettelheim, R., Mansi, J.L. et al. (1988). The relationship between micrometastases in the bone marrow, histopathological features of the primary tumour in breast cancer and prognosis. *American Journal of Clinical Pathology*, 90, 1–6.

Blichert-Toft, M., Rose, C., Andersen, J.A. et al. (1992). Danish randomized trial comparing breast conservation therapy with mastectomy: six years of life-table analysis. *Monographs of the National Cancer Institute*, 11, 19–25.

Boova, R., Bonanni, R., Rosato, F. (1982). Patterns of axillary nodal involvement in breast cancer: predictability of level I dissection. *Annals of Surgery*, 196, 642–4.

Borgstein, P.J., Pijpers, R., Comans, E.F. et al. (1998). Sentinel lymph node biopsy in breast cancer: guidelines and pitfalls of lymphoscintigraphy and gamma probe detection. *Journal of the Americal College of Surgeons*, 186, 275–83.

Bracke, M.E., Charlier, C., Bruyneel, E.A. et al. (1993). Insulin-like growth factor I activates the invasion supressor function of E-cadherin in MCF-7 human mammary carcinoma cells in vitro. *British Journal of Cancer*, 68, 282–9.

Braun, S., Pantel, K., Müller, P. et al. (2000). Cytokeratin-positive cells in the bone marrow and survival of patients with stage I, II or III breast cancer. *The New England Journal of Medicine*, 342(8), 525–33.

Brinkley, D. & Haybittle, J.L. (1966). Treatment of stage II carcinoma of the female breast. *Lancet*, 2, 291–5.

Bruce, J. (1971). Operable cancer of the breast. A controlled clinical trial. *Cancer*, 28, 1443–52.

Bryant, H. & Brasher, P. (1995). Breast implants and breast cancer – reanalysis of a linkage study. *New England Journal of Medicine*, 332, 1535–9.

Cabanes, R.M. (1977). An approach for the treatment of penile carcinoma. *Cancer*, 39, 456–66.

Cady, B. (1994). The need to re-examine axillary lymph node dissection in invasive breast cancer. *Cancer*, 73, 505–8.

Calle, R., Pilleron, J.P., Schlienger, P. & Vilcoq, J.R. (1978). Conservative management of operable breast cancer. *Cancer*, 42, 2045–53.

Cancer Research Campaign Working Party (1980). Cancer Research Campaign (King's/Cambridge) Trial for Early Breast Cancer: a detailed update at the tenth year. *Lancet*, 2, 55–60.

Choy, A. & McCulloch, P. (1996). Induction of tumour cell shedding into effluent venous blood during breast cancer surgery. *British Journal of Cancer*, 73, 79–82.

Cote, R.J., Peterseon, H.F., Chalwun, B. et al. (1999). Role of immunohistochemical detection of lymph-node metastases in management of breast cancer. *Lancet*, 354, 896–900.

Cox, C.E., Pendas, S., Cox, J.M. et al. (1998). Guidelines for sentinel node biopsy and lymphatic mapping of patients with breast cancer. *Annals of Surgery*, 227, 645–53.

Cuzick, J., Stewart, H., Peto, R. et al. (1987). Overview of randomized trials of postoperative adjuvant radiotherapy in breast cancer. *Cancer Treatment Reports*, 71, 15–29.

Cuzick, J., Stewart, H., Rutqvist, L. et al. (1994). Cause specific mortality in long term survivors of breast cancer who participated in trials of radiotherapy. *Journal of Clinical Oncology*, 12, 447–53.

Dahl-Iverson, E. & Tobiassen, T. (1969). Radical mastectomy with parasternal and supraclavicular dissection for mammary carcinoma. *Annals of Surgery*, 170, 889–91.

Davidson, T. (1995). Why I favour axillary node clearance in the management of breast cancer. *European Journal of Surgical Oncology*, 21, 5–7.

Dearnaley, D.P., Sloane, J.P., Ormerod, M.G. et al. (1981). Increased detection of mammary carcinoma cells in marrow smears using antisera to epithelial membrane antigen. *British Journal of Cancer*, 44, 85–90.

Diel, I.J., Kaufmann, M., Costa, S.D. et al. (1996). Micrometastatic breast cancer cells in bone marrow at primary surgery: prognostic value in comparison with nodal status. *Journal of the National Cancer Institute*, 88, 1652–8.

Dixon, J.M. (1995). Surgery and radiotherapy for early breast cancer. *British Medical Journal*, 311, 1515–16.

Dixon, J.M., Mamman, U. & Thomas, J. (1999). Accuracy of intraoperative frozen-section analysis of axillary lymph nodes. *British Journal of Surgery*, 86, 392–5.

Durand, J.C., Pojicak, M., Lefrang, J.P. & Pilleron, J.P. (1984). Wide excision of the tumour, axillary dissection and postoperative radiotherapy as treatment of small breast cancers. *Cancer*, 53, 2439–43.

Engell, H. C. (1955). Cancer cells in the circulating blood: clinical study on occurrence of cancer cells in peripheral blood and in venous blood draining tumour area at operation. *Acta Chirurgica Scandinavia*, Suppl. 201, 1–70.

Fentiman, I.S. & Mansel, R.E. (1991). The axilla: not a no-go zone. *Lancet*, 337, 221–3.

Fentiman, I.S., Gregory, W.M. & Richards, M.A. (1994). Effect of menstrual cycle phase on surgical treatment of breast cancer. *Lancet*, 344, 402.

Fisher, B. & Fisher, E.R. (1966). The interrelationship of haematogenous and lymphatic tumour cell dissemination. *Surgery, Gynaecology and Obstetrics*, 122, 791–8.

Fisher, B. & Fisher, E.R. (1967). Barrier function of lymph node to tumour cells and erythrocytes. I. Normal nodes. *Cancer*, 20, 1907–13.

Fisher, B., Montague, E., Redmond, C. et al. (1977). Comparison of radical mastectomy with alternative treatments for primary breast cancer. *Cancer*, 39, 2827–39.

Fisher, E.R., Swamidoss, S., Lee, C.H. et al. (1978). Detection and significance of occult axillary lymph node metastases in patients with invasive breast cancer. *Cancer*, 42, 2025–31.

Fisher, B., Bauer, M., Margolese, R. et al. (1985a). Five year results of a randomized clinical trial comparing total mastectomy and segmental mastectomy with or without radiation in the treatment of breast cancer. *New England Journal of Medicine*, 312, 665–73.

Fisher, B., Redmond, C., Fisher, E.R. et al. (1985b). Ten-year results of a randomized clinical trial comparing radical mastectomy and total mastectomy with or without radiation. *New England Journal of Medicine*, 312, 674–81.

Fisher, B., Redmond, C., Poisson, R. et al. (1989). Eight year results of a randomized clinical trial comparing total mastectomy and lumpectomy with or without irradiation in the treatment of breast cancer. *New England Journal of Medicine*, 320, 822–8.

Flett, M., Stanton, P.D. & Cooke, T.G. (1998). Lymphatic mapping and sentinel lymph node biopsy in breast cancer. *British Journal of Surgery*, 85, 991–3.

Folscher, D.J., Langman, G., Panieri, E. et al. (1997). Sentinel axillary lymph node biopsy: helpful in axillary management in patients with breast cancer? *British Journal of Surgery*, 84, 1586, Abstract.

Forrest, A.P.M., Stewart, H.J., Roberts, M.M., Steele, R.J.C. (1982). Simple mastectomy and axillary node sampling (pectoral node biopsy) in the management of primary breast cancer. *Annals of Surgery*, 196, 371–7.

Giuliano, A.E., Kirgan, D.M., Guenther, J.M., Morton, D.L. (1994). Lymphatic mapping and sentinel lymphadenectomy for breast cancer. *Annals of Surgery*, 220, 391–401.

Giuliano, A.E., Dale, P.S., Turner, R.R. et al. (1995). Improved axillary staging of breast cancer with sentinel lymphadenectomy. *Annals of Surgery*, 222, 394–401.

Gore, S.M. Come, S.E., Griem, K. et al. (1987). Influence of the sequencing of chemotherapy and radiation therapy in node-negative breast cancer patients treated by conservative surgery and radiation therapy. In: *Adjuvant Therapy of Cancer V*, ed. S.E. Salmon, pp. 365–73. Orlando, FL: Grune & Stratton.

Gray, J.H. (1938–39). The relation of lymphatic vessels to the spread of cancer. *British Journal of Surgery*, 26, 462–95.

Greenall, M.J. (1995). Why I favour axillary node sampling in the management of breast cancer. *European Journal of Surgical Oncology*, 21, 2–5.

Gui, G.P.H., Puddefoot, J.R., Vinson, G.P. et al. (1995). In vitro regulation of human breast cancer cell adhesion and invasion via integrin receptors to the extracellular matrix. *British Journal of Surgery*, 82, 1192–6.

Haagensen, C.D. (1971). In: *Diseases of the Breast*, 2nd edn, p. 622. Philadelphia: W.B. Saunders.

Halsted, W.S. (1894–95). The results of operations for the cure of cancer of the breast performed at the Johns Hopkins Hospital from June 1889 to January 1894. *Johns Hopkins Hospital Reports*, 4, 297–351.

Handley, W.S. (1922). In: *Cancer of the Breast and its Treatment*, 2nd edn, p. 256. London: John Murray.

Handley, R.S. & Thackray, A.C. (1969). Conservative radical mastectomy (Patey's operation). *Annals of Surgery*, 170, 880–2.

Harris, J.R., Hellman, S. & Silen, W. (1983). In: *Conservative Management of Breast Cancer: New Surgical and Radiotherapeutic Techniques*. Philadelphia: J.B. Lippincott.

Harris, J.R., Schnitt, S.J., Connolly, J.L. & Silen, W. (1987). Conservative surgery and radiation therapy for early breast cancer. *Archives of Surgery*, 122, 754–5.

Harris, J.R., Lippman, M.E., Veronesi, U. & Willett, W. (1992). Breast cancer. *New England Journal of Medicine*, 327, 390–8.

Hayward, J. & Caleffi, M. (1987). The significance of local control in the primary treatment of breast cancer. *Archives of Surgery*, 122, 1244–7.

Heidenhain, L. (1889). Ueber die Ursachen der localen Krebsrecidive nach Amputation mammae. *Verhandlungen der Deutschen Gesellschaft fur Chirurgie*. Berlin.

Hellman, S., Harris, J.R. & Levene, M.B. (1980). Radiation therapy of early carcinoma of the breast without mastectomy. *Cancer*, 45, 988–94.

Hochman, A. & Robinson, E. (1960). Eighty-two cases of mammary cancer treated exclusively with roentgen therapy. *Cancer*, 13, 670–3.

Holland, R., Veling, S.H., Mravunac, M. & Hendriks, J.H. (1985). Histologic multifocality of Tis, T1-2 breast carcinomas: implications for clinical trials of breast-conserving surgery. *Cancer*, 56, 979–90.

Holland, R., Connolly, J.L., Gelman, R. et al. (1991). The presence of an extensive intraductal component following a limited excision correlates with prominent residual disease in the remainder of the breast. *Journal of Clinical Oncology*, 8, 113–18.

Huggins, C. & Bergenstal, D.M. (1951). Influence of bilateral adrenalectomy, adrenocorticotrophin and cortisone acetate on certain human tumours. *Science*, 114, 482.

Hynes, R.O. (1992). Integrins: versatility modulation and signalling in cell adhesion. *Cell*, 69, 11–25.

Independent Review Group (1998). Silicon Gel Breast Implants. London.

Janicke, F., Schmitt, M. & Graeff, H. (1991). Clinical relevance of the urokinase-type and tissue-type plasminogen activators and of their type I inhibitor in breast cancer. *Seminars in Thrombosis and Haemostasis*, 17, 303–12.

Jensen, E.V., DeSombre, E.R. & Jungblut, P.W. (1967). Estrogen receptors in hormone respon-. sive tissues and tumours. In: *Endogenous Factors Influencing Host–Tumor Balance*, ed. R.W. Wissler, Y.L. Dao & S. Wood, p. 15. Chicago, IL: University of Chicago Press.

Joensuu, H. Toikkanen, S. & Isola, J. (1995). Stromal cell Cathepsin D expression and long term survival in breast cancer. *British Journal of Cancer*, 71, 155–9.

Kaae, S. & Johansen, H. (1969). Simple mastectomy plus postoperative irradiation by the method of McWhirter for mammary carcinoma. *Annals of Surgery*, 170, 895–9.

Keynes, G. (1937). Conservative treatment of cancer of the breast. *British Medical Journal*, ii, 643–7.

Krag, D.N., Meijer, S.J., Weaver, D.L. et al. (1995). Minimal-access surgery for staging of malignant melanoma. *Archives of Surgery*, 130, 654–8.

Küster, E. (1883). Zur Behandlung des Brustkrabses. *Archiv für Klinische Chirurgie*, 29, 723.

Lacour, J., Bucalossi, P., Cacers, E. et al. (1976). Radical mastectomy versus radical mastectomy plus internal mammary dissection. *Cancer*, 37, 206–14.

Leather, A.J.M., Gallegos, N.C., Kocjan, G. et al. (1993). Detection and enumeration of circulating tumour cells in colorectal cancer. *British Journal of Surgery*, 80, 777–80.

Le Dran, H.F. (1757). Memoire avec un précis de plusieurs observations sur le cancer. *Mémoires de l'Académie royal de chirurgie*, 3, 1–21.

Levene, M.B., Harris, J.R. & Hellman, S. (1977). Treatment of carcinoma of the breast by radiation therapy. *Cancer*, 39, 2840–5.

Lewis, D. & Rienhoff, W.F. Jr (1932). A study of the results of operations for cure of cancer of the breast. *Annals of Surgery*, 95, 336–400.

Lichter, A.S., Lippman, M.E., Danforth, D.N. et al. (1992). Mastectomy versus breast conserving therapy in the treatment of stage I & II carcinoma of the breast: a randomized trial at the National Cancer Institute. *Journal of Clinical Oncology*, 10, 976–83.

Liotta, L., Kleinerman, J. & Saidel, G.M. (1976). The significance of haematogenous tumour cell clumps in the metastatic process. *Cancer Research*, 36, 889–94.

Liotta, L.A. & Stetler-Stevenson, W.G. (1991). Tumour invasion and metastasis: an imbalance of positive and negative regulation. *Cancer Research*, 51, 5054–95.

Luft, R. & Olivecrona, H. (1953). Experiences with hypophysectomy in man. *Journal of Neurosurgery*, 10, 301–16.

Madden, J.L. (1965). Modified radical mastectomy. *Surgery, Gynaecology and Obstetrics*, 121, 1221–30.

Mansi, J.L., Berger, U., Easton, D. et al. (1987). Bone marrow micrometastases in patients with primary breast cancer: an early predictor of bone metastases. *British Medical Journal*, 295, 1093–6.

Mansi, J.L., Berger, U., McDonnell, T. et al. (1989). The fate of bone marrow micrometastases in patients with primary breast cancer. *Journal of Clinical Oncology*, 7, 445–9.

Mansi, J.L., Gogas, H., Bliss, J.M. et al. (1999). Outcome of primary-breast-cancer patients with micrometastases: a long-term follow-up study. *Lancet*, 354, 197–202.

Mansour, E.G., Ravdin, P.M. & Dressler, L. (1994). Prognostic factors in early breast carcinoma. *Cancer*, 74, 381–400.

Marcel, M., Bracke, M. & van Roy F. (1994). Invasion promoter versus invasion suppressor molecules: the paradigm of E-cadherin. *Molecular Biology Reports*, 19, 45–67.

McCormick, B. (1997). Radiotherapy plus chemotherapy: concomitant or sequential therapy. In: *Textbook of Breast Cancer: A Clinical Guide to Therapy*, ed. G. Bonadonna, G.N. Hortobagyi & A.M. Gianni, pp. 195–206. London: Martin Dunitz.

McCulloch, P., Choy, A. & Martin, L. (1995). Association between tumour angiogenesis and tumour cell shedding into effluent venous blood during breast cancer surgery. *Lancet*, 346, 1334–5.

McGuckin, M.A., Cummings, M.C., Walsh, M.D. et al. (1996). Occult axillary node metastases in breast cancer: their detection and prognostic significance. *British Journal of Cancer*, 73, 88–95.

McIntosh, S.A. & Purushotham, A.D. (1998). Lymphatic mapping and sentinel node biopsy in breast cancer. *British Journal of Surgery*, 85, 1347–56.

McWhirter, R. (1948). The value of simple mastectomy and radiotherapy in the treatment of cancer of the breast. *British Journal of Radiology*, 21, 599–610.

Meyer, W. (1894). An improved method of the radical operation for carcinoma of the breast. *Medical Record*, 46, 746–51.

Miller, W.R., Ellis, I.O., Sainsbury, J.R.C. & Dixon, J.M. (1994). ABC of breast diseases: prognostic factors. *British Medical Journal*, 309, 1573–6.

Moore, C.H. (1867). On the influence of inadequate operations on the theory of cancer. *Royal Medical and Chirurgical Society*, 32, 245–80.

Morton, D.L., Wen, D.-R., Wong, J.H. et al. (1992). Technical details of intraoperative lymphatic mapping for early stage melanoma. *Archives of Surgery*, 127, 392–9.

Murray, J.G., MacIntyre, J., Simpson, J.S. et al. (1977). Cancer research campaign study of the management of 'early' breast cancer. *World Journal of Surgery*, 1, 317–9.

Nigam, A. & Pignatelli, M. (1993). Adhesion and the cancer jigsaw. *British Medical Journal*, 307, 3–4.

Noguchi, S., Aihara, T., Motomura, K. et al. (1996). Detection of breast cancer micrometastases in axillary lymph nodes by means of reverse transcriptase polymerase chain reaction. *American Journal of Pathology*, 148, 649–56.

Offodile, R., Hoh, C., Barsky, S.H. et al. (1998). Minimally invasive breast carcinoma staging using lymphatic mapping with radiolabeled dextran. *Cancer*, 82, 1704–8.

O'Hea, B.J., Hill, A.D.K., El-Shirbiny, A.M. et al. (1998). Sentinel lymph node biopsy in breast cancer: initial experience at Memorial Sloan-Kettering Cancer Center. *Journal of the American College of Surgeons*, 186, 423–7.

Overgaard, M., Hansen, P.S., Overgaard, J. et al. (1997). Postoperative radiotherapy in high-risk premenopausal women with breast cancer who receive adjuvant chemotherapy. *New England Journal of Medicine*, 337, 949–55.

Overgaard, M., Jensen, M.-J. Overgaard, J. et al. (1999). Postoperative radiotherapy in high-risk postmenopausal breast cancer patients given adjuvant tamoxifen: Danish Breast Cancer Cooperative Group DBCG 82c randomized trial. *Lancet*, 353, 1641–8.

Pantel, K., Izbicki, J. R., Angstwurn, M. et al. (1993). Immunocytological detection of bone-marrow micrometastases in operable small cell lung cancer. *Cancer Research*, 53, 1027–31.

Paterson, R. & Russell, M.H. (1959). Clinical trials in malignant disease. Part III. Breast cancer: evaluation of postoperative radiotherapy. *Journal of the Faculty of Radiologists*, 10, 175–8.

Patey, D.H. (1967). A review of 146 cases of carcinoma of the breast operated on between 1930 and 1943. *British Journal of Cancer*, 21, 260–9.

Patey, D.H. & Dyson W.H. (1948). The prognosis of carcinoma of the breast in relation to the type of operation performed. *British Journal of Cancer*, 2, 7–13.

Peters, M.V. (1977). Wedge resection with or without radiation in early breast cancer. *International Journal of Radiation Oncology, Biology and Physics*, 2, 1151–6.

Pfahler, G.E. (1932). Results of radiation therapy in 1022 private cases of carcinoma of the breast from 1902 to 1928. *American Journal of Roentgenology and Radiation Therapy*, 27, 497–508.

Pierquin, B., Owen, R., Maylin, C. et al. (1980). Radical radiation of breast cancer. *International Journal of Radiation Oncology Biology and Physics*, 6, 17–24.

Pigott, J., Nichols, R., Maddox, W., Balch, C. (1984). Metastases to the upper levels of the axillary nodes in carcinoma of the breast and its implications for nodal sampling procedures. *Surgery, Gynecology and Obstetrics*, 158, 255–9.

Pijpers, R., Meijer, S., Hoekstra, O.S. et al. (1997). Impact of lymphoscintigraphy on sentinel node identification with technetium-99m-colloidal albumin in breast cancer. *Journal of Nuclear Medicine*, 38, 366–8.

Power, D. (1934–35). The history of the amputation of the breast to 1904. *Liverpool Medical-Chirurgical Journal*, 42/43, 29–56.

Prudente, A. (1949). L'amputation inter-scapulo-mammothoracique (technique et resultats). *Journal de Chirurgie*, 65, 729–35.

Ragaz, J., Jackson, S.M., Le N. et al. (1997). Adjuvant radiotherapy and chemotherapy in node-positive premenopausal women with breast cancer. *New England Journal of Medicine*, 337, 956–62.

Ratajzak, H.V., Sothern, R.B. & Hrushevsky, W.J.M. (1988). Estrous influence on surgical cure of breast cancer. *Journal of Experimental Medicine*, 168, 73–83.

Rayter, Z. (1998). Early experience of the nipple/areola tattoo after breast reconstruction. *European Journal of Surgical Oncology*, 24, 629–30.

Rayter, Z., Gazet, J.-C., Ford, H.T. et al. (1990). Comparison of conservative surgery and radiotherapy with mastectomy in the treatment of early breast cancer. *European Journal of Surgical Oncology*, 16, 486–92.

Recht, A., Come, S.E., Gelman, R.S. et al. (1991). Integration of conservative surgery, radiotherapy and chemotherapy for the treatment of early stage, node positive breast cancer: sequencing, timing and outcome. *Journal of Clinical Oncology*, 9, 1662–7.

Recht, A., Come, S.E., Henderson, I.C. et al. (1996). The sequencing of chemotherapy and radiation therapy after conservative surgery for early-stage breast cancer. *New England Journal of Medicine*, 334, 1350–6.

Rosen, P.P., Lesser, M.L., Kinne, D.W., Beattie, E.J. (1983). Discontinuous or 'skip' metastases in breast carcinoma: analysis of 1228 axillary dissections. *Annals of Surgery*, 197, 276–83.

Rosen, P.P., Groshen, S., Kinne, D.W. (1991). Prognosis in $T_2N_0M_0$ stage I breast carcinoma: a 20-year follow up study. *Journal of Clinical Oncology*, 9, 1650–61.

Roumen, R.M.H., Valkenburg, J.G.M., Geuskens, L.M. (1997). Lymphoscintigraphy and feasibility of sentinel node biopsy in 83 patients with primary breast cancer. *European Journal of Surgical Oncology*, 23, 495–502.

Royds, J.A., Stephenson, T.J., Rees, R.C. et al. (1993). Nm 23 protein expression in ductal carcinoma in situ and invasive human breast carcinoma. *Journal of the National Cancer Institute*, 85, 723–31.

Sanchez-Guerrero, J., Colditz, G.A., Karlson, E.W. et al. (1995). Silicone breast implants and the risk of connective-tissue diseases and symptoms. *New England Journal of Medicine*, 332, 1666–70.

Sarrazin, D., Le, M.G., Rouesse, J. et al. (1984). Conservative treatment versus mastectomy in breast cancer tumours with microscopic diameter of 20 mm or less. *Cancer*, 53, 1209–13.

Sarrazin, D., Le, M.G., Arriagada, R. et al. (1989). Ten-year results of a randomized trial comparing a conservative treatment to mastectomy in early breast cancer. *Radiotherapy and Oncology*, 14, 177–84.

Schain, W.S., Jacobs, E. & Wellisch, D.K. (1984). Psychosocial issues in breast reconstruction: intrapsychic, interpersonal and practical concerns. *Clinics in Plastic Surgery*, 11, 237–51.

Schmid, H. (1887). Zue Statistick der Mammacarcinomie und deren Heilung. *Deutsche Zeitschrift fur Chirurgie*, 26, 139–45.

Senie, R.T., Rosen, P.P., Rhodes, P., Lesser, M.L. (1991). Timing of breast cancer excision during the menstrual cycle influences duration of disease free survival. *Annals of Internal Medicine*, 115, 337–42.

Silverstein, M.J., Gierson, E.D., Waisman, J.R. et al. (1994). Axillary lymph node dissection for T1a breast carcinoma: is it indicated? *Cancer*, 73, 664–7.

Smith, B.M., Slade, M.J., English, J. et al. (2000). Response of circulating tumor cells to systemic therapy in patients with metastatic breast cancer: comparison of quantitative polymerase chain reaction and immunocytochemical techniques. *Journal of Clinical Oncology*, 18(7), 1432–9.

Sugarbaker, E.D. (1953). Radical mastectomy combined with in-continuity resection of the homolateral internal mammary node chain. *Cancer*, 6, 969–79.

Taylor, M.E., Perez, C.A., Halverson, K.J. et al. (1995). Factors influencing cosmetic results after conservative surgery for breast cancer. *International Journal of Radiation Oncology Biology and Physics*, 31, 753–64.

Turner, R.R., Ollila, D.W., Krasne, D.L., Giuliano, A.E. (1997). Histopathological validation of the sentinel node hypothesis for breast cancer. *Annals of Surgery*, 226, 271–8.

Tyzzer, E.E. (1913). Factors in the production and growth of tumour metastases. *Journal of Medical Research*, 28, 309–22.

Urban, J.A. (1964). Surgical excision of internal mammary nodes for breast cancer. *British Journal of Surgery*, 51, 209–12.

Uren, R.F., Howman-Giles, R.B., Thompson, J.F. et al. (1997). Mammary lymphoscintigraphy in breast cancer. *Journal of Nuclear Medicine*, 36, 1775–80.

van der Veen, H., Hoekstra, O.S., Paul, M.A. et al. (1994). Gamma probe-guided sentinel node biopsy to select patients with melanoma for lymphadenectomy. *British Journal of Surgery*, 81, 1769–70.

Veronesi, U. & Valagussa, P. (1981). Inefficacy of internal mammary node dissection in breast cancer surgery. *Cancer*, 47, 170–5.

Veronesi, U., Saccozzi, R., Del Vecchio, M. et al. (1981). Comparing radical mastectomy with quadrantectomy, axillary dissection and radiotherapy in patients with small cancers of the breast. *New England Journal of Medicine*, 305, 6–11.

Veronesi, U., Cascinelli, N., Bufalino, R. et al. (1983). Risk of internal mammary lymph node metastases and its relevance on prognosis in breast cancer. *Annals of Surgery*, 198, 681–4.

Veronesi, U., Banfi, A., Salvadori, B. et al. (1990a). Breast conservation is the treatment of choice in small breast cancer: long-term results of a randomized trial. *European Journal of Cancer*, 26, 668–70.

Veronesi, U., Luini, A., Galimberti, V. et al. (1990b). Extent of metastatic involvement in 1446 cases of breast cancer. *European Journal of Surgical Oncology*, 127–33.

Veronesi, U., Luini, A., Del Vecchio, M. et al. (1993). Radiotherapy after breast-preserving surgery in women with localized cancer of the breast. *New England Journal of Medicine*, 328, 1587–91.

Veronesi, U., Luini, A., Mariani et al. (1994). Effect of menstrual phase on surgical treatment of breast cancer. *Lancet*, 343, 1544–6.

Veronesi, U., Paganelli, G., Galimberti, V. et al. (1997). Sentinel node biopsy to avoid axillary dissection in breast cancer with clinically negative lymph nodes. *Lancet*, 349, 1864–7.

Wangensteen, O.H., Lewis, F.J. & Arhelger, S.W. (1956). The extended or super-radical mastectomy for carcinoma of the breast. *Surgical Clinics of North America*, 36, 1051.

Wazer, D.E., DiPetrillo, T., Schmidt-Ullrich, R., et al. (1992). Factors affecting cosmetic outcome and complication risk after conservative surgery and radiotherapy for early-stage breast carcinoma. *Journal of Clinical Oncology*, 10, 356–63.

Wells, C.A., Heryet, A., Brochier, J. et al. (1984). The immunocytochemical detection of axillary micrometastases in breast cancer. *British Journal of Cancer*, 73, 88–95.

2

Chemoprevention of breast cancer

Tamas Hickish

Poole General Hospital, Longfleet Road, Poole, Dorset

Introduction

At present we are in an era of controlled clinical trials evaluating chemoendocrine agents in the prevention of breast cancer. Although breast cancer deaths (in the UK and USA) have now started to decline (Peto et al., 2000), the commitment to this approach originated in the recognition that early diagnosis and improvements in treatment had not translated into an order of magnitude step-down in mortality figures. Research directed at primary prevention of breast cancer has become a priority, especially for those women who are at increased risk of developing the disease. This is further enhanced by the emerging detail of breast cancer genetics, heralded with the identification of *BRCA1* and *BRCA2*, and the consequent ability to refine risk assessment, along with developments in the understanding of breast cancer biology, the oestrogen receptor (ER) and the availability of new selective oestrogen receptor modulators (SERMs).

In the early months of the year 2000 there was intense pressure on these prevention trials. Tamoxifen in the National Surgical Adjuvant Breast and Bowel Project (NSABP) P1 Breast Cancer Prevention Trial has been reported to reduce the incidence of invasive (and noninvasive) breast cancer when compared to placebo (Fisher et al., 1998), and as a consequence the Food and Drug Administration (FDA) have approved tamoxifen for breast cancer risk reduction in high-risk women. In contradistinction, the preliminary analyses of the Royal Marsden, London, UK and Italian tamoxifen randomized chemoprevention trials (Powles et al., 1998a; Veronesi et al., 1998) yielded null results. The NSABP, based on P1 and the observation that raloxifene in a placebo-controlled osteoporosis prevention trial (Multiple Outcomes of Raloxifene Evaluation [MORE]) was associated, as a secondary end-point, with a reduced incidence of invasive breast cancer (Cummings et al., 1999) have initiated a tamoxifen versus raloxifene prevention trial – STAR (Study of Tamoxifen and Raloxifene), whilst in Europe the placebo-controlled International Breast Cancer Prevention Study (IBIS) trial continues accrual. Given this apparent polarization, at this time, is tamoxifen chemoprevention of breast cancer standard for women at high risk or can continuation of the placebo-controlled trials be endorsed? Below we review these trials preceded by a consideration of chemoprevention.

Chemoprevention as a strategy in breast cancer

Chemoprevention as a strategy is based on the premise that multistep epithelial carcinogenesis is not inevitable once activated and can be halted (or reversed) in its preinvasive stages and that this effect will hold across multiple potentially malignant foci (field carcinogenesis) in a tissue. Furthermore, pending the development of chemopreventive agents tailored to a particular molecular defect(s) responsible for risk, the chosen agent should have activity whatever the carcinogenic pathway.

The justification for a randomized placebo-controlled trial may appear tenuous when an individual is considered to be at very high risk. It might be argued that such individuals should have any treatment that may be of benefit. This ignores the opposing issue of the risks of treatment itself and, futhermore, for breast cancer, a very strong family history occurs in just 10% of cases and therefore a prevention initiative dedicated to women at high risk would impact only on a minority of cancers. Ideally then, the outcomes from an intervention should be applicable to the larger population of women at lower risk since the overriding strategy is to develop a treatment that may safely be used by all well women. A stark example of the play of these issues is given by a consideration of bilateral prophylactic mastectomy which appears to be effective in preventing breast cancer. A recent retrospective study from the Mayo Clinic of 639 women with a well-defined family history of breast cancer who underwent bilateral prophylactic mastectomy and their untreated sisters, who served as controls, found that with a follow-up of 14 years, mastectomy was associated with a reduction of at least 90% in both the incidence of breast cancer and the risk of death from this disease; equating in this study to 2 deaths rather than the expected 20 (Hartmann et al., 1999). This can be viewed as encouraging for those women who wish to, or have undergone, such surgery. Equally, however, 621 women who would likely have not died from breast cancer have undergone an intervention which may carry substantial psychological sequelae (Eisen & Weber, 1999).

Primary chemoprevention is directed towards healthy individuals and therefore chemoprevention trials differ from conventional drug trials in cancer patients in that both acute and long-term toxicity must be minimal. The effectiveness and safety of a chemopreventive agent can only be assessed in prospective controlled clinical trials. The number of participants needed in such trials depends on the risk level for cancer development of the participants, the degree of 'protection' afforded and compliance. Even to detect a major prevention effect the study population required may need to be large. For breast cancer with a relative risk of 5, a total of 250–300 cancers would be expected in 5000 women over a 10-year period.

Therefore 10 000 women are required for a placebo-controlled trial to detect a 25% reduction in breast cancer incidence with 95% confidence limits. Compliance with allocated treatment is of great importance in maintaining the statistical power of the study, for example 50% compliance requires a fourfold increase in number of subjects. Follow-up over years is required to determine both the level of protection afforded by the tested agent(s) and any differences in the natural history of those cancers which do develop, along with monitoring for adverse effects. As such, it is clear that the resources necesssary to conduct a randomized prevention trial are substantial. Futhermore, in the context of a rationally evolving chemoprevention programme for breast cancer it may take years to build upon the results of trials if the end point is disease-specific mortality. Surrogate end points for efficacy are urgently required and it is likely these will be developed as the current chemoprevention programmes proceed.

Rationale for tamoxifen chemoprevention trials

That tamoxifen may act to prevent or delay breast cancer development was indicated by experimental and clinical data. By 1977 it was established that tamoxifen inhibits the oestrogen-dependent proliferation of MCF7 (a breast cancer cell line) cells in vitro. In animal models of breast cancer, tamoxifen treatment prevents the development of carcinogen (dimethylbenzanthracene) initiated ER-positive, but not ER-negative, mammary tumours in the rat and tumours in mice infected with the mouse mammary tumour virus. In 1985 Cuzick and Baum first noted that tamoxifen reduced the incidence of contralateral breast cancer in an adjuvant tamoxifen trial which has been confirmed as a 47% reduction in risk in a meta-analysis of all tamoxifen trials (Early Breast Cancer Trialists' Collaborative Group, 1998).

These observations when set in the context of the general low toxicity profile associated with tamoxifen – less than 5% of patients withdrawing from adjuvant trials because of drug-related acute toxicity – encouraged the testing of tamoxifen in the prevention of breast cancer.

The Royal Marsden Tamoxifen Prevention Trial

The first step in the evaluation of tamoxifen in the chemoprevention of breast cancer was undertaken in 1986 when a feasibility trial was initiated at The Royal Marsden Hospital, London, UK. This was designed to assess the logistic problems of a full-scale tamoxifen prevention trial in healthy women recruited from screening and symptomatic breast clinics involving a 1 : 1 randomization to tamoxifen or placebo. Participants had at least one first-degree relative aged under 50 years with breast cancer, or one first-degree relative with bilateral breast cancer, or more than one first-degree relative of any age, or a first-degree relative of any age together with a second-degree relative with breast cancer; these criteria equate to an estimated relative age-related risk of developing breast cancer of approximately fourfold that in the general population. Women with a past history of venous thrombosis, any previous malignancy or an estimated life expectancy of less than 10 years were excluded. Women who had not completed their families or were at pregnancy risk or taking the oral contraceptive pill were not eligible. Post-menopausal women were not excluded if they were receiving hormone replacement therapy (HRT) at the time of entry to the trial and usage of HRT during the trial was recorded. Initially the planned duration of medication was 5 years but subsequently this was extended to 8 years. During follow-up, clinical examination and assessment of toxicity (by an oral check list) were performed every 6 months and mammography repeated annually. Safety monitoring involved assessment of coagulation factors, lipids, bone mineral density, ovarian cysts and uterine thickness.

By 1991, the first women randomized into the feasibility programme had received 5 years of medication and a review of acute toxicity, safety (in particular, the reduction in cholesterol levels) and compliance data prompted extension of the initial feasibility study into a pilot programme of 2500 healthy women (Powles et al., 1994). At this time it was estimated that by 1998 there would be a 90% chance of detecting a 50% reduction in breast cancer incidence. The study closed for accrual in April 1996 with randomization of 2494 healthy women. An interim analysis was reported in 1998 of the 2471 eligible participants with a median follow-up of 70 months (Powles et al., 1998a) (Table 2.1). The two arms of the study were evenly matched for baseline characteristics. Compliance, assessed by questioning, was in excess of 78% for both tamoxifen and placebo and consistent with measurements of cholesterol and tamoxifen metabolites from subsets of the participants. Allocated treatment was prematurely discontinued by 877 participants either due to side-effects or nontoxic reasons (tamoxifen 320, placebo 176, $p < 0.0005$). The frequency of breast cancer was the same for tamoxifen and placebo (tamoxifen 34, placebo 36 $p = 0.8$). HRT was taken during the trial by 26% of participants (tamoxifen 336, placebo 305) but taken for only 13% of the time while on tamoxifen; there was no evidence of any negative interaction between tamoxifen and HRT with 12 cancers in the 523 participants who took HRT and 13 in the 507 on placebo ($p = 0.6$).

Table 2.1. Summary of reported placebo-controlled studies of tamoxifen for breast cancer

Trial	No. of participants	No. of breast cancer median follow-up	Participant characteristics	Results
NSABP P1	13 388	358 42 months	Increased risk by Gail model ($>1.66\%$ for 5-year risk) or age over 60 or LCIS; no concurrent HRT, 39% <50 years old	49% overall reduction in breast cancers ($p<0.00001$) in tamoxifen; no effect on incidence of ER-negative cancers
Italian Study	5408	41 46 months	Low-risk population; prior hysterectomy required; concurrent HRT allowed; 38% <50 years old	No difference in breast cancer between groups; (subgroup analysis – reduction in breast cancers in tamoxifen plus HRT group ($p=0.02$))
Royal Marsden Study	2471	70 70 months	Increased risk by family history 96% with first-degree relative; pedigree analysis indicates 36% *BRCA1/2* carriers; concurrent HRT allowed; 62% <50 years old	No difference in breast cancers between groups

Breast cancer events include both invasive and noninvasive new breast cancers.

LCIS – lobular carcinoma in situ; ER – oestrogen receptor; HRT – hormone replacement therapy.

The NSABP-P1 trial

The NSABP-P1 trial opened for accrual in 1991 and randomized between placebo or tamoxifen 20 mg daily for 5 years. The primary objective was to determine whether 5 years of tamoxifen therapy would reduce the incidence of invasive breast cancer in participants who had a 5-year predicted risk of breast cancer of equal to or greater than 1.66%, as assessed by the Gail model, or had a biopsy of lobular carcinoma in situ, or who were over 60 years of age. The Gail model factors age, number of first-degree relatives with breast cancer, number of previous biopsies, presence of atypical hyperplasia, age of first live birth and age of menarche (Gail et al., 1989; Costantino et al., 1999). HRT was an exclusion criterion. In total, 13 388 women were randomized with an average risk of breast cancer derived by the Gail model of 3.2%; 78% of participants continued on treatment throughout the trial.

In March 1998, the trials' independent Data Monitoring Committee concluded that the primary end point of the trial had been reached; that tamoxifen treatment resulted in a 45% reduction in breast cancer risk (Table 2.1). Subsequently, with 13 175 women analysed and a median of 42 months follow-up the figure was updated to a 49% reduction in breast cancer risk ($p > 0.00001$) (Fisher et al., 1998). Tamoxifen-treated women had a 1.3% risk of breast cancer at 5 years compared to 2.6% for the placebo-treated group with an absolute risk reduction of 1.3%. The impact of tamoxifen treatment appeared to be limited to ER-positive cancers. Furthermore, tamoxifen treatment was associated with a 50% reduction (tamoxifen 35, placebo 69), in cases of noninvasive breast cancer ($p < 0.002$). The reduction in risk held for all age groups but was somewhat greater for women 60 years or older (49 years or younger, 44% reduction; 50–59 years, 51% reduction; 60 years or older, 55% reduction). Reduction in breast cancer risk varied according to risk level as determined by the Gail algorithm. Statistically significant reduction only occurred in the lowest ($< 2\%$ in 5 years) and highest ($> 5.01\%$ in 5 years) risk groups.

The Italian Tamoxifen Prevention Study

The Italian Tamoxifen Prevention Study, based upon the identified increase of endometrial cancer with tamoxifen, elected to include only women who had had a total hysterectomy, with only 26% of women having conservation of their ovaries. Increased risk of breast cancer by virtue of family history or other factors was not a requirement. HRT was not an exclusion criterion and participants who commenced HRT during the study were not withdrawn from the study. Recruitment to this trial began in 1992 with participants randomized to tamoxifen 20 mg daily or placebo, with allocated treatment to continue for 5 years. In 1997, after review by the Data Monitoring Committee, recruitment was ended early because of the number of participants 'dropping out' of the study; 5408 healthy women were randomized and with a median follow-up of 46 months 41 cases of breast cancer were identified; there was no difference in breast cancer frequency between the two treatment groups (tamoxifen 19, placebo 22). Of the women who were taking HRT (placebo 390, tamoxifen 362), 8 breast cancers developed in the placebo group as compared to 1 in tamoxifen-treated participants (95% CI: 0.02–1.02 HR 0.13; $p = 0.02$) (Table 2.1). Allocated treatment was discontinued by 26% of participants, most within the first year. Of these, 1027 did so of their own accord and 239 withdrew because of an adverse event. The absolute level of breast cancer in this population was low, probably because most women had had bilateral oophorectomies, an intervention known to reduce the risk of breast cancer, both in low and high-risk women (Parazzini et al., 1997; Rebbeck et al., 1999). This could have compromised any tamoxifen chemoprevention effect (apart from those women who also received HRT) and thereby negated the overall effect.

Overview of the reported tamoxifen breast cancer prevention trials

Based on the results of the P1 trial, the FDA have approved tamoxifen 20 mg daily to reduce the early incidence of breast cancer in women at risk as defined by the Gail model. This form of wording has been used, since the P1 trial has not shown a reduction in breast cancer mortality in these at-risk women, and, since closure of the trial, tamoxifen was offered to the placebo group of participants thereby making it impossible to gain any further morbidity data. Controversy exists as to whether, in P1, tamoxifen can be considered to treat or prevent breast cancer development (Bruzzi, 1998; Pritchard, 1998). Within the terms of P1 – that a reduction in the early incidence of invasive breast cancer over the period of the study indicates prevention (Fisher et al., 1998; Lippman & Brown, 1999) – the trial has proved the principle of chemoprevention for that particular study population. However, the distinction between prevention and treatment of occult tumours is important given the relatively limited follow-up in P1. The tamoxifen-associated reduction in breast cancer incidence will disappear with time if the effect is due to treatment of occult disease whereas, with prevention of the development of malignant disease, the benefit would be expected to persist. Although mathematical modelling and computer simulation of tumour growth seem to indicate that, in P1, tamoxifen has reduced breast cancer incidence by both treating occult disease and prevention of new tumour development and growth (Radmacher & Simon, 2000), ultimately this is not a substitute for longer follow-up with a range of efficacy endpoints including all-cause mortality. The IBIS trial remains open and has enrolled over 6100 participants with a target of 7000. This study will have sufficient statistical power to detect a survival advantage for tamoxifen treatment. Furthermore, a meta-analysis of the reported prevention trials is scheduled for later in 2000. At this time, however, there are a number of differences between the trials that may account for the differences in the apparent efficacy, or lack of it, of tamoxifen in chemoprevention.

Compliance and statistical power

If the same magnitude of the effect of tamoxifen prevention identified in P1 recurred in the Royal Marsden trial, there is just a 10% chance it would not have been detected. It is unclear whether differences in compliance explain the different outcomes of the trials. The rate of noncompliers in the first year of the Italian trial may have compromised the power of the trial to detect tamoxifen prevention (Pritchard, 1998).

The differences between the trials in terms of risk of breast cancer among the participants

The most likely explanation for the differences between the trial outcomes lies with differences in the subjects. For the Royal Marsden trial, eligibility criteria were predominantly derived from a strong family history with a consequent increased risk of inheriting *BRCA1* or *BRCA2*. Pedigree analysis indicates that approximately 36% of all participants and over 60% of those who developed breast cancer have a greater than 80% likelihood of carrying *BRCA1* or *BRCA2* – whereas, in P1, factors other than dominant genetic lesions are more probably involved. There are significant biological, pathological and clinical differences between non-*BRCA* and *BRCA1* and *BRCA2* cancers. Whereas 30–40% of sporadic cancers are ER negative, 70–80% of breast cancers that develop in *BRCA1* carriers are ER negative and high grade (Lakhani et al., 1999). Similarly, *BRCA1* and *BRCA2* cancers generally lack progesterone receptors (Osin et al., 1998). Moreover, ER changes in breast carcinogenesis are incompletely understood. If, in the development of an ER-negative invasive cancer there is an ER-positive stage then there would be the potential for prevention by treatment with tamoxifen. However, that such an ER-positive stage may not occur is indicated by the observation that ductal carcinoma in situ (DCIS), which is usually ER positive, is mostly ER negative in *BRCA1* mutation carriers (Osin et al., 1998). Furthermore, the possibility exists that any intermediate ER-positive stage is tamoxifen resistant. Therefore, assuming any chemoprevention effect exerted by tamoxifen is via opposition at the ER, tamoxifen would not be likely to prevent the majority of *BRCA1* and *BRCA2* related cancers. As such, the relatively large number of predicted ER-negative cancers in the Royal Marsden trial may have 'diluted' any prevention effect. In contradistinction, in the Italian trial, in which participants had a low risk and therefore perhaps were more likely to develop ER-positive cancers, there was a trend ($p = 0.16$) to fewer breast cancers in those randomized to tamoxifen in the group of participants who took allocated treatment for at least one year, perhaps consistent with tamoxifen prevention of ER-positive cancers.

Taken together, the reported tamoxifen prevention trials do not show any reduction in the risk of ER-negative disease and this is consistent with the action of tamoxifen at the ER. ER-negative invasive disease is a significant burden and is a major issue for women at highest genetic risk. The relevance of tamoxifen/SERM exposure to the prevention of ER-negative disease should become clearer from the emerging detail of carcinogenesis, including the interaction between ER and *BRCA1* and 2.

The use of HRT

The Royal Marsden and Italian trials allowed for the use of HRT. However, in neither was there evidence that HRT attenuated the effect of tamoxifen. Indeed, in the Italian trial, subgroup analysis indicated a reduction in breast cancer incidence in patients allocated tamoxifen who also took HRT throughout the duration of the study. The numbers of participants and duration of HRT usage was low in the Royal Marsden study but there was no evidence of any differences in surrogates of tamoxifen activity – cholesterol, bone mineral density and uterine changes – between those receiving HRT or not, and cholesterol was reduced in those receiving tamoxifen who developed breast cancer.

Adverse effects of tamoxifen in the breast cancer prevention trials

Taken together, the profile of adverse effects in the Royal Marsden trial, P1 and Italian Tamoxifen Prevention trials is broadly consistent with experience of tamoxifen usage in patients with established breast cancer and essentially derive from the action of tamoxifen as a SERM.

Menopausal symptoms and anxiety

In the Royal Marsden trial significantly more women discontinued tamoxifen due to side-effects (tamoxifen 320, placebo 176, $p < 0.0005$) and these were most commonly hot flushes, other vasomotor symptoms and gynaecological problems. Similarly in a cohort of 11 064 women recruited over the first 24 months of the P1 study, a health related quality of life analysis was performed at baseline and the first 36 months of follow-up and this identified an increase in vasomotor and gynaecological symptoms in the tamoxifen group. The proportion of women on tamoxifen reporting difficulties with sexual functioning, at a definite or serious level, was greater in the tamoxifen group although the overall rates of sexual activity in both groups were similar. There was no difference between the quality of life measurements using the centre for epidemiological studies (depression scale or the medical outcome study 36 item short form health status survey) (Day et al., 1999). An analysis of anxiety amongst a cohort of women participating in the Royal Marsden trial in comparision to women offered screening mammography through the UK National Breast Screening Programme found no excess of anxiety in the prevention trial women, although there is no breakdown for tamoxifen versus placebo (Thirlaway et al., 1996).

Vascular events

In the Royal Marsden trial the incidence of vascular events (pulmonary embolism, stroke, venous thrombosis) was low and equivalent for tamoxifen and placebo. However, in both the P1 and the Italian trials there were more vascular events in the tamoxifen-treated participants. In P1, the risk of vascular events collectively was increased approximately threefold with pulmonary embolism and stroke being of greatest concern, although the increase of each was not statistically significant. Pulmonary embolism in the tamoxifen group was increased threefold compared with placebo (RR 3.01; 95% CI: 1.15–9.27). The incidence of strokes in the tamoxifen group was approximately double that receiving placebo (women ≥ 50 years, RR 1.75; 95% CI: 0.98–3.2: average annual incidence per 1000 women; placebo 0.92, tamoxifen 1.45). In the Italian trial vascular events occurred significantly more frequently with tamoxifen (tamoxifen 38, placebo 18, $p = 0.0053$). However, most of these were superficial phlebitis and there were just two reports of pulmonary embolus (tamoxifen 1, placebo 1) and 14 reports of stroke (tamoxifen 9, placebo 5, $p = 0.27$).

The level of risk for thromboembolic events equates to that observed with oestrogen and other SERMs (Grodstein et al., 1996; Cummings et al., 1998; Hulley et al., 1998). The mechanism for this effect is uncertain. A detailed analysis of coagulation parameters in a sequential subset of women in the Royal Marsden trial found no sustained changes in coagulation parameters (Protein S, Protein C or cross-linked fibrinogen degradation products (Jones et al., 1992). Developments in pharmacogenetics are likely to enable the identification of those prone to thromboembolism.

Endometrial cancer

The P1 trial was consistant with experience in established breast cancer (Fisher et al., 1994), in that the rate of endometrial cancer was increased in the tamoxifen group (RR = 2.53; 95% CI: 1.35–4.97). There were three cases of endometrial cancer on tamoxifen treatment compared with one on placebo in the Royal Marsden trial. The EBCTCG 1998 overview indicates that use of tamoxifen increases the risk of endometrial cancer twofold for those on tamoxifen for 2 years and fourfold for those on it for 5 years. Postmenopausal women are chiefly at risk of endometrial cancer as a result of tamoxifen exposure and this is thought to result from its sustained oestrogenic action which is not abrogated by menstruation.

In P1 all the endometrial cancers were FIGO stage I. The increased awareness of tamoxifen associated endometrial cancer with prompt intervention in symptomatic participants may account for the early stage of these tumours. However, concerns remain, particularly with regard to the histological type (Bergman et al., 2000; Gelmon, 2000). Protocols for screening need to be derived.

Experience in breast cancer patients receiving adjuvant tamoxifen indicates routine surveillance with ultrasonography and/or endometrial biopsy is likely to be of limited value (Barakat, 1999; Barakat et al., 2000; Gerber et al., 2000).

Analysis of women participating in the Royal Marsden trial noted that premenopausal women at the start of tamoxifen treatment who developed amenorrhoea may be at risk of endometrial carcinoma, especially in the presence of endometrial thickening, low plasma oestradiol levels or gynaecological symptoms (Chang et al., 1998).

Ocular effects

In the P1 trial, in comparison to the placebo group, women treated with tamoxifen were significantly more likely to develop cataracts (RR 1.14; 95% CI 1.01–1.29) and to undergo cataract surgery (RR 1.57; 95% CI 1.16–2.14). No such effects were detected in the Royal Marsden and Italian trials. Of note, tamoxifen at high dose (180 mg/day), has been associated with retinopathy as well as keratopathy. However, the data regarding ocular toxicity generally is conflicting at conventional doses. Tamoxifen induced retinopathy appears to be reversible if diagnosed early and women in prevention and adjuvant trials should be monitored for new symptoms of visual impairment on tamoxifen (Kaiser-Kupfer & Lippmann, 1978; McKeown et al., 1981; Longstaff et al., 1989; Pavlidis et al., 1992).

Cardiovascular disease

ER is present in liver and SERMs influence lipid profiles. Consistent with cholesterol, lipid and lipoprotein analyses in postmenopausal women receiving adjuvant tamoxifen (e.g. Love et al., 1990; Morales et al., 1996), in the Royal Marsden trial tamoxifen treatment was associated with a reduction in total plasma cholesterol in pre and postmenopausal women which occured within 3 months of treatment and which was sustained over at least 5 years (Powles et al., 1998a). Of note in the Royal Marsden trial, there was a smaller but significant reduction in plasma cholesterol in women receiving placebo which is not explained, although it is possible that increased awareness of breast cancer risks may be associated with changes in dietary patterns and a lower fat intake. An analysis of other lipid and lipoprotein fractions in a subset of women in the Royal Marsden trial detected a decrease in low-density lipoprotein cholesterol (LDLC) and no change in apolipoproteins A & B or high-density lipoprotein cholesterol (HDLC) (Powles et al., 1994). A fall in LDLC as part of a reduction in total cholesterol is thought to be a strong independent predictor for reduction of cardiovascular disease in women. Such changes are found with HRT in healthy postmenopausal women, yet in the placebo-controlled HERS trial (Hulley et al., 1998) oestrogen/progestin treatment was associated with an increased risk of cardiovascular events at one year which fell to below that for placebo thereafter. However, the Royal Marsden P1 (Reis et al., 2001) and Italian trials did not detect a difference in the rate of cardiovascular disease between participants receiving tamoxifen and placebo. Although cardiovascular morbidity and mortality have not been defined end points in the adjuvant tamoxifen studies, these and the EBCTCG overview have not clearly demonstrated a reduced risk with tamoxifen treatment (EBCTCG, 1998). Triglycerides were not specifically monitored in the Italian study but an unexpected finding was of an apparent excess of instances of hypertriglyceridaemia in tamoxifen-treated women (tamoxifen 15, placebo 2, $p = 0.0013$). This observation requires further evaluation.

Bone density and fractures

Data on bone mineral density (BMD) was collected prospectively on a cohort of participants in the Royal Marsden trial. Consistent with data from studies of BMD in patients receiving adjuvant tamoxifen (Love et al., 1992), tamoxifen treatment in postmenopausal women was associated with a mean annual increase in BMD of approximately 1.5% (spine 1.17% $p < 0.005$; hip 1.71% $p < 0.001$) compared with a nonsignificant loss for women on placebo. A novel observation was that in premenopausal women receiving tamoxifen, BMD decreased progressively with a mean annnual loss of approximately 1.5% (spine $p < 0.001$, hip $p < 0.05$) (Powles et al., 1996). The mechanism(s) that explain the apparent opposite effect of tamoxifen on pre and postmenopausal bone have not been defined but presumably relate to a difference in the setting of ER in the pre and postmenopausal oestrogen environments. In the P1 trial, data on mechanism and site of fracture was collated prospectively. Fractures of the hip and wrist (Colles') and subsequently spine and lower radius, were considered to be indicative of osteoporosis. With 40% of the study population being 35–49 years of age and therefore at low risk of osteoporotic fracture, there was a trend to fewer fracture events (tamoxifen 111 vs. 137 placebo, RR 0.81; 95% CI 0.63–1.05). Data on bone-related events in the Italian study have not been reported.

Risk–benefit calculation

The quantitative estimation and meaning of individualized risk is notoriously difficult, yet it is central to any assessment of benefit from tamoxifen treatment as prevention (Chlebowski et al., 1999). In a general Western population, the number of breast cancer deaths in women in a birth cohort of 1000 is low; for example, 3 deaths would be expected in those aged 60–64, 4 deaths in those aged 65–69 years and 5 deaths in those aged 70–74 years – such women were eligible for P1 by virtue of age alone. This compares to deaths from cardiovascular disease for these age groups respectively of 9, 16 and 28. Even as risk increases with age, the risk of breast cancer in any decade of life never exceeds 1 in 34 (Phillips et al., 1999). The relative level of competing health risks may not be clearly appreciated. A survey of 1000 women aged 45–64 years by the National Council on Ageing of the USA found that 61% feared cancer, chiefly breast cancer, with just 9% fearing the leading cause of death, cardiovascular disease (National Council on Ageing, 1997).

A methodology for a risk–benefit analysis to identify categories of healthy women for whom benefits of tamoxifen may outweigh risks has been developed by Gail and colleagues (Gail et al., 1999). A review of data from outside P1 was used to estimate the background incidence of invasive breast cancer and of in situ lesions with respect to ethnic group as well as other pathology: endometrial cancer, vascular events, fractures and ocular disease. Data from P1 was used to estimate the effect of tamoxifen treatment on these same factors so as to provide an individualized calculation of the impact of tamoxifen on health outcomes. Their analysis indicates that tamoxifen is most beneficial for younger women with a projected 5-year risk of breast cancer ranging from 1.5% to 7%. For women with an intact uterus, negative health outcomes appear to exceed benefits unless the projected 5-year risk of invasive breast cancer is greater than 3% for those over 50 years and greater than 6% for those over 60 years.

There are, however, substantial information gaps. Representation of black women and other ethnic minorities was low in the P1 trial with just 469 included, and therefore whether the findings of this study can be translated to these ethnic minority groups is unknown (Taylor et al., 1999). Furthermore, other potentially deleterious effects of tamoxifen have not yet been quantified. For example, mutations of *BRCA1* and/or *2* might impair DNA repair and a genotoxic potential of tamoxifen in this setting may be harmful (Scully et al., 1997). The results of tamoxifen treatment on *BRCA1* or *2* mutation carriers will need to be carefully evaluated over the long term. BMD is not a risk factor in the Gail model but there is a strong positive association between BMD and breast cancer risk: prospective observational studies have found that in comparison to those in the lowest quartile of BMD, women in the highest quartile have a twofold to sevenfold increased relative risk (Cauley et al., 1996; Zhang et al., 1997). Set against this, the impact of tamoxifen on osteoporosis has not been evaluated prospectively and so in risk–benefit calculations of tamoxifen usage, the influence of BMD is unknown. Likewise the implication of premenopausal BMD loss with tamoxifen treatment requires further evaluation but conceivably may be a negative influence on the risk–benefit calculations (as currently formulated by Gail et al. (1999) the trend to a reduced risk of fracture is considered to hold whatever the age).

Other long-term risks of tamoxifen may exist and any reports of experimental or clinical toxicity of tamoxifen would warrant reappraisal of tamoxifen chemoprevention and the implementation of appropriate safety monitoring.

ER is present in brain and oestrogen deficiency is associated with accelerated progression of dementia. The effect of tamoxifen on the brain and cognitive function remains to be fully categorized. Although testing for depression and aspects of mental function by questionnaires did not detect any adverse effect of tamoxifen in P1, formal evaluation is now underway with more sensitive psychometric tests and neuroimaging (e.g. Ratner et al., 2000).

The potential for genotoxicity remains a concern with tamoxifen (Powles & Hickish, 1995). There is evidence for tamoxifen as a promotor of hepatic carcinogenesis in rats and this is thought to be a genotoxic rather than an oestrogenic effect. Tamoxifen can cause stable DNA adducts in rat and hamster liver even after short exposure to doses of tamoxifen as low as 1 mg/kg/day; however, the significance of this in man is unknown. To date there is no evidence for an excess of hepatocellular cancers in the adjuvant studies, although the median follow-up is relatively short.

For premenopausal women the question of teratogenesis is important and although there have been no reports of teratogenesis with tamoxifen, the use of tamoxifen as a chemopreventative agent would be contraindicated in women at pregnancy risk.

Could tamoxifen-related risk be reduced so as to favourably influence the balance of risk and benefit? If toxicity is related to tamoxifen dose, an option may be to reduce dose. Studies in vitro show that once ER is saturated the dose-response curve reaches a plateau (Coezy et al., 1982). Perhaps consistent with this observation, the EBCTCG 1998 has demonstrated equivalence in reduction of recurrence and death in adjuvant studies of tamoxifen at doses ranging from 20, 30 and 40 mg/day. However, there is no analysis with respect to the development of contralateral tumours. The antitumour effect of lower doses of tamoxifen has not been tested. However, low-dose tamoxifen has bioactivity as demonstrated in a placebo-controlled study in healthy women in which a dose of 10 mg on alternate days was comparable to 20 mg/day in its effect on a range of oestrogen-sensitive biomarkers including lipid profile and insulin-like growth factor 1 – elevated levels are associated with increased breast cancer risk (Hankinson et al., 1998), yet with an 80% reduction in blood concentration of tamoxifen and its main metabolites (Decensi et al., 1999). These observations cannot be readily extrapolated to tamoxifen chemoprevention (Jordan, 1999). At low doses, in experimental models, tamoxifen displays more oestrogenic activity promoting both breast cancer cell proliferation in vitro (Reddel & Sutherland, 1984) and endometrial cancers in athymic mice (O'Regan et al., 1998). Given the uncertanties surrounding efficacy and toxicity, a low-dose tamoxifen option would require full evaluation in a controlled trial.

Another approach to reduce the risks of tamoxifen might be to mitigate its effect on the uterus in postmenopausal women. Postmenopausal women in the Royal Marsden trial who had persistent endometrial thickening (>8 mm) (tamoxifen 56, placebo 5) were offered oral norethisterone 2.5 mg daily for 21 of 28 days for three consecutive cycles (Powles et al., 1998b). After norethisterone treatment, 39 of 47 women on tamoxifen had persistent ultrasound changes – cysts, polyps and endometrial thickening – however, 45 had a progesterone withdrawal bleed. Whether norethisterone would protect the uterus in post-menopausal women treated with tamoxifen would need to be tested in a clinical trial. Current data would caution against this approach since there may be a detrimental effect on breast tissue (Schairer et al., 2000). An alternative approach, to limit any potential adverse systemic effects of progestagens, would be to treat topically using intrauterine delivery.

A randomized study of endometrial surveillance alone compared to surveillance combined with application of a levonorgestrel intrauterine system in 122 post-menopausal women who had received at least 1 year of adjuvant tamoxifen found a 100% decidualization of the endometrium and prevention of endometrial polyp development (Gardner et al., 2000). The effects of intrauterine levonorgestrel on lipids and breast cancer and uterine cancer events needs to be evaluated (Neven, 2000).

Could treatment duration with tamoxifen be altered to lessen toxicity and maintain efficacy? The NSABP B14 trial of adjuvant study of stage 1 ER-positive cancers suggests 5 years as compared to 10 years of tamoxifen usage is associated with a reduced risk of endometrial cancer and vascular events but is equivalent in protecting against contralateral breast cancer development (Fisher et al., 1996). The EBCTCG 1998 indicates that the incidence of contralateral breast cancers is proportional to duration of adjuvant tamoxifen treatment from 1 to 5 years. As such, based on 5-year data it seems unlikely that trials of tamoxifen treatment other than for 5 years will beneficially alter the balance of risks and benefits.

HRT usage was excluded from P1 but allowed in the Royal Marsden and Italian trials. While there was no evidence that HRT usage accounted for the lack of a tamoxifen prevention effect in these studies the possibility of an interaction between HRT and tamoxifen (or any SERM that produces menopausal symptoms) warrants exploration. Vasomotor and other menopausal symptoms were a significant cause for discontinuing tamoxifen in all three trials and not being able to take HRT was a major reason for women declining enrollment in P1 (Yeomans Kinney et al., 1998). If HRT does not adversely interact with tamoxifen then accrual to tamoxifen/SERM prevention studies may be improved and unpleasant menopausal symptoms abrogated.

Evolving chemoprevention

The process of building upon the tamoxifen-led breast cancer prevention trials is under way even pending definitive evidence of a reduction in mortality and overall health benefit. This includes the evaluation of nongenotoxic SERMs with established toxicity profiles, such as toremifene which is now the subject of a placebo-controlled pilot study at the Royal Marsden (Powles, 1999). Like tamoxifen, such compounds may also have other healthcare benefits in terms of cardiovascular disease, preservation of BMD and perhaps fertility control.

Raloxifene

In the forefront of this approach is raloxifene. Raloxifene is a SERM which, like tamoxifen, opposes oestrogen in breast tissue and has oestrogen-like activity in bone. Unlike tamoxifen it does not have a uterotrophic effect (Boss et al., 1997; Delmas et al., 1997).

Experience with raloxifene in the treatment of breast cancer is very limited with just two small studies in advanced breast cancer. In one study of just 14 patients with tamoxifen-resistant disease there were no responses following treatment with a dose of 200 mg/day. In the other study at a dose of raloxifene 300 mg/day, there were three objective responses in 18 patients with ER-positive disease (Buzdar et al., 1988; Gradishar et al., 1997).

The agonist action on bone in postmenopausal women and the absence of an antagonist effect in the uterus encouraged the evaluation of raloxifene in postmenopaual women with osteoporosis in the MORE trial. This study is a multicentre randomized trial in which 7705 women were randomized to receive either raloxifene 60 mg/day, raloxifene 120 mg/day or placebo. Additionally, all women received calcium supplementation along with vitamin D. To be eligible, women were under 80 years of age, postmenopausal, and had osteoporosis as defined by a spine and/or hip fracture or spine bone density at least 2.5 standard deviations below that considered normal for young Caucasian women. Women who were taking oestrogen, or who had prior breast cancer or endometrial cancer or any abnormal uterine bleeding were excluded. The primary end point was vertebral fracture, secondary end points included breast cancer and thrombotic events.

Three year follow-up data has shown at least one new vertebral fracture in 10.1% of women receiving placebo, in 6.6% of patients receiving raloxifene 60 mg/day and in 4% in patients receiving raloxifene 120 mg/day (Ettinger et al., 1999).

With both doses of raloxifene, over the 3-year treatment period, the overall risk of newly diagnosed invasive breast cancer was reduced by 76% with no apparent effect on ER-negative disease (Cummings et al., 1999). Similarly, in a meta-analysis of nine raloxifene trials involving 10 575 patients, raloxifene treatment was associated with a 55% reduction in the risk of developing invasive breast cancer (Jordan et al., 1998). Again this effect was seen for ER-positive tumours only.

Analysis of other secondary end points have shown a threefold increase in the incidence of vascular events including pulmonary emboli but no measurable uterine effects.

In 1997 raloxifene received FDA approval as a treatment for osteoporosis in postmenopausal women. Based on the encouraging risk–benefit data for raloxifene, the NSABP have initiated a large phase III breast cancer prevention trial of tamoxifen 20 mg/day versus raloxifene 60 mg/day – the STAR or P2 trial – with the hypothesis that raloxifene treatment will have a superior therapeutic index than tamoxifen due to a reduction in uterine events. P2 plans to accrue 22 000 postmenopausal women. At present, premenopausal women are excluded due the lack of sufficient safety data. Additionally, in comparision to P1, there are stricter vascular exclusions and breast cancer risk calculations for women over 60 years of age.

There is limited experience with raloxifene and the newer SERMs in premenopausal women. Yet for *BRCA1* and *2* mutation carriers the risk-of-penetrance curve starts to rise from age 35 years. Hence strategies are required for evaluating chemoprevention with SERMs in such high-risk premenopausal women (Eeles & Powles, 2000). A pilot trial will shortly commence in the UK and Australia in women aged 35–45 with a risk of breast cancer, judged by family history, exceeding that in the tamoxifen prevention studies, which will initially assess compliance and quality of life matters resulting from ovarian suppression with Zoladex combined with raloxifene; the RAZOR study – Raloxifene and Zoladex Research Study.

Nutriceuticals – breast cancer prevention with phyto-oestrogens

The concept that 'natural' and therefore potentially nontoxic substances may protect against breast cancer is exemplified by the phyto-oestrogens. Phyto-oestrogens are plant-based diphenolic molecules which as a result of digestion develop oestrogeneic properties. The term covers a wide range of plant constituents, plant extracts and synthetic products. In vitro phyto-oestrogens appear to have an antiproliferative effect on breast cells. Epidemiological studies have indicated that a diet rich in phyto-oestrogens may be associated with a reduced risk of breast cancer (Messina et al., 1994), possibly along with a protective effect against osteoporosis and cardiovascular disease. These observations and some evidence indicating that phyto-oestrogens interact with the ER (Kuiper et al., 1998), indicate they may be environmental or natural SERMs. This in turn encourages the evaluation of phyto-oestrogens in breast cancer prevention. However, just as with drugs, these mechanistically complex molecules will require formal evaluation as they may have adverse effects either by virtue of their properties as SERMs (if indeed they prove to be) or via other paths (Ginsburg & Prelevic, 2000; Sirtori, 2000).

Fenretinide breast cancer prevention

The nuclear retinoid receptors, retinoic acid receptor (RAR) and retinoid X receptor (RXR), are transcription factors and belong to the same intracellular receptor family as ER. Fenretinide is a synthetic derivative of all-*trans*-retinoic acid. It has a high therapeutic index in preventing chemically induced murine breast cancer. It has activity in ER-positive and ER-negative cell lines and selectively induces apoptosis perhaps by modulating the retinoid receptor to inhibit proliferative signals (Fanjul et al., 1996). In clinical studies it accumulates in breast tissue. Finally, and crucially, it has a favourable toxicity profile. On this basis, in 1987, the Italian National Cancer Institute initiated a randomized phase III trial of fenretinide 200 mg/day for 5 years in the prevention of second (contralateral or ipsilateral) breast cancers following resection of early stage breast cancer or DCIS – the estimated incidence of secondary breast cancer in these women is 0.8% per year. This trial was not placebo controlled. Eligibility criteria included age 30–70 years, T1 N0 breast cancer; 1-node-positive patients were included from July 1991 and 17 such patients were randomized to no adjuvant systemic therapy. Women were eligible up to 10 years following primary therapy in the absence of breast cancer recurrence. The primary endpoint was the incidence of contralateral or ipsilateral breast cancer 7 years after randomization. Compliance was evaluated by counting returned capsules and in a subset (60%) of the study population, by serial estimation of plasma levels. The study was closed for accrual prematurely in July 1993 following the US National Cancer Institute Medical Alert recommending adjuvant therapy for node-negative breast cancer. A total of 2972 women were randomized and with median follow-up of 97 months there was no difference in the incidence of either contralateral ($p = 0.642$) or ipsilateral ($p = 0.177$)

breast cancer (Veronesi et al., 1999). Subgroup analysis indicated a possible reduction in second breast cancer incidence in premenopausal women and an increase in postmenopausal women. With the limitations of a *post hoc* analysis in mind (Piantadosi, 1999), this observation has biological plausability since in premenopausal women fenretinide depresses circulating levels of insulin-like growth factor I but not in postmenopausal women (Torrisi et al., 1998). Fenretinide requires further evaluation in breast cancer chemoprevention and other RXR and RAR targeting molecules are under development.

Conclusion and future directions

The preceeding discusion has emphasized the many unresolved issues surrounding breast cancer prevention, particularly the evaluation of clinical benefit associated with a reduction in early incidence, and the identification of risk groups, which again should benefit from tamoxifen, strategies to improve the balance of risks and benefits that may accrue from use of SERMs and other more selective endocrine interventions and treatment and to the identification of individuals who are likely to benefit from treatment. The key developments in the future will be in the structuring of risk profiles based on genomic analysis and molecular markers (Ellis & Hayes, 1999; Gobbi et al., 1999). The molecular mechanisms of carcinogenesis in the context of particular genetic risk should become clearer, and thereby allow the evaluation of established and new agents that have real potential for selective chemoprevention.

REFERENCES

Barakat, R.R. (1999). Screening for endometrial cancer in the patient receiving tamoxifen for breast cancer. (Editorial.) *Journal of Clinical Oncology*, 17, 1967–8.

Barakat, R.R., Gilewski, T.A., Almadrones, L. et al. (2000). Effect of adjuvant tamoxifen on the endometrium in women with breast cancer: a prospective study using office endometrial biopsy. *Journal of Clinical Oncology*, 18, 3459–63.

Bergman, L., Beelan, M.L.R., Galee, M.P.W. et al. and the Comprehensive Cancer Centres' ALERT Group (2000). Risk and prognosis of endometrial cancer after tamoxifen for breast cancer. *Lancet*, 356, 881–7.

Boss, S.M., Huster, W.J., Neild, J.A. et al. (1997). Effects of raloxifene hydrochloride on the endometrium of postmenopausal women. *American Journal of Obstetrics and Gynecology*, 177, 1458–64.

Bruzzi, P. (1998). Tamoxifen for the prevention of breast cancer: important questions remain unanswered and existing trials should continue. *Lancet*, 351, 1428–9.

Buzdar, A.V., Marcus, C., Holmes, F. et al. (1988). Phase II evaluation of LY 156758 in metastatic breast cancer. *Oncology*, 45, 344–5.

Cauley, J.A., Lucas, F.L., Kuller, L.H. et al. (1996). Bone mineral density and risk of breast cancer in older women: the study of osteoporotic fractures. *Journal of the American Medical Association*, 276, 1404–8.

Chang, J., Powles, T.J., Ashley, S.E. et al. (1998). Variation in endometrial thickening in women with amenorrhoea on tamoxifen. *Breast Cancer Research and Treatment*, 48(1), 81–5.

Chlebowski, R.T., Collyar, D.E., Somerfield, M.R. et al. (1999). American Society of Clinical Oncology Technology Assessment on Breast Cancer Risk Reduction Strategies: tamoxifen and raloxifene. *Journal of Clinical Oncology*, 17(6), 1939–55.

Coezy, E., Borgna, J.L. & Rochefort, H. (1982). Correlation between binding to oestrogen receptor and inhibition of cell growth. *Cancer Research*, 42, 317–23.

Costantino, J.P., Gail, M.H., Pee, D. et al. (1999). Validation studies for models projecting the risk of invasive and total breast cancer incidence. *Journal of the National Cancer Institute*, 91, 1541–8.

Cummings, S.R., Norton, L., Eckert, S. et al. (1998). Raloxifene reduces risk of breast cancer and may decrease the risk of endometrial cancer in postmenopausal women. Two-year findings from the Multiple Outcomes of Raloxifene Evaluation (MORE) trial. *Proceedings of the American Society of Clinical Oncology*, 17(2a), Abstract 3.

Cummings, S.R., Eckert, S., Krueger, K.A. et al. (1999). The effect of raloxifene on risk of breast cancer in postmenopausal women: results from the MORE randomized trial. *Journal of the American Medical Association*, 281, 2189–97.

Day, R., Ganz, P.A., Costantino, J.P. et al. (1999). Health-related quality of life and tamoxifen in breast cancer prevention: a study from the National Surgical Adjuvant Breast and Bowel Project P–1 Study. *Journal of Clinical Oncology*, 17, 2659–69.

Decensi, A., Gandini, S., Guerrieri-Gonzaga, A. et al. (1999). Effect of blood tamoxifen concentrations on surrogate biomarkers in a trial of dose reduction in healthy women. *Journal of Clinical Oncology*, 17, 2633–8.

Delmas, P.D., Bjarnasan, N.G., Mitlak, B.H. et al. (1997). Effects of raloxifene on bone mineral density, serum cholesterol concentrations, and uterine endometrium in postmenopausal women. *New England Journal of Medicine*, 337, 1641–7.

Early Breast Cancer Trialists' Collaborative Group (1998). Tamoxifen for early breast cancer: an overview of the randomised trials. *Lancet*, 351, 1451–67.

Eeles, R.A. & Powles, T.J. (2000). Chemoprevention options for BRCA1 or BRCA2 mutation carriers. *Journal of Clinical Oncology*, 18 (21 Suppl.), 93S–9S.

Eisen, A. & Weber, B.L. (1999). Prophylactic mastectomy – the price of fear. (Editorial.) *New England Journal of Medicine*, 340, 137–8.

Ellis, M.J. & Hayes, D.F. (1999). Refining breast cancer risk assessment with molecular markers: the next step? *Journal of the National Cancer Institute*, 91(24), 2067–9.

Ettinger, B., Black, D.M., Mitlak, B.H. et al. (1999). Reduction of vertebral fracture risk in post menopausal women with osteoporosis treated with raloxifene: results from a 3-year randomised clinical trial. *Journal of the American Medical Association*, 282, 637–45.

Fanjul, A.N., Delia, D., Pierotti, M.A. et al. (1996). 4-Hydroxyphenyl retinamide is a highly selective activator of retinoid receptors [published erratum appears in *Journal of Biological Chemistry* (1996), 271, 33705]. *Journal of Biological Chemistry*, 271, 22 441–6.

Fisher, B., Costantino, J.P., Redmond, C.K. et al. (1994). Endometrial cancer in tamoxifen-treated breast cancer patients: findings from the National Surgical Adjuvant Breast and Bowel Project (NSABP) B-14. *Journal of the National Cancer Institute*, 86, 527–37.

Fisher, B., Dignam, J., Bryant, J. et al. (1996). Five versus more than five years of tamoxifen therapy for breast cancer with negative lymph nodes and estrogen receptor positive tumors. *Journal of the National Cancer Institute*, 88, 1529–42.

Fisher, B., Costantino, J.P., Wickerham, D.L. et al. (1998). Tamoxifen for prevention of breast cancer: report of the National Surgical Adjuvant Breast and Bowel Project P-1 study. *Journal of the National Cancer Institute*, 90, 1371–88.

Gail, M.H., Brinton, L.A., Byar, D.P. et al. (1989). Projecting individualized probabilities of developing breast cancer for white females who are being examined annually. *Journal of the National Cancer Institute*, 81, 1879–86.

Gail, M.H., Costantino, J.P., Bryant, J. et al. (1999). Weghing the risks and benefits of tamoxifen treatment for preventing breast cancer. *Journal of the National Cancer Institute*, 91, 1829–46.

Gardner, F.J.E., Konje, J.C., Abrams, K.R. (2000). Endometrial protection from tamoxifen-stimulated changes by a levonorgestrel-releasing intrauterine system: a randomised controlled trial. *Lancet*, 356, 1711–17.

Gelmon, K. (2000). One step forward or one step back with tamoxifen? (Editorial.) *Lancet*, 356(9233), 868–9.

Gerber, B., Krause, A., Müller, H. et al. (2000). Effects of adjuvant tamoxifen on the endometrium in postmenopausal women with breast cancer: a prospective long-term study using transvaginal ultrasound. *Journal of Clinical Oncology*, 18, 3464–70.

Ginsburg, J. & Prelevic, G.M. (2000). Lack of significant hormonal effects and controlled trials of phyto-oestrogens. (Editorial.) *Lancet*, 355, 163–4.

Gobbi, H., Dupont, W.D., Simpson, J.F. et al. (1999). Transforming growth factor- B and breast cancer risk in women with mammary epithelial hyperplasia. *Journal of the National Cancer Institute*, 91, 2096–101.

Gradisher,W.J., Glusman, J.E., Vogel, C.L. et al. (1997). Raloxifene HCl, a new endocrine agent, is active in estrogen receptor positive (ER+) metastatic breast cancer. *Breast Cancer Research and Treatment: San Antonio Breast Cancer Symposium Proceedings*, 20, 53, Abstract.

Grann, V.R., Panageas, K.S., Whang, W. et al. (1998). Decision analysis of prophylactic mastectomy and oopherectomy in BRCA1-positive or BRCA2-positive patients. *Journal of Clinical Oncology*, 16, 979–85.

Grodstein, F., Stampfer, M.J., Goldhaber, S.Z. et al. (1996). Prospective study of exogenous hormones and risk of pulmonary embolism in women. *Lancet*, 348, 983–7.

Hankinson, S.E., Willett, W.C., Colditz, G.A. et al. (1998). Circulating levels of insulin-like growth factor-I and risk of breast cancer. *Lancet*, 351, 1393–6.

Hartmann, L.C., Schaid, D.J., Woods, J.E. *et al.* (1999). Efficacy of bilateral prophylactic mastectomy in women with a family history of breast cancer. *New England Journal of Medicine*, 340, 77–84.

Hulley, S., Grady, D., Bush, T. et al. (1998). Randomized trial of estrogen plus progestin for secondary prevention of coronary heart disease in postmenopausal women: Heart and

Estrogen/Progestin Replacement Study (HERS) Research Group. *Journal of the American Medical Association*, 280, 605–13.

Jones, A.L., Powles, T.J., Treveaven, J.G. et al. (1992). Haemostatic changes and thromboembolic risk during tamoxifen therapy in normal women. *British Journal of Cancer*, 66(4), 744–7.

Jordan, V.C. (1999). Tamoxifen: too much of a good thing? *Journal of Clinical Oncology*, 17, 2629–30.

Jordan, V.C., Glusman, J.E., Eckert, S. et al. (1998). Incident primary breast cancers are reduced by raloxifene: integrated data from multicenter, double blind, randomized trials in 12,000 postmenopausal women. *Proceedings of the American Society of Clinical Oncology*, 17, 122a, Abstract 466.

Kaiser-Kupfer, M.I & Lippmann, M.E. (1978). Tamoxifen retinopathy. *Cancer Treatment Reports*, 62, 315–20.

Kuiper, G.G., Lemmen, J.G., Carlsson, B. et al. (1998). Interaction of estrogenic chemicals and phytoestrogens with estrogen receptor beta. *Endocrinology*, 139, 4252–63.

Lakhani, S., Sloane, J.P., Gusterson, B.A. et al. (1999). A detailed analysis of the morphological features associated with breast cancer in patients harbouring mutations in BRCA1 and BRCA2 predisposition genes. *Journal of the National Cancer Institute*, 90, 1138–45.

Lippman, S.M. & Brown, P.H. (1999). Tamoxifen prevention of breast cancer: an instance of the Fingerpost. *Journal of the National Cancer Institute*, 91(21), 1809–19.

Longstaff, S., Sigurdsson, H., O'Keeffe, M. et al. (1989). A controlled study of the ocular effects of tamoxifen in conventional dosage in the treatment of breast carcinoma. *European Journal of Cancer and Clinical Oncology*, 25(12), 1805–8.

Love, R.R., Newcomb, P.A., Wiebe, D.A. et al. (1990). Effects of tamoxifen therapy on lipid and lipoprotein levels in postmenopausal patients with node-negative breast cancer. *Journal of the National Cancer Institute*, 82, 1327–32.

Love, R.R., Mazess, R.B., Barden, H.S. et al. (1992). Effects of tamoxifen on bone mineral density in postmenopausal women with breast cancer. *New England Journal of Medicine*, 326, 852–6.

McKeown, C., Swartz, M. & Blom, J. (1981). Tamoxifen retinopathy. *British Journal of Ophthalmology*, 65, 177–9.

Messina, M.J., Persky, V., Setchell, K.D.R. et al. (1994). Soy intake and cancer risk: a review of in vitro and in vivo data. *Nutrition and Cancer*, 21, 113–31.

Morales, M., Santana, N., Soria, A. et al. (1996). Effects of tamoxifen on serum lipid and apolipoprotein levels in postmenopausal patients with breast cancer. *Breast Cancer Research and Treatment*, 40, 265–70.

National Council on Ageing (1997). *Myths and perceptions about ageing and women's health.* Washington, DC.

Neven, P. (2000). Local levonorgestrel to prevent tamoxifen-related endometrial lesions. (Editorial.) *Lancet*, 356, 1698–9.

O'Regan, R.M., England, G., Cisneros, A. et al. (1998). Relationship of tamoxifen dose and the growth of tamoxifen-stimulated tumors. *Proceedings of the American Society of Clinical Oncology*, 17, 109a, Abstract 419.

Osin, P., Crook, T., Powles, T. et al. (1998). Hormone status of *in situ* cancer in BRCA1 and BRCA2 mutation carriers. *Lancet*, 351, 1487.

Parazzini, F., Braga, C., La Vecchia, C. et al. (1997). Hysterectomy, oophorectomy and premenopause and risk of breast cancer. *Obstetrics and Gynecology*, 90, 453–6.

Pavlidis, N., Petris, C., Briassoulis, E. et al. (1992). Clear evidence that long-term low-dose tamoxifen treatment can induce ocular toxicity. *Cancer*, 69, 2961–4.

Peto, R., Boreham, J., Clarke, M. et al. (2000). UK and USA breast cancer deaths down 25% in year 2000 at age 20–69 years. *Lancet*, 355, 1822.

Phillips, K.-A., Glendon, G. & Knight, J.A. (1999). Putting the risk of breast cancer in perspective. *New England Journal of Medicine*, 340, 141–4.

Piantadosi, S. (1999). Vitamin A analogue for breast cancer prevention: a grade F or incomplete? *Journal of National Cancer Institute*, 91, 1794.

Powles, T.J. (1999). Tamoxifen for prevention of breast cancer: report of the National Surgical Adjuvant Breast and Bowel P-1 study. *Journal of the National Cancer Institute*, 91, 730 (letter).

Powles, T.J. & Hickish, T.F. (1995). Tamoxifen therapy and carcinogenic risk. (Editorial.) *Journal of the National Cancer Institute*, 87, 1343–5.

Powles, T., Eeles, R., Ashley, S. et al. (1998a). Interim analysis of the incidence of breast cancer in the Royal Marsden Hospital tamoxifen randomized chemoprevention trial. *Lancet*, 352, 98–101.

Powles, T.J., Bourne, T., Athanaiou, S. et al. (1998b). The effects of norethisterone on endometrial abnormalities identified by transvaginal ultrasound screening of healthy post-menopausal women on tamoxifen or placebo. *British Journal of Cancer*, 78, 272–5.

Powles, T.J., Hickish, T., Kanis, J.A. et al. (1996). Effect of tamoxifen on bone mineral density measured by dual-energy x-ray absorptiometry in health premenopausal and postmenopausal women. *Journal of Clinical Oncology*, 14, 78–84.

Powles, T.J., Jones, A.L., Ashley, S.E. et al. (1994). The Royal Marsden Hospital pilot tamoxifen chemoprevention trial. *Breast Cancer Research and Treatment*, 31, 73–84.

Pritchard, K.L. (1998). Is tamoxifen effective in prevention of breast cancer? *Lancet*, 352, 80–1.

Radmacher, M.D. & Simon, R. (2000). Estimation of tamoxifen's efficacy for preventing the formation and growth of breast tumors. *Journal of the National Cancer Institute*, 92, 1, 48–53.

Ratner, L., Mortimer, J.E., Mintun, M. et al. (2000). Effect of tamoxifen on memory and cognitive functioning – clinical correlation with positron emission tomography. *Proceedings of the American Society of Clinical Oncology*, 19, 644a, Abstract 2543.

Rebbeck, T.R., Levin, A.M., Eisen, A. et al. (1999). Breast cancer risk after bilateral prophylactic oophorectomy in BRCA1 mutation carriers. *Journal of the National Cancer Institute*, 91(17), 1475–9.

Reddel, R.R. & Sutherland, R.L. (1984). Tamoxifen stimulation of human breast cancer cell proliferation in vitro: a possible model for tamoxifen tumor flare. *European Journal of Clinical Oncology*, 20, 1419–24.

Reis, S.E., Costantino, J.P., Wickerham, D.L. et al. (2001). Cardiovascular effect of tamoxifen in women with and without heart disease: Breast Cancer Prevention Trial. *Journal of the National Cancer Institute*, 93, 16–21.

Schairer, C., Lubin, J., Troisi, R. et al. (2000). Menopausal estrogen and estrogen–progestin replacement therapy and breast cancer risk. *Journal of the American Medical Association*, 283(4), 485–91.

Scully, R., Chen, J., Plug, A. et al. (1997). Association of the BRCA1 gene product with Rad51 in meiotic and mitotic cells. *Cell*, 88, 265–75.

Sirtori, C.R. (2000). Dubious benefits and potential risk of soy phyto-oestrogens. *Lancet*, 355, 849 (letter).

Taylor A.L., Adams-Campbell, L.L. & Wright, J.T. (1999). Risk/benefit assessment of tamoxifen to prevent breast cancer – still a work in progress? *Journal of the National Cancer Institute*, 91, 1792–3.

Thirlaway, K., Fallowfield, L., Nunnerley, H. et al. (1996). Anxiety in women 'at risk' of developing breast cancer. *British Journal of Cancer*, 73, 1422–4.

Torrisi, R., Parodi, S., Fontana, V. et al. (1998). Effect of of fenretinide on plasma IGF-I and IGFBP-3 in early breast cancer patients. *International Journal of Cancer*, 76, 787–90.

Veronesi, U., Maisonneuve, P., Costa, A. et al. (1998). Prevention of breast cancer with tamoxifen: preliminary findings from the Italian randomised trial among hysterectomised women. Italian Tamoxifen Prevention Study. *Lancet*, 352(9122), 93–7.

Veronesi, U., De Palo, G., Marubini, E. et al. (1999). Randomized trial of fenretinide to prevent second breast malignancy in women with early breast cancer. *Journal of the National Cancer Institute*, 91, 1847–56.

Yeomans Kinney, A., Vernon, S.W., Shui, W. et al. (1998). Validation of a model predicting enrollment status in a chemoprevention trial for breast cancer. *Cancer Epidemiology, Biomarkers and Prevention*, 7, 591–5.

Zhang, Y., Kiel, D.P., Kreger, B.E. et al. (1997). Bone mass and the risk of breast cancer among post menopausal women. *New England Journal of Medicine*, 336, 611–16.

3

Familial breast cancer

H. Gogas and V. Murday

St George's Hospital, Blackshaw Road, London

Introduction

Breast cancer affects about 1 in 12 women and the annual incidence of breast cancer in the UK is 25 000. Of the known risk factors for breast cancer a positive family history appears to be the most important.

The recurrence of breast cancer in families may be a result of genetic factors, environmental factors or coincidence. Given the high frequency of breast cancer in Western populations most families in which two cases have occurred will be as a result of a coincidence. Population studies have suggested that most of the excess genetic risk is due to high penetrance autosomal dominant genes. Members of such families usually have cancer at an early age, an excess of bilateral, multifocal breast cancer and sometimes other related cancers such as of the ovary, prostate and colon. Inherited susceptibility accounts for only about 5% of all breast cancer cases (Claus et al., 1991), but about 25% of early onset cases ($<$30 years). Since there is such a strong association with early age of onset and the presence of a genetic susceptibility this is a strong indicator of risk in families where more than one case has occurred.

BRCA1

In October 1994 the first gene for susceptibility to breast cancer, *BRCA1*, was identified (Miki et al., 1994). *BRCA1* had been localized previously on chromosome 17q21 in 1990 by linkage analysis studies (Hall et al., 1990). Mutations of the *BRCA1* gene are thought to account for approximately 45% of families with a high incidence of breast cancer and at least 80% of families with increased incidence of both early onset breast cancer and ovarian cancer. Estimates of the penetrance from families collected from linkage studies worldwide have shown the risk of breast cancer in carriers to be 59% by the age of 50 years and 82% by the age of 70, and the risk of ovarian cancer to be about 42% by age 70 (Easton et al., 1993). The lifetime risk of breast cancer is 80% to 90% and of ovarian cancer 40% to 50%. The ovarian cancer risk varies greatly between families (Easton et al., 1995). It is estimated that 89% of families have a relatively low risk of ovarian cancer (26% by age 70) and the remaining have a much higher risk at 85%. The presumed explanation for this finding is that different mutations may confer inherently different risks of ovarian cancer. There is some evidence that mutations in the 3' third of the gene have a lower risk of ovarian cancers (Shattuck-Eidens et al., 1995). However, the variability between families does not appear to be due solely to the type or site of the mutation, as different families with the same mutation seem to vary in their risk of ovarian cancer. This may be due either to modifying genes or environmental factors.

BRCA1 mutation-carrier rates are estimated between 1 in 2000 to 1 in 500 women (Easton et al., 1994). Hundreds of distinct mutations have been found, and three specific mutations appear relatively common, 185delAG, 5382insC, and 4184del4 (Shattuck-Eidens et al., 1995). The 185delAG frameshift mutation has been found to be common in Ashkenasi Jewish breast/ovarian families (of Eastern European origin) (Struewing et al., 1995a; Takahashi et al., 1995; Tonin et al., 1995). The carrier frequency of this mutation is 0.9% in Ashkenasi individuals (Struewing et al., 1995b), which is several times higher than the expected frequency of all *BRCA1* mutations combined in the general population of 1 in 800 (Mitchell & Eeles, 1999). Interestingly, the penetrance of this mutation in Ashkenasi population studies has been lower than that calculated from the families collected in the linkage consortium (Struewing et al., 1997). This may reflect the bias of ascertainment of the high-risk families who may have other modifying risk factors that have ensured their ascertainment.

Tumour analysis has demonstrated somatic loss of heterozygosity in the region of *BRCA1* in about 30–60% of sporadic breast cancers and 60% of ovarian cancers, which suggest that cancer-predisposing mutations can also be acquired within somatic cells during neoplastic transformation (Sato et al., 1991; Futreal et al., 1992). Significant excesses of colon and prostatic cancer were observed in *BRCA1* carriers, a fourfold and threefold increase respectively (Ford et al., 1994). This gene has 22 exons and it codes for a protein of 1863 amino acids. It shows no homology to other known genes with the exception of a 126 nucleotide sequence at the amino terminus which encodes a *RING* finger motif (a configuration characteristic of the *RING-1* gene), a motif which may be involved in protein–protein interactions (Bertwhistle & Ashworth, 1998).

BRCA2

A second susceptibility locus, *BRCA2* was mapped on chromosome 13q12–13 (Wooster et al., 1994) and has now been identified (Wooster et al., 1995). This gene has 27 exons and encodes a protein of 3418 amino acids with an estimated molecular weight of 384 kDa (Bertwhistle & Ashworth, 1998). It is thought to be a tumour suppressor gene, as analysis of tumours taken from *BRCA2* linked families have shown loss of the wild-type chromosome in the tumours (Smith et al., 1992). It accounts for about as many familial breast cancer cases as does *BRCA1*. It appears to confer a high risk of early onset breast cancer with a risk of 87% by age 80. The risk of ovarian cancer may be lower than that for *BRCA1* but the risk of breast cancer in men is greater. Studies in the Icelandic population, who have a founder mutation 999*del*5, indicate that the male breast cancer risk varies from family to family with the same mutation suggesting possible modifiers (Thorlacius et al., 1998). However, as with *BRCA1*, there appears to be some phenotype/genotype correlation in relation to the risk of ovarian cancer, truncations in the 3′ and 5′ regions being associated with a lower risk. Examination of sporadic tumours shows loss of heterozygosity to be common around *BRCA2*, which suggests again that *BRCA2* is also a tumour suppressor gene (Collins et al., 1995).

   BRCA1 and *BRCA2* have a number of similarities including similar expression patterns. They are transcribed at late G1/early S phase of the cell cycle. Both have sites for interaction with Rad51, a protein thought to have a role in the repair of chromosomal breaks by homologous recombination (Scully et al., 1997). *BRCA1* copurifies with RNA polymerase II holoenzyme as does Rad51. The suggestion is, therefore, that *BRCA1* and *BRCA2* may be involved in double stranded DNA repair and recombination (Bertwhistle & Ashworth, 1998).

Other genes associated with increased risk of breast cancer

Most of the identified mutations in *BRCA1* and *BRCA2* result in truncated protein product although missense mutations have been found in the Ring finger of *BRCA1* (Bertwhiste & Ashworth, 1998). Linkage studies to *BRCA1* and *BRCA2* loci have suggested the existence of at least one other breast cancer susceptibility gene as some families appear to be unlinked to these two loci (Sobol et al., 1994). Other genes associated with increased risk of breast cancer are *P53* on chromosome 17p which is implicated in about one half of the Li–Fraumeni syndrome families (a rare cancer syndrome) (Malkin et al., 1990), the gene for ataxia telangiectasia (AT) (Swift et al., 1991) on chromosome 11q, and the mismatch repair genes *MSH2* and *MLH1* for Muir–Torre syndrome (Hall et al., 1992). About 1% of women diagnosed with breast cancer before age 30 years have germline mutations in the *P53* tumour suppressor gene. In addition to premenopausal breast cancer, families with the Li–Fraumeni syndrome have extremely high rates of brain tumours, sarcomas and adrenocortical cancers among children with a mutant *P53* allele. Fibroblasts from Li–Fraumeni patients have increased transforming ability and reduced radiosensitivity in culture, so irradiation of *P53* heterozygotes could increase the risk of second malignancy because radiation damage will be tolerated by the irradiated cells.

Heterozygotes at the AT locus on chromosome 11q have been reported to have a sixfold increased risk for breast cancer. The population frequency of AT heterozygotes is estimated to be 1.4% and on this basis AT could account for 7% of all breast cancer cases. AT homozygotes have severely adverse response to ionizing radiation with marked normal tissue necrosis. It has been reported in case control studies of relatives with AT that blood-related female relatives with breast cancer were significantly more likely to have been exposed to selected sources of ionizing radiation than the controls without cancer, therefore there should be concern over the use of screening mammography in known AT heterozygotes. Furthermore, a rare point mutation in the androgen receptor gene on the X chromosome can lead to breast cancer and androgen insufficiency with genitourinary abnormalities in males (Wooster et al., 1992). Breast cancer is also more commonly found in men with Klinefelter syndrome (XXY karyotype) (Everson et al., 1976). Klinefelter males typically have features of androgen insufficiency and may have decreased expression of the androgen receptor.

Referral, assessment and clinical management of women for familial breast cancer

Referral

The following guidelines have been developed to aid healthcare professionals in making a decision to refer a family member to a Family History FH/Genetics Clinic for evaluation: in this context 'first-degree relative' refers to a mother, father, sister or daughter whilst a 'second-degree relative' denotes an aunt, grandmother or granddaughter.

- Not at significantly increased risk (about 90% of all women)
  (1) No family history.
  (2) One first-degree relative diagnosed with breast cancer over 35 (or 40), or one second-degree relative of any age.
  Lifetime risk (to age 75) is between 1 in 12 (7.5%) and 1 in 8 (12.5%). No referral indicated.
- Suitable for consideration for clinical screening only in FH clinic
  (1) One first-degree relative diagnosed with breast cancer <35 years.
  (2) One first-degree relative with bilateral breast cancer <60 years.
  (3) Two first- or one first- and one second-degree relative on the same side of the family diagnosed with breast cancer >50 years but <60 years.
  Lifetime risk (to age 75) is between 1 in 8 (12.5%) and 1 in 4 (25%). Referral

indicated for screening.

Women with a significant family history of breast cancer should be referred to a Family History Breast Clinic for examination and/or screening mammography.

- Suitable for consideration for clinical screening and genetic screening
  (1) First-degree relatives of Ashkenazi Jewish women affected with breast cancer <40 years old or ovarian cancer at any age. (Ashkenazi Jewish women may have specific mutations in *BRCA1* and *BRCA2* for which it is easy to test.)
  (2) Two first- or second-degree relatives on the same side of the family, one diagnosed with breast cancer <50 and one with ovarian cancer at any age. A single family member with breast <50 and ovarian cancer also fits this criterion.
  (3) Three family members on the same side of the family with breast cancer <70 years.
  (4) Breast and/or ovarian cancer diagnosed in four or more relatives on the same side of the family.
  (5) One male with breast cancer ± female breast or ovarian cancer.
  (6) Breast cancer <40 and a relative with juvenile sarcoma on the same side of the family.

  Lifetime risk (to age 75) is greater than 1 in 4 (25%).

Assessment

Obtaining and interpreting an accurate and detailed family history remain the most important methods of risk assessment, both for deciding if there is likely to be a susceptibility in the family but also the risk to the individual. This remains the situation because there is no clinical phenotype. There are, however, a number of rare Mendelian disorders with an increased risk of breast cancer that can be diagnosed in the affected individual by the associated phenotype. Diagnosis requires enquiry about known associated problems and a careful clinical examination for any dysmorphism, taking particular care over the examination of the skin. Making a specific diagnosis enables a more accurate risk of breast cancer to be given to the individual (an example of this would be Cowden's syndrome, the multiple hamartoma syndrome, in which there is a risk of benign and malignant disease of the thyroid and the risk of breast cancer is about one in three). This condition is recognized not only from the tumour spectrum but also because of the associated macrocephaly and skin manifestations of acral keratoses and trichilemmomas.

The family history must include first- and second-degree relatives and if positive extended as far as is possible. The age at diagnosis of the affected

Table 3.1. Breast cancer risk estimates for members of moderate risk families

Affected relative	Age	Cumulative breast cancer risk by age 80 (%)
One first degree	<50	13–21
	≥50	9–11
One second degree	<50	10–14
	≥50	8–9
Two first degree	Both <50	35–48
	Both ≥50	11–24
Two second degree[a]	Both <50	21–26
	Both ≥50	9–16

Adapted from Claus et al. (1991).

Risk estimates are derived by including age extremes from the risk tables calculated by Claus. For example, for affected relatives younger than 50 years, the lower limit is the calculated risk if the affected relative is in the 40–49-year age group and the upper limit is the calculated risk for a relative in the 20–29-year age group. Thus, these figures represent the range of risk based on age and are not confidence intervals.

[a]Both paternal or maternal.

individuals and the age of all relatives should be recorded. In addition, reproductive history and information about any other serious illnesses should be ascertained. It is useful to collect information about the hospital in which relatives were treated and dates to enable confirmation of diagnoses.

In some families there is clear dominant inheritance, with four or more relatives with breast cancer or breast and ovarian cancer. However, when there are fewer individuals affected in the family it becomes more difficult to decide if there is a susceptibility in the family or not. Since breast cancer is common there will be families where breast cancer has recurred or occurred by chance alone. However, an early age of onset is associated with an increased chance of susceptibility. There have now been a number of genetic epidemiological studies that enable risks to relatives to be calculated using information on the number and age of their affected relatives (Table 3.1). In addition, information from some of these studies has been used to produce graphs that are useful for rapid assessment of risk. These tables and graphs have also been useful for developing guidelines for referral to family history clinics (Eccles et al., 2000).

The ability to identify mutations in affected individuals from families enables the confirmation of a genetic susceptibility in the family and, in addition, allows unaffected individuals to have predictive testing. However, currently it is not technically possible to identify a mutation in all *BRCA1* and *2* families although with time this will improve. In addition there may be other genes causing breast cancer, which are as yet unidentified.

Establishing a molecular diagnosis in a family provides much more accurate risk information for family members, including information on the risk for other cancers such as ovarian cancer. In addition, individual mutations may produce variable risks and more information will be gained over the next few years.

Predictive genetic testing should only be offered in a cancer family clinic setting. All consulting women should be precounselled for ambiguous or uninformative results, and should be aware that a negative result does not preclude the risk due to the background of sporadic cancers or other susceptibility genes. At present, failure to find a mutation in an at-risk individual is only useful clinically if a *BRCA1* or *BRCA2* mutation has been identified in an affected first-degree relative.

Genetic testing is indicated in individuals with a higher chance of carrying the gene. For instance, families in which at least four members had either breast or ovarian cancer with at least two of the breast cancers diagnosed before age 50, or women of Ashkenasi descent where the carrier frequency of the *BRCA1* 185*del*AG mutation is approximately 1%. It is unknown what proportion of women will wish to take up the offer of predictive testing, or what the psychological sequelae of testing are going to be. Predictive testing should be undertaken using established protocols and with appropriate genetic counselling facilities. Following the disclosure of the result patients should be seen at suitable intervals to ensure that they are coping with the result. If they are having problems referral for formal counselling is indicated.

The existence of allelic heterogeneity and the incomplete penetrance should be further addressed through prospective follow-up of relatives of patients with identified mutations. Moreover, research studies assessing new screening and prevention programmes, as well as benefits of genetic testing, are urgently needed.

Family members should be offered annual screening from the age of 25 by breast examination at appropriate intervals. Uncertainty about the use of screening mammography in young women exists as its value is unproven in this cohort of patients, however many groups offer mammography from the age of 35 years (Eccles et al., 2000). After the age of 50 women in groups 1–3 will be discharged to the National Screening Programme.

Screening for ovarian cancer may include physical examination, serum CA125, abdominal or transvaginal ultrasound in combination with colour Doppler flow imaging. So far it is not known whether these techniques have any impact on mortality. Because of the uncertain benefits of screening of ovarian cancer, prophylactic oophorectomy should be offered. However, subsequent development of disseminated intra-abdominal carcinomatosis, indistinguishable from ovarian carcinoma, has been reported, and is not infrequent (Tobachman et al., 1982; Piver et al., 1993).

Clinical management

As current strategies for breast cancer prevention in high-risk women are inadequate, subcutaneous prophylactic mastectomy may be discussed with women from dominant families, particularly if they are considering predictive testing. Subcutaneous mastectomy has been followed in some cases by breast cancer, so total mastectomy including removal of the nipple is an alternative. Any woman requesting mastectomy should, if possible, have a predictive test prior to surgery, so that unnecessary surgery can be avoided. A recent study from the Mayo Clinic of prophylactic mastectomy in women from breast cancer families suggests up to a 90% reduction in incidence of breast cancer (Hartmann et al., 1999). It is still unknown whether this will translate into a sufficiently reduced mortality from breast cancer compared to screening to justify such an invasive procedure. The treatment of breast cancer is now very successful whilst the complication rate in terms of reoperation and problems with reconstruction are significant in prophylactic surgery. All individuals undergoing surgery should be sent for counselling first to have this explained, particularly as many women may suffer emotionally if inadequately prepared.

More recently, the results of prophylactic oophorectomy are being reported and these are very encouraging. As well as offering good protection against the risk of ovarian cancer (up to 94% (Weber et al., 2000)), it is becoming apparent that oophorectomy also reduces the risk of breast cancer by about 50% (Rebbeck et al., 1999). The greatest protection will be achieved by removal of the ovaries before the age of 40 years, (Eisen et al., 2000).

Other ways that women may possibly reduce their risk of breast cancer include:
(1) possible dietary means such as restriction of alcohol intake, increase of vitamin A, carotenoids, vitamin C, E or fibre intake, reduction of fat in the diet to 30%
(2) high levels of physical activity since it has been shown to modify levels of endogenous hormones
(3) breast feeding for at least 3 months
(4) sparing use of hormone replacement therapy and oral contraceptives even though there may be some benefit, as long-term use of oral contraceptives is associated with reduced risk of ovarian cancer
(5) childbearing before the age of 35.

Finally, women at high risk because of their family histories might benefit from entering into prevention trials. The results from these trials have recently been published (see Chapter 2) (Fisher et al., 1998; Powles et al., 1998; Veronesi et al.,

1998). A number of other randomized placebo controlled trials in healthy women at increased risk of breast cancer (many with a positive family history) are also in progress. Tamoxifen has been used in the majority of these studies, although other antioestrogens are also being evaluated. Fenretinide, a vitamin A analogue, which shows preferential accumulation in breast is being evaluated in Italy in a placebo-controlled trial to prevent contralateral breast cancer. This trial is still ongoing and not reported (Costa et al., 1994). In addition, the development of an oral contraceptive pill using a gonadotrophin-releasing hormone agonist, which aims to prevent both breast and ovarian cancer, is awaited with interest (Pike & Spicer, 1993).

Conclusion

Since the identification of the dominantly inherited genes *BRCA1* and *2* we are more able to identify those at high risk of developing familial breast and ovarian cancer. Screening, both clinical and genetic, is now available for those at risk and evidence is accumulating that prevention by surgery is effective in reducing the risk from the gene in mutation carriers. The speed with which information is accumulating should lead both to better management of individuals with inherited cancers and prevention for their relatives.

REFERENCES

Bertwhistle, D. & Ashworth, A. (1998). Functions of the BRCA1 and BRCA2 genes. *Current Opinion in Genetics and Development*, 8, 14–20.

Claus, E.B., Rish, N. & Thompson, W.D. (1991). Genetic analysis of breast cancer in the Cancer and Steroid Hormone Study. *American Journal of Human Genetics*, 48, 232–42.

Collins, N., McManus, R., Wooster, R. et al. (1995). Consistent loss of the wild type allele in breast cancers from a family linked to the BRCA2 gene on chromosome 13q12–13. *Oncogene*, 10(8), 1673–5.

Costa, A., Formelli, F., Chiesa, F. et al. (1994). Prospects of chemoprevention of human cancers with the synthetic retinoid fenretinide. *Cancer Research*, (Suppl.) 54, 2032s–7s.

Easton, D.F., Bishop, D.T., Ford, D. et al. (1993). Breast Cancer Linkage Consortium: genetic linkage analysis in familial breast and ovarian cancer: results from families. *American Journal of Human Genetics*, 52, 678–701.

Easton, D.F., Narod, S.A., Ford, D. et al. (1994). The genetic epidemiology of BRCA1. *Lancet*, 344, 761.

Easton, D.F., Ford, D. & Bishop, D.T. (1995). Breast Cancer Linkage Consortium: breast and ovarian cancer incidence in BRCA1 mutation carriers. *American Journal of Human Genetics*, 56, 265–71.

Eccles, D.M., Evans, D.G.R. & Mackay, J. (2000). On behalf of the UK Cancer Family Study

Group. Guidelines for a genetic risk based approach to advising women with a family history of breast cancer. *Journal of Medical Genetics*, 37, 0–6.

Eisen A., Rebbeck, T.R., Lynch, H.T., Lerman, C. et al. (2000). Reduction in breast cancer risk following bilateral prophylactic oophorectomy in BRCA1 And BRCA2 mutation carriers. *The American Journal of Human Genetics*, 67, 58, Abstract 250.

Everson, R.B., Fraumeni, J.F., Wilson, R.E. et al. (1976). Familial male breast cancer. *Lancet*, l, 9–12.

Fisher, B., Costantino, J.P., Wickerham, D.L. et al. (1998). Tamoxifen for the prevention of breast cancer: report of the National Surgical Adjuvent Breast and Bowel Project P-1 Study. *Journal of the National Cancer Institute*, 90, 1371–88.

Ford, D., Easton, D.F., Bishop, T. et al. (1994). Breast Cancer Linkage Consortium: Risks of cancer in BRCA1 mutation carriers. *Lancet*, 343, 692–5.

Futreal, P.A., Soderkrist, P., Marks, J.R. et al. (1992). Detection of frequent allelic loss on proximal chromosome 17p in sporadic breast carcinoma using microsatellite length polymorphisms. *Cancer Research*, 52, 2624–7.

Hall, J.M., Lee, M.K., Newman, B. et al. (1990). Linkage of early onset familial breast cancer to chromosome 17q21. *Science*, 250, 1684–9.

Hall, N.R., Murday, V.A. & Chapman, P. (1992). Genetic linkage in Muir–Torre syndrome to the same chromosomal region as cancer family syndrome. *European Journal of Cancer*, 30A, 180–2.

Hartmann, L.C., Schaid, D.J., Woods, J.E. et al. (1999). Efficacy of bilateral prophylactic mastectomy in women with a family history of breast cancer. *New England Journal of Medicine*, 340, 77–84.

Malkin, D., Li, F.P., Strong, L.C. et al. (1990). Germline p53 mutations in a familial syndrome of breast cancer, sarcomas, and other neoplasms. *Science*, 250, 1233–8.

Miki, Y., Swensen, J., Shattuck-Eidens, D. et al. (1994). A strong candidate for the breast and ovarian cancer susceptibility gene BRCA1. *Science*, 26, 66–71.

Mitchell, G. & Eeles, R. (1999). The breast cancer predisposition genes BRCA1 and BRCA2: cancer risks and predictive genetic testing. *Cancer Topics*, 11, 1–7.

Pike, M.C. & Spicer, D.V. (1993). The chemoprevention of breast cancer by reducing sex steroid exposure: perspectives from epidemiology. *Journal of Cellular Biochemistry*, Supplement 17G, 26–36.

Piver, M.S., Barlow, J.J., Sawyer, D.M. et al. (1993). Primary peritoneal cancer after prophylactic oophorectomy in women with a family history of ovarian cancer. *Cancer*, 71, 2751–5.

Powles, T., Eeles, R., Ashley, S. et al. (1998). Interim analysis of the incidence of breast cancer in the Royal Marsden Hospital tamoxifen randomised chemoprevention trial. *Lancet*, 352, 98–101.

Rebbeck, T.R.R., Levin, A.M., Eisen, A. et al. (1999). Breast cancer risk after bilateral prophylactic oophorectomy in BRCA1 mutation carriers. *Journal of the National Cancer Institute*, 91(17), 1475–9.

Sato, T., Akiyama, F., Sakamoto, G. et al. (1991). Accumulation of genetic alterations and progression of primary breast cancer. *Cancer Research*, 51, 5794–9.

Scully, R.S., Chen, J., Plug, et al. (1997). Association of BRCA1 with Rad51 in mitotic and meiotic cells. *Cell*, 88, 265–75.

Shattuck-Eidens, D., McClure, M., Simard, J. et al. (1995). A collaborative survey of 80 mutations in the BRCA1 breast and ovarian cancer susceptibility gene: implications for presymptomatic testing and screening. *Journal of the American Medical Association*, 273(7), 535–41.

Smith, S.A., Easton, D.F., Evans, D.G.R. et al. (1992). Allele losses in the region 17q12–21 in familial breast and ovarian cancer involve the wild-type chromosome. *Nature Genetics*, 2, 128–31.

Sobol, H., Birnhaum, D. & Eisinger, F. (1994). Evidence for a third breast cancer susceptibility gene. *Lancet*, 344, 1151–2.

Struewing, J.P., Brody, L.C., Erdos, M.R. et al. (1995a). Detection of eight BRCA1 mutations in 10 breast/ovarian cancer families, including one family with male breast cancer. *American Journal of Human Genetics*, 57, 1–7.

Struewing, J.P., Abeliovich, D., Peretz, T. et al. (1995b). The carrier frequency of the BRCA1 185delAG mutation is approximately per cent in Ashkenasi Jewish individuals. *Nature Genetics*, 11, 198–200.

Struewing, J.P., Hartge, P., Wacholder, S. et al. (1997). The risk of cancer associated with specific mutations of BRCA1 and BRCA2 among Ashkenasi Jews. *New England Journal of Medicine*, 336, 1401–8.

Swift, M., Morrell, D., Massey, R.B. et al. (1991). Incidence of cancer in 161 families affected by the ataxia telangectasia. *New England Journal of Medicine*, 325, 1831–6.

Takahashi, H., Behbakht, K., McGovern, P.E. et al. (1995). Mutation analysis of the BRCA1 gene in ovarian cancers. *Cancer Research*, 55, 2998–3002.

Thorlacius, S., Struewing, J.P., Hartge, P. et al. (1998). Population-based study of the risk of breast cancer in carriers of BRCA2 mutation. *Lancet*, 352, 1337–9.

Tobachman, J.K., Greene, M.H., Tucker, M.A. et al. (1982). Intraabdominal carcinomatosis after prophylactic oophorectomy in ovarian cancer prone families. *Lancet*, ii, 795–7.

Tonin, P., Serova, O., Lenoir, G. et al. (1995). BRCA1 mutations in Ashkenasi Jewish women. *American Journal of Human Genetics*, 57, 189.

Veronesi, U., Maisonneuve, P., Costa, A. et al. (1998). Prevention of breast cancer with tamoxifen: preliminary findings from the Italian randomised trial among hysterectomised women. *Lancet*, 352, 93–7.

Weber, B.L., Punzalan, C., Eisen, A. et al. (2000). Ovarian cancer risk reduction after prophylactic oophorectomy in BRCA1 and BRCA2 mutation carriers. *American Journal of Human Genetics*, 67, 59, Abstract 251.

Wooster, R., Mangion, J., Eeles, R. et al. (1992). A germline mutation in the androgen receptor gene in two brothers with breast cancer and Reifenstein syndrome. *Nature Genetics*, 2, 132–4.

Wooster, R., Neuhausen, S.L., Mangion, J. et al. (1994). Localisation of a breast cancer susceptibility gene, BRCA2, to chromosome 13q12–13. *Science*, 265, 2088–90.

Wooster, R., Bignell, G., Lancaster, J. et al. (1995). Identification of the breast cancer susceptibility gene BRCA2. *Nature*, 378, 789–92.

4

Hormone replacement therapy and breast cancer

J. Marsden and N.P.M. Sacks

The Royal Marsden and St George's Hospital Trusts, London

Introduction

The cessation of menstruation is termed the menopause, the median age of which is 51 years in the United Kingdom, whereas the climacteric (or perimenopause) is the transitional period leading up to this during which ovarian function ceases and symptoms of ovarian failure may become manifest. This usually predates the menopause by approximately two to three years in the majority of women. Ovarian failure arises as a result of a reduction in ovarian responsiveness to gonadotrophin stimulation combined with an exhaustion of viable oocytes. As oestradiol production is predominantly dependent on oocyte maturation with an increase in anovulatory cycles, serum levels subsequently fall, endometrial stimulation fails to occur and amenorrhoea results. The short and long-term sequelae of this decline in ovarian oestrogen production are summarized in Table 4.1.

Vasomotor symptoms and their psychological sequelae can severely impair a women's quality of life (Daly et al., 1993). Symptoms are experienced by 75% of climacteric and early postmenopausal women but are usually self-limiting, lasting two to three years, although they can be life-long in a minority of women (Belchetz, 1994). Vaginal dryness and the subsequent superficial dyspareunia experienced by a proportion of women may contribute to loss of libido. Coronary artery disease is the most common cause of morbidity and mortality in women in many countries including the United Kingdom (Office for National Statistics Population and Health Monitor, 1997) and is the most frequent non-neoplastic cause of death in node-negative breast cancer survivors (Rosen et al., 1993). The morbidity and mortality associated with osteoporosis is substantial, accounting for an estimated annual cost to the NHS of £750 million (Compston, 1996).

Hormone replacement therapy (HRT) is prescribed to alleviate these consequences of oestrogen deficiency. It consists of either oestrogen alone, or a combination of an oestrogen and a progestin. Synthetic progestins are added to post-

Table 4.1. Acute, intermediate and long-term consequences of the menopause

Symptom/disease	Time of onset	
Hot flushes	Acute	
Night sweats		months
Mood changes		
Anxiety/irritability	Menstruation	
Poor memory/concentration	ceases	
Genital tract atrophy		
		months
Dyspareunia		
Loss of libido		
Urethral syndrome		
Skin thinning		
? Joint aches and pains		
Cerebrovascular accident		years
Coronary heart disease		
Osteoporosis	Skeletal	

Reproduced from Whitehead and Godfree (1992) with permission.

menopausal oestrogen replacement therapy to reduce the tenfold increase in risk of developing endometrial carcinoma observed with the use of long-term unopposed oestrogen replacement therapy in nonhysterectomized women (Pike et al., 1997). With combined HRT preparations, the progestin may be prescribed for 10–14 days of the 28 day cycle (i.e. sequential combined HRT). Here, three-quarters of women will experience a monthly withdrawal bleed, which incidentally, is the commonest cause of noncompliance (Ellerington et al., 1992). Alternatively, a low dose of progestin is combined with oestrogen and both are taken for 28 days (i.e. continuous combined HRT). However, whilst HRT is very effective, concern that the oestrogen component may increase the risk of developing breast cancer, or stimulate disease recurrence, has prevented its more widespread use.

The importance of endogenous oestrogens in the aetiology of breast cancer originated with the original hypothesis of Schinzinger (1889) that bilateral oophorectomy, by hastening breast atrophy, may inhibit tumour growth. Several years later, George Beatson (1896) described partial clinical responses in three premenopausal women with advanced breast cancer following surgical oophorectomy. Over the intervening 100 years, experiments on mammary tumour cell lines in vitro and in vivo have led to the development of endocrine therapy aimed at inhibiting the synthesis or action of endogenous oestrogens (Howell et al., 1997). This, in conjunction with the demonstration that ovarian ablation and tamoxifen (a mixed oestrogen antagonist and agonist) increase the survival of breast cancer patients (Early Breast Cancer Trialists' Collaborative Group, 1996 and 1998a), clearly implicate endogenous oestrogens in promoting the growth of breast cancer. Based on this evidence it would appear justified to exercise caution in the prescription of HRT and to avoid its use in breast cancer survivors. However, despite a lack of any controlled data demonstrating that HRT is safe in breast cancer survivors, it is being prescribed increasingly on an *ad hoc* basis as many women experience iatrogenic oestrogen deficiency symptoms in response to their breast cancer therapy. Observational data has not demonstrated that HRT has an adverse effect on the prognosis of breast cancer survivors but uncertainty will prevail in the absence of controlled, prospective trials. Ethical and scientific arguments exist for conducting such randomized trials and necessitate scrutiny of existing clinical data on the use of HRT in healthy women, those at high risk of breast cancer and women who have been treated for the disease (Cobleigh et al., 1994; Consensus Statement, 1998). It is the aim of this review to summarize this evidence.

The incidence of oestrogen deficiency symptoms in women with breast cancer

It can be very difficult to determine whether oestrogen deficiency symptoms in breast cancer patients are naturally occurring or iatrogenic as the median age of onset of the climacteric or menopause in women in the United Kingdom often coincides with the time of breast cancer diagnosis and treatment. The abrupt withdrawal of HRT when breast cancer is diagnosed may further exacerbate pre-existing symptoms. However, it is acknowledged that many women experience symptoms as a direct consequence of their breast cancer therapy. Cross-sectional surveys suggest that oestrogen deficiency symptoms are the most common adverse effect of adjuvant therapy, occurring in up to 66% of women at any one time (Canney & Hatton, 1994; Couzi et al., 1995). Canney and Hatton (1994) observed that 69% of postmenopausal women treated with adjuvant tamoxifen and 93% treated with ovarian suppression experienced moderate to severe symptoms in comparison with 20% of women who have never received any adjuvant therapy. Furthermore, iatrogenic symptoms have been reported to be more bothersome and persist for longer in postmenopausal breast cancer survivors compared with healthy postmenopausal women (Carpenter et al., 1998). In randomized trials, tamoxifen significantly increases the severity of hot flushes in pre and postmenopausal women but the mechanism underlying this has not yet been elucidated (Love et al., 1991; Powles et al., 1994). Chemical castration with chemotherapy and gonadotrophin-releasing agonists (GHRH-a) can also contribute towards the occurrence of oestrogen deficiency symptoms and in younger women may induce a premature menopause. Older age and systemic chemotherapy appear to be the strongest predictors of menopause during the first year after breast cancer diagnosis. The use of cyclophosphamide-based polychemotherapy regimens increase the risk of menopause in a 40-year-old women from less than 5% to more than 40% (Goodwin et al., 1999). Loss of sexual interest is another frequently reported symptom that may accompany endocrine breast cancer therapy (Fallowfield et al., 1999). Chemotherapy and GHRH-a may induce vaginal dryness, which along with decreased emotional well-being are important predictors of sexual health in breast cancer survivors (Ganz et al., 1999). Whilst vaginal dryness and dyspareunia are less frequent in women taking tamoxifen, problems with sexual interest, arousal and orgasm are reported with its use (Couzi et al., 1995; Day et al., 1999). The importance of the management of oestrogen deficiency in women with breast cancer therefore, cannot be emphasized too strongly. It is anticipated that the prevalence of treatment-induced oestrogen deficiency symptoms and premature menopause is likely to increase with the more widespread use of tamoxifen, chemotherapy and ovarian ablation following the clear survival benefits shown in the most recent worldwide overviews of adjuvant therapy trials (Early Breast Cancer Trialists' Collaborative Group, 1996, 1998a, 1998b).

Alternatives to HRT for the management of postmenopausal oestrogen deficiency

Most of the currently available alternatives to HRT do not share its wide range of short and long-term clinical benefits. Of the nonhormonal alternatives advocated for symptom relief, those which have been evaluated in controlled studies (i.e. evening primrose oil, vitamin E) have not been shown to be any more effective than placebo alone (Chenoy et al., 1992; Barton et al., 1998). There is some evidence that in the very short term (i.e. 4 weeks) the antihypertensive, clonidine, may relieve symptoms but unpleasant side-effects have been reported by women if they are normotensive (Laufer et al., 1982; Pandya et al., 2000). Serotonin-uptake inhibitors have been reported to reduce hot flushes by 50% but there is no long-term data on their efficacy or side-effect profile (Loprinzi et al., 2000). As sexual dysfunctioning is reported with chronic use of this family of antidepressants, this may affect prolonged continuance in breast cancer survivors. The use of naturally occurring soy phyto-oestrogens, which contain weakly oestrogenic plant steroids, for symptom relief has not been substantiated by a recent placebo-controlled study (Quella et al., 1999). Furthermore, increased soy intake has been positively correlated with an increase in the number of hyperplastic epithelial cells in breast fluid suggesting that the oestrogenic effect of phyto-oestrogens on the breast may not be negligible as its proponents imply (Finkel, 1999).

For women troubled with distressing vaginal symptoms, low-dose topical oestrogen preparations may be beneficial and do not appear to be associated with any significant absorption across the vaginal epithelium. They are therefore unlikely to exert any oestrogenic effect on the breast or endometrium (Bachmann, 1998). They provide better symptom control than simple vaginal moisturisers or Replens, an acidic, polycarbophil-based, bioadhesive vaginal moisturiser which restores the vaginal pH and hydrates cells (Schaffer & Fantl, 1996; Loprinzi et al., 1997). None of the other complementary therapies advocated for the treatment of oestrogen deficiency symptoms (e.g. acupuncture), have been evaluated in prospective trials.

Low-dose progestins and the synthetic gonadomimetic agent, tibolone, which has weak oestrogen, progestogen and androgen-like activity, are hormonal preparations which are being prescribed to breast cancer patients as safe alternatives to HRT. Short-term use (i.e. 3 months) of medroxyprogesterone acetate and megestrol acetate in daily dosages of ≥ 20 mg or 40 mg respectively, appear to significantly reduce vasomotor symptoms (Loprinzi et al., 1994; Rees et al., 1996). The use of depot meroxyprogesterone acetate (500 mg i.m. every two weeks) has also been reported to be as effective as low-dose oral progestins for the control of symptoms (Bertilli et al., 1999). Whilst it has been claimed that low-dose progestins provide effective long-term symptom relief, the only study published to date consists of an uncontrolled follow-up of 18 breast cancer patients for 3 years where nearly 40% of women were still symptomatic on treatment (Quella et al., 1998). Although only a small progestin dose was prescribed (i.e. megestrol acetate 20 mg/day), side-effects were common, including vaginal bleeding, episodes of chills, appetite stimulation and depressive mood. In randomized trials directly comparing tibolone (2.5 mg) and HRT, both appear to be equally efficacious in the control of oestrogen deficiency symptoms and tibolone also has an oestrogenic effect on the vaginal epithelium which appears to provide relief of vaginal dryness (Milner et al., 1996; Rymer et al., 1994a).

There are now a growing list of alternatives to HRT which have been demonstrated in randomized trials to reduce vertebral fractures (e.g. bisphosphonates, calcium and calcitonin) but none have been compared directly with HRT (Kanis, 1998). Low-dose progestins reduce bone mineral loss in postmenopausal women, although not to the same extent as oestrogen replacement and the underlying mechanism is unknown (Horowitz et al., 1993). Whilst tibolone preserves bone mineral density in the spine and hip (Rymer et al., 1994b), there is no long-term randomized data demonstrating an associated reduction in the incidence of osteoporotic fractures. Animal studies have shown that this bone-sparing effect is prevented by antioestrogens suggesting that it may not be a useful intervention in women treated concomitantly with tamoxifen or other antioestrogens (Ederveen & Kloosterboer, 2001). This contrasts with preliminary data from The Royal Marsden Hospital chemoprevention trial where no antagonism has been reported, results suggesting that with tamoxifen and HRT in combination, the annual increase in femoral bone mineral density may be as much as 4% (Chang et al., 1996).

Of the many factors influencing cardiovascular disease risk, some cannot be modified (e.g. age, sex or family history) but others, including smoking, excessive alcohol intake and hypertension, can be. Observational data suggests that postmenopausal HRT reduces the risk of arterial disease by 20–50% (Grodstein et al., 1997). Whilst a recent randomized trial of combined sequential HRT in women with pre-existing arterial disease found no protection (Hulley et al., 1998), it is still considered likely that postmenopausal HRT will reduce the risk of arterial disease in the setting of primary prevention. Simvastatin, a 3-hydroxy-3-methylglutaryl coenzyme A reductase inhibitor which lowers LDL cholesterol and HRT appears to exert a similar cardioprotective lipid-lowering effect in hypercholesterolaemic women, but no direct comparisons of the two on cardiovascular events have been undertaken (Darling et al., 1997). Tibolone reduces HDL cholesterol which could theoretically be detrimental but it also has favourable effects on the fibrinolytic system which may offset this risk (Cortes-Prieto, 1987; Rymer et al., 1994c). Again, long-term trials evaluating cardiovascular events, rather than surrogate outcomes, are necessary to clarify any potential role of tibolone in these circumstances.

Whilst low-dose progestins and tibolone appear to offer both short-and long-term benefits for oestrogen deficient women, their safety and efficacy in breast cancer survivors still requires more detailed, controlled investigation. The debate about which type of progestin may, or may not, place women at increased risk of developing breast cancer recurrence is ongoing and discussed in greater detail later. As tibolone has been shown to inhibit the conversion of estrone sulphate to oestradiol in MCF-7 and T-47D breast cancer cell lines, and in vivo not to induce changes in circulating oestradiol in postmenopausal women, it has been suggested that it will protect against breast cancer recurrence (Milner et al., 1996; Pasqualini et al., 1998). However, its relative oestrogenic and androgenic activities have been observed to increase with the higher dosages that are sometimes required for symptom control, particularly in prematurely menopausal women (Kicovic et al., 1996; Howell & Rose, 1997).

A series of agents described as SERMs (selective oestrogen receptor modulators), which are mostly analogues of tamoxifen (e.g. raloxifene, idoxifene) are under development as alternatives to HRT for treating osteoporosis. These have oestrogenic effects on some tissues (e.g. bone and lipid) and antioestrogenic effects on others such as the breast and endometrium. One of these, raloxifene, has been reported to significantly reduce the incidence of postmenopausal oestrogen-receptor (ER) positive breast cancer in a meta-analysis of data from nine randomized, placebo controlled trials (RR 0.46, 95% CI 0.28–0.75), (Jordan et al., 1998). Recent data from the ongoing Multiple Outcomes of Raloxifene Evaluation (MORE) study has reported a relative risk of developing breast cancer of 0.35 (95% CI 0.21–0.58) with a mean follow-up of 40 months (Cauley et al., 1999a). However, these results should be treated with caution as osteoporosis prevention and not breast cancer incidence was the primary end point of these trials. A breast cancer chemoprevention trial comparing tamoxifen and raloxifene has just started in the United States, where breast cancer incidence and mortality will be the main outcome measures (Study of Tamoxifen and Raloxifene – the STAR or NSABP-P2 Trial). In common with tamoxifen and other SERMs under development, raloxifene is ineffective in treating oestrogen deficiency symptoms and may even induce them and therefore has no role in the treatment of vasomotor symptoms in breast cancer patients (Glusman et al., 1997).

Is serum oestradiol an important indicator of the risk of developing breast cancer recurrence?

Current understanding of endocrine therapy for breast cancer relies on the acceptance that tumours are deprived of oestrogen derived from the plasma or synthesized locally in the breast tissue itself (Dowsett, 1997). However, mean oestradiol concentrations in breast cancers are similar in pre and postmenopausal women despite the fact that their serum hormone levels are significantly different (Thijssen & Blankenstein, 1989). Oestrogen and progestogen are required for the differentiation of breast ductules and lobules respectively but other, permissive factors are essential for the complete maturation of breast tissue to occur (e.g. thyroid and growth hormone, insulin and cortisol) (DiSaia, 1993). Whilst it is probable that the initiation and promotion of breast cancer is not dependent on a single mitogen, concern exists that increasing circulating serum oestradiol will promote the growth of breast cancer cells.

Prospective observational studies have demonstrated an association between elevated serum levels of endogenous oestrogens and the risk of developing breast cancer in postmenopausal women (Toniolo et al., 1995; Berrino et al., 1996; Thomas et al., 1997; Hankinson et al., 1998; Cauley et al., 1999b). The range of serum oestrogen over which statistically significant increases in the risk of breast cancer have been calculated in these studies however, are very small and all lie within the normal postmenopausal range (i.e. <100 pmol/l). For example, Toniolo et al. (1995) reported a large increase in the relative risk of developing breast cancer from 1.0 to 5.03 (95% CI 2.02–12.49) with a change in serum oestradiol from only <30.7 pmol/l to >41.0 pmol/l. It has been suggested that the amount of biologically available serum oestradiol is the most important factor in determining risk, and in support of this, inverse relationships of breast cancer risk with oestradiol bound to sex hormone binding globulins (SHBG) have been reported (Toniolo et al., 1995). However, a protective role of SHBG has not been demonstrated in prospective observational studies. These studies are largely limited by the fact that the numbers of breast cancer cases have often been very small. An inverse relationship between the disease-free interval in women with breast cancer and serum levels of oestradiol, oestrone sulphate and serum ratios of oestradiol/oestrone and oestrone sulphate/oestrone, has been reported but again the recorded plasma levels over which differences in associated risk were observed all fell within the low postmenopausal range (Lønning et al., 1996).

Collectively, these studies imply that HRT will increase the risk of developing breast cancer and promote disease recurrence as the serum oestradiol levels achieved with the use of either oral, transdermal or low-dose implant (i.e. 25 μg oestradiol) replacement therapy range from a mean of 200 pmol/l to 360 pmol/l, exceeding those observed in postmenopausal women (Whitehead & Godfree, 1992). However, if the risk of developing breast cancer was related simply to levels of circulating oestrogens, it is surprising that the calculated relative risk of developing breast cancer with exposure to HRT has been reported to be so small in several meta-analyses and, most recently, in the comprehensive reanalysis of worldwide observational HRT studies (Table 4.2, Collaborative Group on Hormonal Factors for Breast Cancer, 1997). The collaborative reanalysis calculated that current, long-term HRT (for a median of 11 years) was associated with a lifetime breast cancer relative risk of 1.35 (95% CI 1.21–1.49). These overviews and the recent reanalysis have been based on data accrued from individual observational, case-controlled and cohort studies which have yielded contradictory findings. It is probable that the lack of appropriate randomized controlled groups in these studies accounts for their inconsistency. Certainly, bias associated with the collection of retrospective data (e.g. recall bias, interviewer bias, nonresponse bias), patient selection and surveillance limit the reliability of the results obtained. Whilst the small, calculated increase in the risk of developing breast cancer with long-term HRT exposure reported in some individual studies and overview analyses could be considered significant, the lower limits of the associated 95% confidence intervals have not been greater than two. Epidemiologists concur that risk is only likely to be significant and not accounted for by bias if the lower limit of the 95% confidence interval is at least doubled (Taubes, 1995). Only one small, prospective, placebo-controlled randomized trial has been published and this did not demonstrate an increase in breast cancer with exposure to HRT.

Table 4.2. Meta-analyses of HRT and breast cancer risk

Reference	No. of studies	Any HRT use (RR, 95% CI)	Duration of use (RR, 95% CI)
Armstrong, 1988	—	1.01 (0.95–1.08)	—
Dupont & Page, 1991	28	1.07 (1.00–1.05)	—
Steinberg et al., 1991	16	1.0	> 15 years, 1.30 (1.20–1.60)
Grady & Ernster, 1991	10	1.0	≥ 10 years, 1.23 (1.04–1.51)
Sillero-Arenas et al., 1992	37	1.06 (1.00–1.12)	≥ 8 years, 1.20 (no CI stated)
	Combined HRT, 3 studies	0.99 (0.72–1.36), ever use	
Colditz et al., 1993	31	1.40 (1.20–1.63), current use	> 10 years, 1.23 (1.08–1.40)
	Combined HRT, 4 studies	1.13 (0.78–1.64), ever use	
Collaborative Group on Hormonal Factors in Breast Cancer, 1997	51		> 5 years, 1.35 (1.21–1.49)
	Combined HRT, ? no. of studies		≥ 5 years, 1.53 (SE 0.33)

RR = relative risk; CI = confidence interval; SE = standard error.

Here, 84 matched pairs of postmenopausal women institutionalized for chronic medical disease, were randomly assigned combined sequential HRT (i.e. conjugated oestrogens [2.5 mg/day] and medroxyprogesterone acetate [10 mg/day]) and followed up for 10 years. Participants were then given the option to stop, continue or commence HRT and observed for a further 12 years. Despite the statistically significant reduction in breast cancer incidence in women who had been exposed to HRT and the long overall follow-up of 22 years, patient numbers are too small for the results to be considered conclusive (Nachtigall et al., 1992).

Large, prospective, randomized trials of HRT are now under way in the United Kingdom (the MRC WISDOM Study; Women's International Study of Long Duration Oestrogen use after Menopause) and in the United States (the Women's Health Initiative, which was set up by the National Institutes of Health). These will ultimately provide more reliable data on the long-term benefits and risks of HRT but obviously results will not be available for several years. In the intervening period clinicians will still have to rely on data from observational studies and further meta-analyses of these studies, the limitations and biases implicit as a result of their design must be borne in mind when one is interpreting their findings.

Indirect evidence that HRT may not have an adverse effect in breast cancer survivors

The assumption that oestrogens alone are responsible for development and progression of breast cancer is further questioned in consideration of the paradoxical behaviour of breast cancer when exposed to high serum levels of exogenous, or endogenous oestrogen, examples of which follow. In isolation, none of these arguments are sufficient to justify the use of HRT for women with a previous history of breast cancer but they suggest that the disruption of the endocrine environment of a breast cancer, one way or the other, may not always have an adverse effect on prognosis and may even be of clinical benefit.

Unopposed oestrogen replacement therapy (i.e. Premarin 2.5–3.75 mg, or oestradiol valerate 2 mg with oestriol 1 mg), has been prescribed to women with advanced breast cancer in an attempt to increase the growth fraction of breast cancer cells and thus enhance the clinical response to subsequently administered palliative chemotherapy (Horn et al., 1994; Hug et al., 1994). Irrespective of tumour ER status, no association between the time to disease progression and either the percentage change of basal oestrogen level or peak oestrogen levels was detected. As tumour growth did not appear to be stimulated with these higher HRT dosages, the corollary is that standard replacement therapy may not significantly influence the growth of occult metastatic disease. Pharmacological doses of oestrogens are a proven, effective palliative therapy in postmenopausal women with advanced stage disease (Carter et al., 1977). The high levels of serum oestradiol induced by tamoxifen in premenopausal breast cancer patients, which can exceed those observed during the peak phase of the follicular phase of the menstrual cycle by two or threefold, do not appear to reduce the efficacy of tamoxifen in women with ER-positive tumours (Yasumura et al., 1990; Early Breast Cancer Trialists' Collaborative Group, 1998a).

Pregnancy induces high circulating levels of endogenous oestrogens but this does not appear to adversely affect breast cancer prognosis. Whilst pregnancy has been suggested to be a poor prognostic factor, conferring an increased relative risk of death from breast cancer of 3.1 (Tretli et al., 1988), similar 5- and 10-year survival rates have been reported in women with pregnancy or non-pregnancy-associated breast cancer when matched for age and stage (Petrek et al., 1991). Controlling for stage of disease, evidence suggests that the prognosis of women becoming pregnant subsequent to a diagnosis of breast cancer may be improved with lower recurrence (28% compared to 46%) and death rates (69% 5-year survival compared with 27% 5-year survival), (Peters, 1968; Cooper & Butterfield, 1970; Ribeiro et al., 1986; Sutton et al., 1990; von Scholtz et al., 1995). The fact that adjustment for stage of disease may have been incomplete and women with more advanced disease may not have contemplated or been advised against planning a pregnancy, or had reduced fertility as a result of their breast cancer therapy (e.g. chemotherapy or ovarian ablation), may however, have biased these results.

Whilst both the oral contraceptive pill (OCP), and HRT contain oestrogen, they differ in that the synthetic oestrogens (e.g. ethinyl oestradiol) prescribed in the OCP produce substances with pharmacological oestrogenic activity, suppressing FSH secretion and ovulation. These are far more potent than the natural oestrogens contained in HRT which produce oestrogens identical to those produced by the premenopausal ovary, achieving physiological levels of plasma oestrone or oestradiol. Prior exposure to the OCP does not have an obvious adverse effect on the disease-free or overall survival of breast cancer patients, irrespective of duration of use, latency or recent use. In common with HRT, breast tumours arising in women with a history of prior OCP use have been reported to be less clinically advanced and supports the contention that exogenous oestrogens are unlikely to have a significant effect on breast cancer outcome (Spencer et al., 1978; Matthews et al., 1981; Vessey et al., 1983, Rosner & Lane, 1986; Millard et al., 1987; Collaborative Group on Hormonal Factors for Breast Cancer, 1996). However, in these studies evaluating HRT and the OCP, it is not possible to determine whether this is a true, favourable effect on breast cancer growth or a manifestation of detection bias as information on the frequency of mammography and breast examination have not always been collected. When surveillance mammography has been controlled for, the number of small or impalpable tumours and a nonsignificant increase in the proportion of grade I breast cancers have been reported in women using HRT (Bonnier et al., 1998).

The dose of oral oestrogen prescribed in HRT (i.e. 0.625–1.25 mg conjugated equine oestrogens, 2 mg of oestradiol valerate) has been shown, like tamoxifen, to reduce insulin-like growth factor-I (IGF-I), levels by 20–30%, which in vitro is a potent breast cancer mitogen. Furthermore, SHBG levels are increased (Campagnoli et al., 1995). Elevations in SHBG reduce free testosterone which may have a role in the development of postmenopausal breast cancer. These hepatocellular effects may, therefore, theoretically protect against breast cancer recurrence.

HRT, breast density and mammography

Breast cancer risk has been reported to be increased if more than 75% of the total breast area is dense on mammography (relative risk 4.35, 95% CI: 3.1–6.1, Byrne et al., 1995). Data from the randomized Postmenopausal Estrogen/Progestin

Intervention (PEPI) Trial has confirmed the findings of numerous observational studies proporting an increase in mammographic breast density with exposure to HRT and furthermore demonstrated that combined replacement therapy induces greater density increases than oestrogen alone (Greendale et al., 1999). It may be inappropriate though to assume that density increases incurred by HRT confer an equivalent degree of risk as those which are naturally occurring. A potential problem with HRT is that its current use does appear to reduce the sensitivity of mammographic breast cancer screening (Kavanagh et al., 2000). However, the prognostic features of interval cancers which were probably missed at initial screening due to HRT use, do not appear to be more adverse, suggesting that prolonged exposure of a breast cancer to HRT may not have a detrimental effect on overall survival (Kavanagh et al., 2000; Stallard et al., 2000). The Million Women Study that was launched recently in the United Kingdom is a survey of HRT use in women attending for mammographic breast cancer screening. Whilst this will undoubtedly provide useful information about current HRT usage and the effects of HRT on mammography, it will not provide definitive data about breast cancer risk in the absence of a randomized control group for comparison. There is no evidence that healthy women on HRT require more frequent mammograms than are received through the National NHS Breast Cancer Screening Programme (British Association of Surgical Oncology: Breast Speciality Group, 1998). Whilst the ideal frequency for mammographic follow-up of women with breast cancer is not established, and current practice is variable, there is no evidence to support it being performed more often than annually if women are taking HRT.

HRT and its effect on tumour biology and breast cancer mortality

The small increase in the risk of *developing* breast cancer, related to the duration of HRT use that was reported in the recent collaborative reanalysis, disappears completely within five years of it being stopped. This suggests that HRT may be promoting the growth of pre-existing breast cancer cells rather than initiating carcinogenic change in the breast. Case reports of breast tumour regression following withdrawal of HRT and the observation that breast cancers arising in women taking HRT tend to be better differentiated and have a more favourable prognosis have been quoted as evidence in support of the hypothesis that HRT may only stimulate the growth of ER-positive tumours (Henderson et al., 1991; Powles & Hickish, 1995; Dhodapkar et al., 1995; Harvey et al., 1996; Collaborative Group on Hormonal Factors in Breast Cancer, 1997). Whilst there is no evidence that HRT has any influence at all on the determination of breast tumour ER expression, when taken up to the day of tissue analysis, it has been shown to induce progesterone receptor (PgR) content and inhibit proliferation (assessed by Ki67 and S-phase fraction) in normal breast tissue and that taken from breast cancers, particularly those which are ER positive (Hargreaves et al., 1998; Holli et al., 1998). Given that the mean range of serum oestradiol achieved with standard dosages of oral HRT of 200–360 pmol/l is significantly lower than that observed in premenopausal women, this lack of any discernible effect of HRT on the ER content of breast tumours is indirectly supported by the observation that the ER content of breast tumour tissue from premenopausal women is stable throughout the menstrual cycle despite large fluctuations in serum oestrogens (Markopoulous et al., 1988). The identification of two distinct subtypes of the ER, ERα and ERβ, in the rat, mouse and human have resulted in a revaluation of the molecular basis for oestrogen activity. At present, the significance of their different tissue distributions and ligand selectivities are unknown and requires further extensive study (Speirs et al., 1999). How this will influence our understanding of the effect of HRT on breast cell proliferation is open to speculation.

With the exception of one study, breast cancer mortality does not appear to be decreased in women with a prior history of HRT exposure (Table 4.3). Whilst the majority of studies have reported a reduction in breast cancer mortality with previous exposure to HRT, in most, this reduction has not been statistically significant. These results may also be influenced by the fact that women with breast cancer are not usually prescribed HRT and will be amongst the nonusers in observational studies, and that women requesting HRT tend to have more of an interest in general disease prevention activities such as breast cancer surveillance (Seeley, 1994). However, if confirmed, this suggests that even if HRT increases the incidence of breast cancer or promotes disease recurrence, that it may not have a detrimental effect on breast cancer compared with all cause mortality, which is really the important end point.

HRT and breast cancer risk in women at high risk of developing breast cancer

Familial breast cancer

Approximately half of the familial breast cancers (i.e. 5% of all breast cancers) are due to an inherited genetic mutation and are characterized by an early age of onset (i.e. < 40 years) and clustering of breast (often bilateral), ovarian, gastrointestinal and endometrial cancers within affected families. The recent collaborative reanalysis reported that breast cancer risk in women with a family history exposed to HRT was no greater than that of women without a positive family history, but the 99% confidence intervals were very wide and all encompassed unity (Collaborative Group on Hormonal Factors in Breast Cancer, 1997). Furthermore, HRT has been reported to significantly reduce total mortality in women developing breast cancer

Table 4.3. Mortality in breast cancer patients with a history of previous HRT exposure: observational studies

Reference	Overall cancer mortality (RR, 95% CI)	HRT characteristics	Breast cancer mortality (RR, 95% CI, P value)
Gambrell, 1984	—		0.53 (CI not stated) (P < 0.007)
Criqui et al., 1988	0.22 (no CI)		0.73 (0.44–1.22)
Berkqvist et al., 1989	—		0.68 (0.52–0.87)
Hunt et al., 1990	0.70 (0.55–0.85)		0.76 (0.45–1.06)
Henderson et al., 1991	0.80 (NS)		0.81 (CI not stated) (P > 0.05)
Ewertz et al., 1991	—		1.07 (0.88–1.30)
Strickland et al., 1992	—	No reduction (P ≤ 0.01)	
Colditz et al., 1995	—	Past use	0.80 (0.60–1.07)
		Current use	1.14 (0.85–1.51)
		⇔5 years use	0.99 (0.66–1.48)
		> 5 years use	1.45 (1.01–2.09)
Folsom et al., 1995	—	< 5 years use	0.75 (0.48–1.17)
		> 5 years use	0.79 (0.83–1.67)
Persson et al., 1996	—	Overall reduction	0.5 (0.4–0.6)
		< 5 years use	0.2 (0.1–0.3)
		5–9 years use	0.7 (0.5–0.9)
		≥ 10 years use	0.7 (0.5–0.9)
Willis et al., 1996	—	0.84 (0.75–0.94)	
		Natural menopause < 40 years	0.59 (0.40–0.87)
		Surgical menopause < 40 years	0.76 (0.54–1.09)
Sellers et al., 1997	0.55 (0.28–1.07) FH of breast cancer	Ever use HRT – no FH	1.91 (0.64–5.96)
	0.84 (0.67–1.06) no FH	Ever use HRT – FH of breast cancer	0.92 (0.55–1.54)

RR = relative risk; CI = confidence interval; FH = family history; NS = not significant.

who have a family history of the disease (Sellers et al., 1997). It is extremely difficult to interpret these findings as review of the published data reveals that the family histories of women studied were not documented accurately, rendering it impossible to determine whether the women investigated were at an increased risk or not. None of these studies, for instance, have recorded the age at diagnosis of breast cancer in affected first-degree relatives. In the absence of conclusive evidence it is recommended that HRT should be avoided in women with a significant family history of breast cancer (Evans et al., 1994). However, tumours arising in women with inherited mutations of the *BRCA1* and *BRCA2* genes, which account for 75% of familial disease, appear to have a hormone-resistant phenotype in that they are usually high grade, ER and PgR negative and resistant to tamoxifen therapy (Osin et al., 1998). HRT may not therefore have an adverse effect on the prognosis of women with a strong family history of breast cancer who develop breast cancer. This is supported by a recent study, which reported that whilst bilateral oophorectomy protected against the development of breast cancer in women with *BRCA1* mutations, the use of 'add-back' HRT to relieve subsequent problems relating to oestrogen deficiency did not appear to reduce the benefit accrued from castration (Rebbeck et al., 1999). However, patient numbers were small and confirmation of these preliminary findings is necessary.

Benign breast disease

Clinical benign breast disease encompasses a wide range of histopathological conditions of the breast, of which only atypical ductal, or lobular hyperplasia is associated with a significantly increased four to fivefold increase in the relative risk of developing subsequent breast cancer. The few studies evaluating the effect of HRT in women with a history of benign disease have not demonstrated any obvious detrimental effect (Dupont & Page, 1991). One trial reported that long-term use of HRT for more than 10 years increased the risk of developing breast cancer threefold, however there was no significant difference in the 5-year survival between HRT users and controls (Brinton et al., 1986). In common with the studies on family history and HRT, it is not possible to determine whether the women evaluated in these studies were at an increased risk of developing breast cancer as the type of benign breast disease was not defined. The only study in which benign disease has been categorized has failed to show that risk is significantly influenced by exposure to estrogen replacement therapy (atypical hyperplasia [RR 2.87, 95% CI: 1.3–6.3 vs. RR 2.53, 95% CI: 1.0–6.3 in controls]; proliferative disease without atypia [RR 1.37, 95% CI: 0.88–2.1 vs. 1.13, 95% CI: 0.69–1.9 in controls], non-proliferative benign disease [RR 1.52, 95% CI: 1.0–2.3 vs. 1.27, 95% CI: 0.8–2.0 in controls], Dupont et al., 1999). This study is of interest in the light of the report that the incidence of proliferative breast disease, including atypia, is increased in postmenopausal women with a history of exposure to HRT (Cahn et al., 1997). Whilst this latter study was retrospective and patient numbers were small ($N = 156$), if HRT is associated with an increased risk of developing proliferative breast lesions, it would not appear to have a significant influence on the subsequent risk of breast cancer development. Prospective data would be necessary to confirm this.

Observational studies of HRT in breast cancer survivors

Given the lack of a proven causal relationship between HRT and breast cancer risk and the known benefits of HRT in relieving menopausal symptoms, it has increasingly been prescribed to individual breast cancer patients on an *ad hoc* basis. Published data from a small number of observational trials of HRT in breast cancer survivors with both early and advanced stage disease, to date, have not demonstrated any increase in disease progression or death from breast cancer, suggesting that it may not adversely affect prognosis, even in those women whose tumours were ER positive (Table 4.4). However, in the absence of any appropriate, randomized control groups for comparison, reliable statements about the safety of HRT in breast cancer patients cannot be made.

The findings of a fivefold increase in the relative risk of developing breast cancer in women with luteal phase progesterone deficiency (Cowan et al., 1981) and a potential survival advantage if premenopausal breast cancer patients are operated on during the luteal rather than the follicular phase of the menstrual cycle (Badwe et al., 1991; Fentiman et al., 1994), has led to the suggestion that only combined oestrogen and progestin replacement therapy should be prescribed to breast cancer survivors, irrespective of whether they have had a hysterectomy. Further-more, it has been postulated that the administration of progestin should be continuous rather than sequential if protection against recurrent breast cancer is to be obtained (Wren, 1995). This is based on the observation that in vitro, after inducing an initial round of cell replication, the continuous application of proges-tin inhibits the proliferation of breast cancer cells, thereby rendering them less susceptible to the subsequent effects of initiating carcinogens (Clarke & Suther-land, 1990). This appears to be achieved by a variety of cellular pathways including an increase in the enzymatic conversion of oestradiol to oestrone sulphate, promotion of apoptosis, inhibition of the proto-oncogenes c-*myc* and c-*fos* and a decrease in the breast cancer growth factor, cathepsin D (Anderson, 1986; Clarke & Sutherland, 1990; Musgrove & Sutherland, 1991; Kutten et al., 1993; Jones et al., 1994). As progestins down-regulate cellular PgR which could theoretically reduce this inhibitory effect, it has been suggested that oestrogens, which increase cellular PgR content, should be administered concomitantly (Wren, 1995).

Table 4.4. HRT use in breast cancer survivors: observational studies

Reference	No. of patients	Stage of disease	Type of HRT	Median duration of use (months	Outcome
Stoll, 1989	unknown	I–II	combined (sequential)	3–6	No relapses reported
Wile et al., 1993	25	I–IV	not stated	35.2 (24–36)	Disease progression in 3 patients, 1 patient died of systemic disease
DiSaia et al., 1993	77	I–IV	combined (sequential) in 83% of patients	27 (1–233)	Disease progression in 3 patients, 3 patients died; 2 from systemic disease 1 from chemotherapy complications
Powles et al., 1993	35	I–IV	combined (sequential) and unopposed oestrogen	14.6 (1–44)	Disease progression in 2 patients
Eden et al., 1995	90	I–II	combined (continuous and sequential); progestin alone; unopposed oestrogen	18 (3–144)	Reduction of recurrence with HRT use (RR 0.4, 95% CI 0.17–0.93)
Vassilopoulou-Sellin et al., 1996	43	I–II	not stated	31 (24–142)	Disease progression in 1 patient
Peters et al., 1996	56	unknown	unopposed oestrogen	94 (1–154)	No relapses reported
Beckmann et al., 1998	64	I–IV	combined (sequential) and unopposed oestrogen	range 6–45	9% recurrence , 6% death rate with HRT 14% recurrence, 13% death rate if no HRT
Bluming et al., 1999	189	I–III	not stated	>41 (1–>76)[a]	Disease progression 12 patients (9 were either ER or PgR positive) 1 death 31 months after HRT stopped

[a]Maximum duration not stated, study indicated that some patients used HRT for more than 76 months.

Data from the Collaborative Group reanalysis, however, suggest that the addition of a progestin to replacement therapy does not confer protection against the development of breast cancer. The Collaborative Group estimated that long-term use of combined HRT may confer a greater risk than oestrogen alone (RR 1.53, standard error 0.23) but as only 5% of women were exposed to a combined preparation, these findings required confirmation. Individual observational studies published subsequent to the reanalysis support its findings but the question of whether risk is increased over and above that observed with oestrogen is unresolved (Colditz & Rosner, 1998; Persson et al., 1999; Magnusson et al., 1999; Schairer et al., 2000; Ross et al., 2000). An important consideration in the interpretation of all these studies is the influence that the formulation of combined HRT may have on risk. In addition to differing according to the timing of progestin prescription (i.e. continuous or cyclical progestin), the class of progestin prescribed may be important. Synthetic progestins are classified as to whether they are structurally related to testosterone (19-nortestosterone derivatives) or to naturally occurring progesterone (21-progestogen derivatives) and vary in their individual progestogenic, oestrogenic, antioestrogenic and androgenic activities. As the 19-nortestosterone derivatives generally exhibit relatively greater androgenic and oestrogenic properties (Jeng et al., 1992; Catherino et al., 1993; Campagnoli et al., 1994), it has been recommended that they be avoided if there is concern about breast cancer risk of recurrence. However, breast cancer risk has been reported to be reduced in women treated with 19-nortestosterone derivatives for benign breast disease or cyclical mastalgia (10 year follow-up, RR 0.48, 95% CI 0.25–0.90; Plu-Bureau et al., 1994) and the 19-nortestosterone derivative, lynestrenol, has been demonstrated to significantly reduce the ER content of cellular aspirates from women with benign breast disease suggesting an inhibition of oestrogen stimulation of breast epithelial cells in vivo (Maudelonde et al., 1991). Whether the biological activity of progestins is altered when they are prescribed in combination with oestrogen is open to speculation but it does appear from oral contraceptive studies that progestins can influence the metabolism, and hence serum levels, of coadministered oestrogens (Jung-Hoffmann et al., 1992).

Whilst recent studies have addressed the question of how risk may be affected by differing combination therapy, lack of direct, controlled comparisons and the small number of incident breast cancer cases in exposed women precludes any firm recommendations from being made. None of the observational studies of HRT in breast cancer survivors have demonstrated any survival advantages for women prescribed continuous combined HRT or any differential effect of the 19-nortestosterone or 21-progesterone progestin derivatives, but again, the small number of patients treated preclude any conclusions being made about optimal therapy in this clinical context.

Potential antagonism between tamoxifen and HRT

Any consideration of the use of HRT in breast cancer survivors has to account for the fact that many patients will already be taking tamoxifen. As the latter is an effective antineoplastic agent in both pre and postmenopausal women with ER-positive disease (Early Breast Cancer Trialists' Collaborative Group, 1998a), concern exists that HRT may eliminate or reduce this beneficial antineoplastic activity. Observational data in breast cancer survivors, at present, does not support this contention but this evidence is uncontrolled and tamoxifen use inadequately documented. Data from the tamoxifen chemoprevention trials are also inconclusive. HRT was an exclusion criteria in the largest of these randomized trials (Fisher et al., 1998) and interim analyses of The Royal Marsden Hospital and the Italian tamoxifen chemoprevention trials are inconsistent. In the former, breast cancer incidence was unaffected by HRT, which was used by 42% of participating women (Powles et al., 1998). In contrast, Veronesi et al. (1998) reported that tamoxifen exerted a preventative effect in the 14% of women who received HRT (hazard ratio 0.13; 95% CI 0.02–1.02). As these two trials have not completed follow-up and the use of HRT in this context was not a primary hypothesis, these preliminary, interim results should be treated with caution.

With the more widespread prescription of tamoxifen for the treatment of breast cancer, it is apparent that it has a complex endocrinological profile, exhibiting both antioestrogenic and partial oestrogen-agonist activities. The partial oestrogenic activity of tamoxifen is presumed to account for the clinical observations of a reduction in arterial disease and preservation of bone mineral density in postmenopausal women (McDonald & Stewart, 1991; Rutqvist & Mattson, 1993; Powles et al., 1996). However, of concern, this biological activity is associated with a very small increase in the risk of thromboembolic disease and a two to threefold increase in the risk of developing endometrial carcinoma with its prolonged use (Early Breast Cancer Trialists' Collaborative Group, 1998a). In the adjuvant setting, these risks are outweighed by the large survival benefits conferred and a significant reduction of 40–50% in the incidence of contralateral breast cancer. Thus, with the exception of its antioestrogenic effect on breast tissue, in postmenopausal women, tamoxifen in other respects mimics oestrogen replacement therapy and it is of relevance to consider the implications of the combined prescription of tamoxifen and HRT on other systems.

Tamoxifen and HRT appear to have a cumulative, beneficial effect on femoral bone mineral density (Chang et al., 1996). However, their oestrogenic effects may not be additive in other situations. Elevated levels of serum oestradiol have been reported to reduce the incidence of tamoxifen-induced endometrial events (Chang et al., 1998), suggesting that the oestrogen component of combined HRT may protect women from developing tamoxifen-associated endometrial pathology. Using changes in serum lipoprotein levels as a surrogate for arterial disease, preliminary data from the tamoxifen chemoprevention trials have found little effect of adding HRT to tamoxifen therapy in healthy postmenopausal women (Chang et al., 1996; Decensi et al., 1998). However, breast cancer patients have a high risk plasma lipoprotein profile (Barclay et al., 1954, 1959; Lane et al., 1995) and to extrapolate from data obtained from healthy women may be inappropriate.

Is a randomized trial of HRT in breast cancer survivors feasible?

Sufficient evidence exists to support the hypothesis that HRT may not have an adverse effect on the prognosis of breast cancer survivors and therefore it has been recommended that randomized controlled trials are undertaken in women with breast cancer who are experiencing oestrogen deficiency symptoms. However, implementation of such trials will be dependent on the prevailing opinions of patients and healthcare professionals. Surveys of women with breast cancer concerning the possible use of HRT have predicted that between 30–50% of patients would use HRT for the relief of oestrogen deficiency symptoms if it was prescribed under medical supervision (Vassilopoulou-Sellin & Zolinski, 1992; Couzi et al., 1995; Harding et al., 1996). Vassilopoulou-Sellin and Theriault (1994) reported that treatment background and menopausal status were important determinants of patients' attitudes towards HRT, with premenopausal women being more willing to consider HRT than postmenopausal women (59% compared with 40%). Clinical decision analysis furthermore suggests that women would be prepared to accept a 33% increase in the relative risk of developing breast cancer recurrence with HRT if they could obtain relief from troublesome oestrogen deficiency symptoms (Ganz et al., 1996). Given this information, it would appear that a randomized trial of HRT, at least for symptomatic benefit, is feasible. However, whilst providing useful insights into women's attitudes about HRT, not all these surveys have questioned symptomatic women or discussed the use of HRT in the context of a randomized trial. Both of these factors may influence individual risk perceptions and the acceptability of any proposed trial. Given the report of poor accrual into a randomized trial instigated in the USA of only 12% (Vassilopoulou-Sellin & Klein, 1996), it was considered appropriate to undertake a pilot randomized study in the United Kingdom.

The authors of this chapter have recently completed a pilot study to ascertain the feasibility of conducting such a trial and, to date, this is the only randomized data on the use of HRT in women with early stage breast cancer (Marsden et al., 2000). Here, with a minimum of 6 months therapy, three women have developed disease recurrence. One did so within 6 weeks of commencing HRT, the other after 2 years continued use. The demonstration of high acceptance (40%) and compliance (>80%) rates in both treatment arms, despite detailed informed consent, has justified the further evaluation of HRT in this group of patients. A national randomized trial of HRT in women with early stage breast cancer has now been set up. Here, symptomatic women will be randomized to HRT for two years. It is anticipated that, in addition to providing reliable data on the effects of HRT use on disease-free and overall survival, the question of potential antagonism between HRT and tamoxifen will be answered.

Conclusion

At present, knowledge of the complex factors involved in the aetiology of breast cancer is incomplete. It is not doubted that breast cancer is a tumour that is sensitive to endogenous oestrogens but the role of exogenous oestrogens still remains unclear. The absence of a clear association between HRT exposure, breast cancer risk or disease progression suggests that if it does have a detrimental effect, then the degree of this effect is likely to be very small. Firm conclusions about HRT cannot be made in the absence of controlled data. Until more reliable evidence is available, the prescription of HRT in breast cancer patients, which should only be undertaken by the specialist in charge of the patient's care, will necessitate extensive counselling. This should involve an explanation of the potential positive benefits of HRT being weighed against the clinical uncertainty that it may increase the risk of breast cancer recurrence.

REFERENCES

Anderson, T.J. (1986). Effects on breast tissue of exogenous estrogen and progestogens. *Acta Obstetrica et Gynaecologia Scandinavia*, 134 (Suppl.), 9–16.

Armstrong, B.K. (1988). Oestrogen therapy after the menopause: boon or bane? *Medical Journal of Australia*, 148, 213–14.

Bachmann, G.A. (1998). The clinical platform for the 17β-estradiol vaginal releasing ring. *American Journal of Obstetrics and Gynaecology*, 178, S257–60.

Badwe, R.A., Gregory, W.M., Chaudary, M.A. et al. (1991). Timing of surgery during menstrual cycle and survival of premenopausal women with operable breast cancer. *Lancet*, 337, 1261–4.

Barclay, M., Cogin, G.F., Escher, G.C. et al. (1954). Human plasma lipoproteins I. In normal women and in women with advanced carcinoma of the breast. *Cancer*, 8, 253–60.

Barclay, M., Calathes, N., DiLorenzo, J.C. et al. (1959). The relationship between plasma lipoproteins and breast carcinoma: effect of degrees of breast disease on plasma lipoproteins and the possible role of lipid metabolic aberrations. *Cancer*, 11, 1163–70.

Barton, D.L., Loprinzi, C.L., Quella, S.K. et al. (1998). Prospective evaluation of vitamin E for hot flashes in breast cancer survivors. *Journal of Clinical Oncology*, 16, 495–500.

BASO Breast Speciality Group (1998). The British Association of Surgical Oncology Guidelines for surgeons in the management of symptomatic breast disease in the UK (1998 revision). *European Journal of Surgical Oncology*, 24, 464–76.

Beatson, G.T. (1896). On the treatment of inoperable carcinoma of the mamma: suggestions for a new method of treatment, with illustrative cases. *Lancet*, 2, 104–7.

Beckmann, M.W., Mohrmann, T., Kuschel, B. et al. (1998). Hormonersatztherapie (HRT) nach Mammakarzinomerkrankung-Ergebnisse einer Beobachtungs-studie. *Geburtsh.u.Frauenheilk*, 58, 193–6.

Belchetz, P.E. (1994). Hormonal treatment of postmenopausal women. *New England Journal of Medicine*, 330, 1062–71.

Berkqvist, L., Adami, H.O., Persson, I. et al. (1989). Prognosis after breast cancer diagnosis in women exposed to oestrogen and oestrogen-progestogen replacement therapy. *American Journal of Epidemiology*, 130, 221–8.

Berrino, F., Muti, P., Micheli, A. et al. (1996). Serum sex hormone levels after menopause and subsequent breast cancer. *Journal of the National Cancer Institute*, 88, 291–6.

Bertilli, G., Venturini, M., Del Mastro, L. et al. (1999). Depot intramuscular medroxyprogesterone acetate (MAP) for the treatment of hot flashes in breast cancer survivors: results of GONO (Gruppo Oncologico Nord Ovest) MIG-4 phase III trial. *Proceedings of the American Society of Clinical Oncology*, 18, A2286 (Abstract).

Bluming, A.Z., Waisman, J.R., Dosik, G.M. et al. (1999). Hormone replacement therapy in women with previously treated primary breast cancer. Update *Proceedings of the American Society of Clinical Oncology*, 18, A471, Abstract.

Bonnier, P., Bessenay, F., Sasco, A.J. et al. (1998). Impact of menopausal hormone-replacement therapy on clinical and laboratory characteristics of breast cancer. *International Journal of Cancer*, 79, 278–82.

Brinton, L.A., Hoover, A.R. & Fraumeni, J.F. (1986). Menopausal oestrogens and breast cancer risk: an expanded case-control study. *British Journal of Cancer*, 54, 825–32.

Byrne, C., Schairer, C., Wolfe, J. et al. (1995). Mammographic features and breast cancer risk: effects with time, age and menopausal status. *Journal of the National Cancer Institute*, 87, 1622–9.

Cahn, M.D., Tran, T., Theur, C.P. et al. (1997). Hormone replacement therapy and the risk of breast lesions that predispose to cancer. *American Surgeon*, 63, 858–60.

Campagnoli, C., Biglia, N., Peris, C. et al. (1994). Potential impact on breast cancer risk of circulating insulin-like growth factor I modifications induced by oral HRT in menopause. *Gynaecological Endocrinology*, 6, 297–9.

Campagnoli, C., Biglia, N., Peris, C. et al. (1995). Potential impact on breast cancer risk of circulating insulin-like growth factor I modifications induced by oral HRT in menopause. *Gynaecological Endocrinology*, 9, 67–74.

Canney, P.A. & Hatton, M.Q.F. (1994). The prevalence of menopausal symptoms in patients treated for breast cancer. *Clinical Oncology*, 6, 297–9.

Carpenter, J.S., Andykowski, M.A., Cordova, M. et al. (1998). Hot flashes in postmenopausal women treated for breast carcinoma. *Cancer*, 82, 1682–91.

Carter, A.C., Sedransk, N., Kelley, R.M. et al. (1977). Diethylstilbestrol: recommended dosages for different categories of breast cancer patients. *Journal of the American Medical Association*, 237, 2079–85.

Catherino, W.H., Jeng, M.H. & Jordan, V.C. (1993). Norgestrel and gestodene stimulate breast cancer cell growth through an oestrogen receptor mediated mechanism. *British Journal of Cancer*, 67, 945–52.

Cauley, J., Krueger, K., Eckert, S. et al. (1999a). Raloxifene reduces breast cancer risk in postmenopausal women with osteoporosis: 40-month data from the MORE trial. *Proceedings of the American Society of Clinical Oncology*, 18, A328, Abstract.

Cauley, J.A., Lucas, F.L., Kuller, L.H. et al. (1999b). Elevated serum estradiol and testosterone concentrations are associated with a high risk for breast cancer. *Annals of Internal Medicine*, 130, 270–7.

Chang, J., Powles, T.J., Ashley, S.E. et al. (1996). The effect of tamoxifen and hormone replacement therapy on serum cholesterol, bone mineral density and coagulation factors in healthy postmenopausal women participating in a randomised, controlled tamoxifen prevention study. *Annals of Oncology*, 7, 671–5.

Chang, J., Powles, T.J., Ashley, S.E. et al. (1998). Variation in endometrial thickening in women with amenorrhoea. *Breast Cancer Research Treatment*, 48, 81–5.

Chenoy, R., Hussain, S., Tayob, V. et al. (1992). Effect of oral gamolenic acid for evening primrose oil on menopausal flushing. *British Medical Journal*, 308, 501–3.

Clarke, C.L. & Sutherland, R.L. (1990). Progestin regulation of cellular proliferation. *Endocrine Reviews*, 11, 266–301.

Cobleigh, M.A, Berris, R.F., Bush, T. et al. for the Breast Cancer Committees of the Eastern Cooperative Group. (1994). Estrogen replacement therapy in breast cancer survivors. *Journal of the American Medical Association*, 272, 540–5.

Colditz, G.A., Egan, K.M. & Stampfer, M.J. (1993). Hormone replacement therapy and risk of breast cancer: results from epidemiological studies. *American Journal of Obstetrics and Gynaecology*, 168, 1473–80.

Colditz, G.A., Hankinson, S.E., Hunter, D.J. et al. (1995). The use of estrogens and progestins and the risk of breast cancer in postmenopausal women. *New England Journal of Medicine*, 332, 1589–93.

Colditz, G.A. & Rosner, B. For the Nurses' Health Study Research Group (1998). Use of estrogen plus progestin is associated with greater risk than estrogen alone. *American Journal of Epidemiology*, 147 (Suppl.), 64S.

Collaborative Group on Hormonal Factors for Breast Cancer (1996). Breast cancer and hormonal contraceptives: collaborative re-analysis of individual data on 53,297 women with and 100,239 women without breast cancer from epidemiological studies. *Lancet*, 347, 1713–27.

Collaborative Group on Hormonal Factors for Breast Cancer (1997). Breast cancer and hormone replacement therapy: collaborative re-analysis from 51 individual epidemiological studies. *Lancet*, 350, 1047–60.

Compston, J. (1996). Bone density measurements and their use in clinical practice. *Journal of the British Menopause Society*, 2, 11–14.

Consensus Statement. (1998). Treatment of estrogen deficiency symptoms in women surviving breast cancer. *Journal of Clinical Endocrinology and Metabolism*, 83, 1993–2000.

Cooper, D.R. & Butterfield, J. (1970). Pregnancy subsequent to mastectomy for carcinoma of the breast. *Annals of Surgery*, 171, 429–33.

Cortes-Prieto, J. (1987). Coagulation and fibrinolysis in postmenopausal women treated with Org OD14. *Maturitas* (Suppl. 1), 67–72.

Couzi, R.J., Helzlsouer, K.J. & Fetting, J.H. (1995). Prevalence of menopausal symptoms among women with a history of breast cancer and attitudes toward estrogen replacement therapy. *Journal of Clinical Oncology*, 13, 2737–44.

Cowan, L.D., Gordis, L., Tonascia, J.A. et al. (1981). Breast cancer incidence in women with progesterone deficiency. *American Journal of Epidemology*, 114, 209–17.

Criqui, M.H., Suarez, L., Barrett-Connor, E.L. et al. (1988). Postmenopausal estrogen use and mortality. *American Journal of Epidemiology*, 128, 606–14.

Daly, E., Grey, A., Barlow, D. et al. (1993). Measuring the impact of menopausal symptoms on quality of life. *British Medical Journal*, 307, 836–40.

Darling, G.M., Johns, J.A., McCloud, P.I. et al. (1997). Estrogen and progestin compared with simvastatin for hypercholesterolaemia in postmenopausal women. *New England Journal of Medicine*, 337, 595–601.

Day, R., Ganz, P.A., Costantino, J.P. et al. (1999). Health-related quality of life and tamoxifen in breast cancer prevention: a report from the National Surgical Adjuvant Breast and Bowel Project P-1 study. *Journal of Clinical Oncology*, 17, 2659–69.

Decensi, A., Robertson, C., Rotmensz, N. et al. (1998). Effect of tamoxifen and transdermal hormone replacement therapy on cardiovascular risk factors in a prevention trial. *British Journal of Cancer*, 78, 572–8.

Dhodapkar, M.V., Ingle, J.N. & Ahmann, D.L. (1995). Estrogen replacement therapy withdrawal and regression of metastatic breast cancer. *Cancer*, 75, 43–6.

DiSaia, P.J. (1993). Hormone replacement therapy in patients with breast cancer. *Cancer Supplements*, 71(4), 1490–500.

DiSaia, P.J., Odicino, F., Grosen, E.A. et al. (1993). Hormone replacement therapy in breast cancer. *Lancet*, 342, 1232.

Dowsett, M. (1997). Aromatase inhibitors: current status and future applications. *Endocrine Related Cancer*, 4, 313–22.

Dupont, W.D. & Page, D.L. (1991). Menopausal estrogen replacement therapy and breast cancer. *Archives of Internal Medicine*, 151, 67–72.

Dupont, W.D., Page, D.l., Parl, F.F. et al. (1999). Estrogen replacement therapy in women with a history of proliferative breast disease. *Cancer*, 85, 1277–83.

Early Breast Cancer Trialists' Collaborative Group. (1996). Ovarian ablation in early breast cancer: overview of the randomised trials. *Lancet*, 348, 1189–96.

Early Breast Cancer Trialists' Collaborative Group. (1998a). Tamoxifen for early breast cancer: an overview of randomised trials. *Lancet*, 351, 1451–67.

Early Breast Cancer Trialists' Collaborative Group. (1998b). Polychemotherapy for early breast cancer: an overview of the randomised trials. *Lancet*, 352, 930–42.

Eden, J.A., Bush, T., Nand, S. et al. (1995). A case-controlled study of combined continuous oestrogen-progestogen replacement therapy amongst women with a personal history of breast cancer. *Menopause – Journal of the North American Menopause Society*, 2, 67–72.

Ederveen, A.G.H. & Kloosterboer, H.J. (2001). Tibolone, exerts its protective effect on trabecular bone loss in ovariectomised rats through the estrogen receptor. *Journal of Bone and Mineral Research*, 16, 1651–7.

Ellerington, M. C., Whitcroft, S.I.J. & Whitehead, M.I. (1992). Developments in therapy. *British Medical Bulletin*, 48, 401–25.

Evans, D.G.R., Fentiman, I.S., McPherson, K. et al. (1994). Familial breast cancer. *British Medical Journal*, 308, 183–7.

Ewertz, M., Gillanders, S., Meyer, L. et al. (1991). Survival of breast cancer patients in relation to factors which affect the risk of developing breast cancer. *International Journal of Cancer*, 49, 526–30.

Fallowfield, L.J., Leaity, S.K., Howell, A. et al. (1999). Assessment of quality of life in women undergoing hormonal therapy for breast cancer; validation of an endocrine symptom sub-scale for the FACT-B. *Breast Cancer Research and Treatment*, 55, 189–99.

Fentiman, I.S., Gregory, W.M. & Richards, M.A. (1994). Effect of menstrual phase on surgical treatment of breast cancer. *Lancet*, 344, 402.

Finkel, E. (1999). Phyto-oestrogens: the way to postmenopausal health? *Lancet*, 352, 1762.

Fisher, B., Costantino, J.P., Wickerham, D.L. et al. (1998). Tamoxifen for prevention of breast cancer: report of the National Surgical Adjuvant Breast and Bowel Project P-1 study. *Journal of the National Cancer Institute*, 90, 1371–88.

Folsom, A.R., Mink, P.J., Sellers, T.A. et al. (1995). Hormonal replacement therapy and morbidity and mortality in a prospective study of postmenopausal women. *American Journal of Public Medicine*, 85, 1128–32.

Gambrell, D.R. (1984). Proposal to decrease the risk and improve the prognosis in breast cancer. *American Journal of Obstetrics and Gynaecology*, 150, 119–28.

Ganz, P.A., Greendale, G., Kahn, B. et al. (1996). Are breast cancer survivors (BCS) willing to take hormone replacement therapy (HRT)? *Proceedings of the American Society of Clinical Oncology*, 15, A102, Abstract.

Ganz, P.A., Desmond, K., Bekin, T.R. et al. (1999). Predictors of sexual health in women after a breast cancer diagnosis. *Journal of Clinical Oncology*, 17, 2371–80.

Glusman, J., Lu, Y., Huster, W. et al. (1997). Raloxifene effects on climacteric symptoms compared with hormone or oestrogen replacement therapy (HRT or ERT). *Proceedings of the North American Menopause Society*, 8th Annual Meeting Programme p65 (Abstract).

Goodwin, P.J., Ennis, M., Pritchard K.I. et al. (1999). Risk of menopause during the first year after breast cancer diagnosis. *Journal of Clinical Oncology*, 17, 2365–70.

Grady, D. & Ernster, V. (1991). Invited commentary: does hormone replacement therapy cause breast cancer? *American Journal of Epidemiology*, 134, 1396–400.

Greendale, G.A., Reboussin, B.A., Sie, A. et al. for the Postmenopausal Estrogen/Progestin Interventions (PEPI) Investigators (1999). Effects of estrogen and estrogen–progestin on mammographic parenchymal density. *Annals of Internal Medicine*, 130, 262–9.

Grodstein, F., Stampfer, M.J., Colditz, G.A. et al. (1997). Postmenopausal hormone therapy and mortality. *New England Journal of Medicine*, 336, 1769–75.

Hankinson, S.E., Willett, W.C., Manson, J.E. et al. (1998). Plasma sex steroid levels and risk of breast cancer in postmenopausal women. *Journal of the National Cancer Institute*, 90, 1292–9.

Harding, C., Knox, F., Faragher, E. et al. (1996). Hormone replacement therapy and tumour grade in breast cancer. Prospective study in a screening unit. *British Medical Journal*, 312, 1646–7.

Hargreaves, D.F., Knox, F., Swindell, R. et al. (1998). Epithelial proliferation and hormone receptor status in the normal postmenopausal breast and the effects of hormone replacement therapy. *British Journal of Cancer*, 78, 945–9.

Harvey, S.C., DiPiro, P.J. & Meyer, J.E. (1996). Marked regression of a non-palpable breast cancer after cessation of HRT. *American Journal of Radiology*, 167, 394–5.

Henderson, B.E., Paganini-Hill, A. & Ross, R.K. (1991). Decreased mortality in users of oestrogen replacement therapy. *Archives of Internal Medicine*, 151, 75–8.

Holli, K., Isola, J. & Cuzick, J. (1998). Low biologic aggressiveness in breast cancer in women using hormone replacement therapy. *Journal of Clinical Oncology*, 16, 3115–20.

Horn, Y., Walach, N., Pavlotsky, A. et al. (1994). Randomised study comparing chemotherapy with and without estrogen priming in advanced breast cancer. *International Journal of Oncology*, 4, 499–501.

Horowitz, M., Wishart, J.M., Need, A.G. et al. (1993). The effects of norethisterone on bone related biochemical variables and forearm bone mineral density in postmenopausal women. *Clinical Endocrinology*, 39, 649–55.

Howell, A., Clarke, R.B. & Anderson, E. (1997). Oestrogens, Beatson and endocrine therapy. *Endocrine Related Cancer*, 4, 371–80.

Howell, R. & Rose, G. (1997). Failure of tibolone to control hypoestrogenic symptoms in premenopausal women undergoing hysterectomy and bilateral salpingoophorectomy. *Journal of Obstetrics and Gynaecology*, 17, 578–9.

Hug, V., Clark, J. & Johnson, D. (1994). The results of modified use of chemotherapy for patients with metastatic breast cancer. *European Journal of Cancer*, 30A, 438–42.

Hulley, S., Grady, D., Bush, T. et al. for the Heart and Estrogen/Progestin Replacement Study (HERS) Research Group. (1998). Randomised trial of estrogen plus progestin for secondary heart disease in postmenopausal women. *Journal of the American Medical Association*, 280, 605–13.

Hunt, K., Vessey, M. & McPherson, K. (1990). Mortality in a cohort of long term users of hormone replacement therapy: an updated analysis. *British Journal of Obstetrics and Gynaecology*, 97, 1080–6.

Jeng, M., Parker, C.J. & Jordan, V.C. (1992). Estrogenic potential in oral contraceptives to stimulate human breast cancer cell proliferation. *Cancer Research*, 52, 6539–46.

Jones, C., Ingram, D., Mattes, E. et al. (1994). The effect of hormone replacement therapy on prognostic indices in women with breast cancer. *Medical Journal of Australia*, 161, 106–10.

Jordan, V.C., Glusman, J.E., Eckert, S. et al. (1998). Raloxifene reduces incident primary breast cancer: integrated data from multicentre, double blind, placebo controlled, randomised trials in postmenopausal women. *Breast Cancer Research Treatment*, 50, 277 (Abstract).

Jung-Hoffmann, C., Storch, A. & Kuhl, H. (1992). Serum concentrations of ethinylestradiol, 3-keto-desogestrel, SHBG, CBG and gonadotrophins during treatment with a biphasic oral contraceptive containing desogestrel. *Hormone Research*, 38, 184–9.

Kanis, J.A. (1998). Bisphosphonates and the rest – non-HRT agents in the treatment of osteoporosis. *Journal of the British Menopause Society*, 4 (Suppl. 1), 9–11.

Kavanagh, A.M., Mitchell, A. & Giles, G.G. (2000). Hormone replacement therapy and accuracy of mammographic screening. *Lancet*, 355, 270–4.

Kicovic, P.M., Empelen, S. & Coelingh Bennick, H.J.T. (1996). Tibolone: dose response analysis of uterine bleeding in a multicentre placebo controlled study. *Proceedings of the 8th International Congress on the Menopause*, P246 (Abstract).

Kutten, F., Malet, C., Leygue, E. et al. (1993). Anti oestrogen action of progestogens in human breast. In: *The Modern Management of the Menopause. Proceedings of 7th International Congress on the Menopause*, pp. 419–33. London: Parthenon.

Lane, D.M., Boatman, K.K. & McConathy, W.J. (1995). Serum lipids and apolipoproteins in women with breast masses. *Breast Cancer Research and Treatment*, 44, 161–9.

Laufer, L.R., Erlik, Y., Meldrum, D.R. et al. (1982). Effect of clonidine on hot flashes in postmenopausal women. *Obstetrics and Gynaecology*, 60, 583–6.

Lønning, P.E., Helle, S.I., Johannessen, D.C. et al. (1996). Influence of plasma oestrogen levels on the length of the disease free interval in postmenopausal women with breast cancer. *British Cancer Research Treatment*, 39, 335–41.

Loprinzi, C.L., Michalak, J.C., Quella, S.K. et al. (1994). Megestrol acetate for the prevention of hot flashes. *New England Journal of Medicine*, 331, 347–52.

Loprinzi, C.L., Alon-Ghazaleh, S., Sloan, J.A. et al. (1997). Phases III randomised double blind study to evaluate the efficacy of a polycarbophil-based vaginal moisturiser in women with breast cancer. *Journal of Clinical Oncology*, 15, 969–73.

Loprinzi, C.L., Kugler, J.W., Mailliard J.A. et al. (2000). Venlafaxine alleviates hot flashes: A North Centre Cancer Treatment Group Trial. *Proceedings of the (36th) Annual Meeting of the American Society of Clinical Oncology*, 2000; 19, Abstract 4.

Love, R.R., Cameron, L., Connell, B.L. et al. (1991). Symptoms associated with tamoxifen treatment in postmenopausal women. *Archives of Internal Medicine*, 151, 1842–7.

Magnusson, C., Baron, J., Correia, N. et al. (1999). Breast cancer risk following long term oestrogen- and oestrogen–progestin-replacement therapy. *International Journal of Cancer*, 81, 339–44.

Markopoulous, C., Berker, U., Wilson, P. et al. (1988). Oestrogen receptor content of normal breast cells and breast carcinomas throughout the menstrual cycle. *British Medical Journal*, 296, 1349–51.

Marsden, J., Sacks, N.P.M., Baum, M. et al. (2000). Are randomised trials of hormone replacement therapy in symptomatic breast cancer patients feasible? *Fertility and Sterility*, 73, 292–9.

Matthews, P.N., Millis, R.R. & Hayward, J.L. (1981). Breast cancer in women who have taken contraceptive steroids. *British Medical Journal*, 282, 774–6.

Maudelonde, T., Lavaud, P., Salazar, G. et al. (1991). Progestin treatment depresses oestrogen receptor but not cathepsin D levels in needle aspirates of benign breast disease. *Breast Cancer Research Treatment*, 19, 95–102.

McDonald, C.C. & Stewert, H.J. for the Scottish Breast Cancer Committee (1991). Fatal myocardial infarction in the Scottish adjuvant tamoxifen trial. *British Medical Journal*, 303, 435–7.

Millard, F.C, Bliss, J.M, Chilvers, C.E.D, et al. (1987). Oral contraceptives and survival in breast cancer. *British Journal of Cancer*, 56, 377–8.

Milner, M., Sinnott, M., Gasparao, D. et al. (1996). Climacteric symptoms, gonadotrophins, sex steroids and binding proteins with conjugated equine estrogen–progestin and tibolone over two years. *Menopause: Journal of the North American Menopause Society*, 4, 208–13.

Musgrove, E.A. & Sutherland, R.L. (1991). Steroids, growth factors and cell cycle controls in breast cancer. *Breast Cancer Research Treatment*, 53, 305–31.

Nachtigall, M.J., Smilen, S.W., Nacthigall, R.D. et al. (1992). Incidence of breast cancer in a 22-year study of women receiving estrogen–progestin replacement therapy. *Obstetrics and Gynaecology*, 80, 827–30.

Office for National Statistics Population and Health Monitor. (1997). *Deaths registered in 1996 by cause, and by area of residence*. Publications Unit, Office for National Statistics, London.

Osin, P., Crook, T., Powles, T.J. et al. (1998). Hormone status of in situ cancer in BRCA1 and BRCA2 mutation carriers. *Lancet*, 351, 1487.

Pandya, K.J., Raubertas, R.F., Flynn, P.S. et al. (2000). Oral clonidine in postmenopausal patients with breast cancer experiencing tamoxifen-induced hot flushes: a University of Rochester Cancer Centre Community Clinical Oncology Program Study. *Annals of Internal Medicine*, 132, 788–93.

Pasqualini, J.R., Kloosterboer, H.J. & Chetrite, G. (1998). Action of tibolone and its metabolites (org-4094, org-20126) on the biosynthesis and metabolism of estradiol in human breast cancer cells. *Breast Cancer Research Treatment*, 50, P363, Abstract.

Pasternack, B.S. (1995). A prospective study of endogenous estrogens and breast cancer in postmenopausal women. *Journal of the National Cancer Institute*, 87(3), 190–7.

Persson, I., Yuen, J., Berqvist, L. and Schairer (1996). Cancer incidence and mortality in women receiving estrogen and estrogen–progestin replacement therapy – long term follow up of a Swedish cohort. *International Journal of Cancer*, 67, 327–32.

Persson, I., Weiderpass, E., Berqkvist, L. et al. (1999). Risks of breast cancer and endometrial cancer after estrogen and estrogen–progestin replacement therapy. *Cancer Causes Control*, 10, 253–60.

Peters, M.V. (1968). The effect of pregnancy in breast cancer. In: *Prognostic factors in breast cancer*, 65–89. Eds. A.P.M. Forrest & P.B. Kunkler. Baltimore: Williams and Wilkins.

Peters, G.N. & Jones, S.E. (1996). Estrogen replacement therapy in breast cancer patients: a time for change (Meeting Abstract). *Proceedings of the American Society of Clinical Oncology*, 15, A148.

Petrek, J.A, Dukoff, R. & Rogato, A. (1991). Prognosis of pregnancy associated breast cancer. *Cancer*, 67, 869–72.

Pike, M.C., Peters, R.K., Cozen, W. et al. (1997). Estrogen–progestin replacement therapy and endometrial cancer. *Journal of the National Cancer Institute*, 89, 1110–16.

Plu-Bureau, G., Le, M.G., Sitruk-Ware, R. et al. (1994). Progestin use and decreased risk of breast cancer in a cohort study of premenopausal women with benign breast disease. *British Journal of Cancer*, 70, 270–7.

Powles, T.J. & Hickish, T. (1995). Breast cancer response to HRT withdrawal. *Lancet*, 345, 1442.

Powles, T.P., Casey, S., O'Brien, M. et al. (1993). Hormone replacement after breast cancer. *Lancet*, 342, 60.

Powles, T.J., Jones, A.L., Ashley, S.E. et al. (1994). The Royal Marsden Hospital chemoprevention trial. *Breast Cancer Research Treatment*, 31, 73–82.

Powles, T.P., Hickish, T., Kanis, J. et al. (1996). Effect of tamoxifen in bone mineral density measured by dual-energy X-ray absorptiometry in healthy premenopausal and post-menopausal women. *Journal of Clinical Oncology*, 14, 78–84.

Powles, T.J., Eeles, R., Ashley, S. et al. (1998). Interim analysis of breast cancer in The Royal Marsden Hospital tamoxifen randomised chemoprevention trial. *Lancet*, 352, 98–101.

Purdie, D.W. (1998). Selective oestrogen receptor modulation. *Journal of the British Menopause Society*, 4 (Suppl. 1), 9.

Quella, S.K., Loprinzi, C.L., Sloan, J.A. et al. (1998). Long term use of megestrol acetate by cancer survivors for the treatment of hot flashes. *Cancer*, 82, 1784–8.

Quella, S.K., Loprinzi, C.L., Barton, D. et al. (1999). Evaluation of soy phytoestrogens for treatment of hot flashes in breast cancer survivors: an NCCTG trial. *Proceedings of the American Society of Clinical Oncology*, 18, A2285, Abstract.

Rebbeck, T.R., Levin, A.M., Eisen, A. et al. (1999). Breast cancer after bilateral prophylactic oophorectomy in BRCA1 mutation carriers. *Journal of the National Cancer Institute*, 91, 1475–9.

Rees, C.M.P., Brockie, J.A., Suffling, K. et al. (1996). Megestrol acetate to treat vasomotor symptoms. *Proceedings of the 8th International Congress on the Menopause*, F146 (Abstract).

Ribeiro, G., Jones, D.A. & Jones, M. (1986). Carcinoma of the breast associated with pregnancy. *British Journal of Surgery*, 73, 607–9.

Rosen, P.P., Groschen, S., Kinne, D.W. et al. (1993). Factors influencing prognosis in node negative breast carcinoma: analysis of 767 T1 N0 M0/T2 N0 M0 patients with long term follow up. *Journal of Clinical Oncology*, 1, 2090–100.

Rosner, D. & Lane, W. (1986). Oral contraceptive use has no adverse effect on the prognosis of breast cancer. *Cancer*, 57, 591–6.

Ross, R.K., Paganini-Hill, A., Wan, P.C. & Pike, M.C. (2000). Effect of hormone replacement therapy and breast cancer risk: estrogen versus estrogen plus progestin. *Journal of the National Cancer Institute*, 92, 328–32.

Rutqvist, L.E. & Mattsson, A. (1993). Cardiac and thromboembolic morbidity among post-menopausal women with early stage breast cancer in a randomised trial of tamoxifen. The Stockholm Breast Cancer Study Group. *Journal of the National Cancer Institute*, 85, 1398–406.

Rymer, J., Chapman, M.G., Fogelman, I. et al. (1994a). A study of the effect of tibolone on the vagina in postmenopausal women. *Maturitas*, 18, 127–33.

Rymer, J.M., Chapman, M.G. & Fogelman, I. (1994b). Effect of tibolone on postmenopausal bone loss. *Osteoporosis International*, 4, 314–19.

Rymer, J.M., Foley, L., Chapman, M.G. et al. (1994c). Tibolone and the long term effect on serum lipids. *International Journal of Obstetrics and Gynaecology*, 46 (Suppl. 2) FC076.2, Abstract.

Schaffer, J. & Fantl, J.A. (1996). Urogenital effects of the menopause. *Ballière's Clinical Obstetrics and Gynaecology*, 10, 401–17.

Schairer, C., Lubin, J., Troisi, R. et al. (2000). Menopausal estrogen and estrogen–progestin replacement therapy and breast cancer risk. *Journal of the American Medical Association*, 283, 485–91.

Schinzinger (1889). Ueger carcinoma mammae. *Centralblatt Chirurgica*, 16, 55–6 (Abstract).

Seeley, T. (1994). Do women taking hormone replacement therapy have a higher uptake of screening mammograms? *Maturitas*, 19, 93–6.

Sellers, T.A., Mink, P.J., Cerhan, J.R. et al. (1997). The role of hormone replacement therapy in the risk for breast cancer and total mortality in women with a family history of breast cancer. *Annals of Internal Medicine*, 127, 973–80.

Sillero-Arenas, M., Delgado-Rodriguez, M., Rodigues-Canteras, R. et al. (1992). Menopausal hormone replacement therapy and breast cancer: a meta-analysis. *Obstetrics and Gynaecology*, 79, 286–94.

Speirs, V., Parkse, A.T., Kerin, M. et al. (1999). Coexpression of estrogen receptor α and β: poor prognostic factors in human breast cancer? *Cancer Research*, 59, 525–8.

Spencer, J.D, Millis, R.R. & Hayward, J.L. (1978). Contraceptive steroids and breast cancer, *British Medical Journal*, 1, 1024–6.

Stallard, S., Litherland, J.C., Cordiner, C.M. et al. (2000). Effect of hormone replacement therapy on the pathological stage of breast cancer: population based, cross-sectional study. *British Medical Journal*, 320, 348–9.

Steinberg, K.K., Thacker, S.B., Smith, J.S. et al. (1991). A meta-analysis of the effect of estrogen replacement therapy on the risk of breast cancer. *Journal of the American Medical Association*, 265, 1985–90.

Stoll, B.A. (1989). Hormone replacement therapy in women treated for breast cancer. *European Journal of Cancer and Clinical Oncology*, 25, 1909–13.

Strickland, D.M., Gambrell, R.D., Butzin, C.A. et al. (1992). The relationship between breast cancer survival and prior postmenopausal estrogen use. *Obstetrics and Gynaecology*, 80, 400–4.

Sutton, R., Buzdar, A.V. & Hortobagyi, G.N. (1990). Pregnancy and offspring after adjuvant chemotherapy in breast cancer patients. *Cancer*, 65, 847–50.

Taubes, G. (1995). Epidemiology faces its limits. *Science*, 269, 164–9.

Thijssen, J.H. & Blankenstein, M.A. (1989). Endogenous oestrogens and androgens in normal and malignant endometrial and mammary tissues. *European Journal of Cancer and Clinical Oncology*, 25, 1953–9.

Thomas, H.V., Key, T.J., Allen, D.S. et al. (1997). A prospective study of endogenous serum hormone concentrations and breast cancer risk in post-menopausal women on the island of Guernsey. *British Journal of Cancer*, 76, 401–5.

Toniolo, P.G., Levitz, M., Zeleniuch-Jacquotte, A. et al. (1995). A prospective study of endogenous estrogens and breast cancer in postmenopausal women. *Journal of the National Cancer Institute*, 87, 190–7.

Tretli, S., Kvalheim, G., Thoresen, S. et al. (1988). Survival of breast cancer patients diagnosed during pregnancy or lactation. *British Journal of Cancer*, 58, 382–4.

Treves, N. & Holleb, A.I. (1958). A report of 549 cases of breast cancer in women 35 years of age or younger. *Surgical Gynaecology and Obstetrics*, 107, 271–83.

Vassilopoulou-Sellin, R. & Zolinski, C. (1992). Estrogen-replacement therapy in women with breast cancer : a survey of patient attitudes. *American Journal of Medical Science*, 304, 145–9.

Vassilopoulou-Sellin, R. & Theriault, R.L. (1994). Randomised prospective trial of estrogen-replacement therapy in women with a history of breast cancer. *Monographs of the National*

Cancer Institute, 16, 153–9.

Vassilopoulou-Sellin, R. & Klein, M.J. (1996). Estrogen replacement therapy after treatment for localised breast carcinoma, patients' responses and opinions. *Cancer*, 78, 1043–8.

Vassilopoulou-Sellin, R., Theriault, R. & Klein, M.J. (1996). Estrogen replacement therapy in women with prior diagnosis and treatment for breast cancer (Meeting abstract). *Proceedings of the American Society of Clinical Oncology*, 15, A50.

Veronesi, U., Maisonneuve, P., Costa, A. et al. (1998). Prevention of breast cancer with tamoxifen: preliminary findings from the Italian randomised trial among hysterectomised women. *Lancet*, 352, 93–7.

Vessey, M., Baron, J., Doll, R. et al. (1983). Oral contraceptives and breast cancer. Final report of an epidemiological study. *British Journal of Cancer*, 47, 455–62.

von Scholtz, E., Johansson, H., Wilking, N. et al. (1995). Influence of prior and subsequent pregnancy on breast cancer prognosis. *Journal of Clinical Oncology*, 13, 430–4.

Whitehead, M.I. & Godfree, V. (1992). Types of HRT available. In: M.I. Whitehead and V. Godfree (eds.), *HRT, your questions answered*, pp. 93–122. Edinburgh: Churchill Livingstone.

Wile, A.G., Opfell, R.W. & Margileth, D.A. (1993). Hormone replacement therapy in previously treated breast cancer patients. *American Journal of Surgery*, 165, 372–5.

Willis, D.B., Calle, E.E., Miracle-McMahill, H.L. et al. (1996). Estrogen replacement therapy and risk of fatal breast cancer in a prospective cohort of postmenopausal women in the United States. *Cancer Causes Control*, 7, 449–57.

Wren, B.G. (1995). Hormonal replacement therapy and breast cancer. *European Journal of the Menopause*, 2, 13–21.

Yasumura, T., Akami, T., Mitsou, M. et al. (1990). The effect of adjuvant therapy with or without tamoxifen on the endocrine function of patients with breast cancer. *Japanese Journal of Surgery*, 20, 369.

5

Screening for breast cancer

Rosalind Given-Wilson

St George's Hospital, Blackshaw Road, London

Introduction

Screening is the application of diagnostic measures to an apparently healthy population in the hope of uncovering serious disease at an early stage when treatment is more likely to be curative than it is at a later stage. A number of countries have national programmes providing mammographic screening for breast cancer, these include the UK, Finland, Sweden, Netherlands and Australia. In other countries such as the USA widespread mammographic screening activity follows national guidance. This chapter describes the basis for breast screening as well as current practice and potential future developments.

Why screen?

The purpose of screening is to reduce the mortality from breast cancer. The value of regular screening in doing this for women over 50 has been demonstrated by randomized controlled trials.

There are a number of risk factors related to breast cancer (see Table 5.1). The strongest risk factors are being female and an older age. Most of the well-established risk factors for breast cancer are not modifiable. Unlike the association between smoking and lung cancer there is no single major cause of breast cancer that can be easily avoided.

Treatment for breast cancer, both local and systemic shows success rates closely linked to the stage of the cancer at presentation (Figure 5.1). (Cancer Research Campaign, 1996). Patients with small tumours which are less than 2 cm in diameter have a greater than 90% chance of surviving 5 years compared with 60% for patients with tumours over 5 cm in diameter. Involvement of axillary nodes indicates a worse prognosis (Miller et al., 1995).

It therefore seems reasonable to think of early detection by screening as a way of reducing breast cancer deaths. The rationale for this is that, as survival after

Table 5.1. Factors associated with an increased risk of developing breast cancer

- Female sex
- Increasing age
- Family history
- Previous history of breast cancer
- Certain types of benign dysplasias proven on biopsy (e.g. atypical ductal hyperplasia, multiple papillomatosis)
- Reproductive factors: early age of menarche, nulliparity, late age at first birth (>30 years), late age at menopause)
- Rare inherited familial syndromes (e.g. Li–Fraumeni syndrome)
- Ionizing radiation

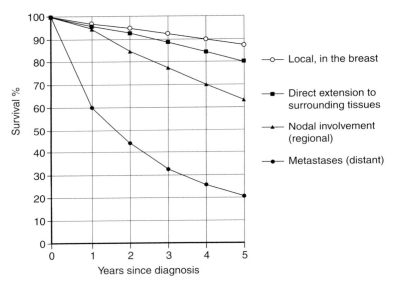

Figure 5.1   Five-year relative survival for patients age 15–74 years diagnosed 1986–89, South East England

treatment and diagnosis is directly related to stage of diagnosis, so the earlier that the breast cancer can be diagnosed, the better the survival rate.

The principles of screening and their application to breast cancer

There are a number of general criteria applying to any screening method which should be satisfied before a screening programme is introduced (Table 5.2). To what extent does mammographic screening for breast cancer fulfil these?

Table 5.2. General principles of screening

- The condition screened for should pose an important health problem
- The natural history of the condition should be well understood
- There should be a recognizable latent or early stage
- Treatment of the disease at an early stage should be of more benefit than treatment started at a later stage
- There should be a suitable test or examination
- The test or examination should be acceptable to the population
- For diseases of insidious onset, screening should be repeated at intervals determined by the natural history of the disease
- There should be adequate facilities available for the diagnosis and treatment of any abnormalities detected
- The chance of physical or psychological harm should be less than the chance of benefit

Adapted from Wilson and Jungner, WHO (1968) and reproduced by permission of the CRC and NHSBSP

- **The condition screened for should pose an important health problem**
  Breast cancer is certainly an important health problem. It is the commonest cancer in women in the UK and the USA where there were an estimated 175 000 new breast cancer cases in 1999. It is estimated that one in twelve women in these countries will develop breast cancer during their lives; 80% of cases occurred in postmenopausal women (CRC, 1996).
- **The natural history of the condition should be well understood**
  The natural history of the disease is not perfectly understood. Breast cancer shows marked variability between individuals in its rate of growth and ability to metastasize. Although we know that in many cases ductal carcinoma in situ (DCIS) will progress to invasive disease with the potential for metastasis, this does not happen in all cases, particularly in women with low grade DCIS. In addition, although size of a tumour together with a number of histological prognostic features may give an indicator of the likelihood of disseminated disease being present, we cannot accurately predict this. Some very low grade or supposedly in situ tumours will actually have metastasized. This makes it difficult to assess the benefit gained by an individual woman from detecting her cancer by screening. Interestingly, there is recent evidence that the presence on mammography of casting type calcification in small invasive tumours indicates a subgroup with a worse prognosis (Tabar et al., 2000).
- **There should be a recognizable latent or early stage**
  Although it is not easy to define what is meant by early breast cancer, the majority of cancers detected on screening are small (more than 50% of the

invasive cancers are less than 15 mm in diameter) or in situ (approximately 20% of screen detected cancer). They are less likely to have metastasized than larger tumours.

- **There should be a suitable test or examination**

  It has been known since the 1960s that mammography is capable of demonstrating breast cancers which are not clinically apparent. Cancers demonstrated by mammography alone tended to be earlier stage than those presenting clinically. It seemed logical to test whether mass population screening by mammography could down stage sufficient numbers of women's breast cancers to reduce the death rate from the disease, which was rising in most countries up to the late 1980s. (Evidence of efficacy of screening trials is considered in the next section).

- **The test or examination should be acceptable to the population**

  Mammography is uncomfortable for the majority of women (81%) and painful for some (56%); 7% classify the pain as severe. However most women feel that this is short lived and bearable (McIlwaine, 1993). Attendance rates for mammography in trials and national programmes is generally over 70%.

- **For diseases with insidious onset screening should be repeated at intervals determined by the natural history of the disease**

  The UK NBSP currently operates with a 3-year screening interval, which is probably the maximum acceptable. This interval was chosen following the success of the Swedish Two County Study which used 24 and 36 months as the screening interval (Tabar et al., 1992). A number of other national programmes such as that in the Netherlands and Australia operate on a 2-year screening interval.

- **There should be adequate facilities available for the diagnosis and treatment of any abnormalities detected**

  Women with potential abnormalities detected on screening are recalled to screening assessment centres staffed by specialist multidisciplinary teams.

- **The chance of physical or psychological harm should be less than the chance of benefit**

  The balance of benefits and disadvantages of breast screening will be covered later.

- **The cost of case finding including diagnosis of subsequent treatment should be economically balanced against the benefit it provides**

  The average cost of screening mammography in the UK is £23.47 (Wald et al., 1995). Breast screening in the UK has been estimated to cost £23 600 per life saved. These costs have to be set against other needs within the Healthcare System.

It can be seen that screening by mammography fulfils most of these criteria.

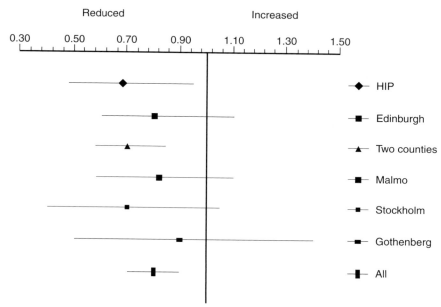

Figure 5.2   Relative risk of mortality from breast cancer in women aged 50–74 invited for screening (RCT)

Evaluation of screening benefit

There is no evidence that screening by clinical examination or teaching breast self-examination reduces the mortality from breast cancer. Screening by mammography, however, was the first screening method for any malignancy shown to be of value in randomized controlled trials (RCT). The use of RCTs for evaluation overcomes the number of potential biases inherent in assessing screening methods.

Bias in survival evaluation

At first look it would seem that if women whose breast cancers are detected by screening live longer they have benefited from screening. This assumption can be misleading however, as it does not take into account lead time bias or length bias.

Lead time bias

This invalidates the use of survival time following detection of cancer to assess screening. When a cancer is detected earlier, the time between detection and death from cancer may be longer either because detection was earlier or because death was deferred. Unless death was deferred the individual has not benefited from screening, she only has had to live longer with the knowledge of her disease. She will appear however, to have had an increased survival time following diagnosis compared with a nonscreened women. Assessment of the overall breast cancer death rate in a screened population compared with nonscreened controls is the only way to avoid lead time bias and truly assess if death is being deferred.

Length bias

Another reason why comparing the survival time after diagnosis of screened and nonscreened women is misleading: length bias arises because screening at regular intervals has a tendency to find more slow growing relatively nonaggressive tumours. The faster growing high-grade tumours which are more likely to kill may increase in size rapidly and present clinically in the interval between screens. If this is the case, screening will have a tendency to preferentially detect better prognosis tumours. The better survival of women with screened detected than nonscreened detected cancers may reflect this selection phenomenon rather than a true effect on mortality.

Randomized controlled trials

The RCT, involving comparison of breast cancer mortality over time in large numbers of women, one group offered regular screening and the other not, avoids length and lead time bias. In order to avoid selection bias it is necessary to assess the outcome in the whole group offered screening whether or not they attend, and compare it with the controls. Otherwise women who have a better prognosis, for instance because they are more health conscious, may preferentially attend for screening causing apparent better survival in the screened group which is not in fact due to the screening process.

Selection bias is also avoided by having truly random allocation of women between control and study groups. If, for instance, women are able to volunteer for the study group they may have a different level of the disease under study from the rest of the population (e.g. women who have breast symptoms and suspect they have breast cancer). This will make the trial nonrandom and it will lack generalizability. Its results will not be applicable to the general population, but only to the study group.

The results of RCTs may be compromised if there is a high level of noncompliance in the study group (women who decline to be screened). This will mean that a significant proportion of women counted as being screened are actually unscreened. Another problem is that of contamination in the control group. These are women who are supposedly nonscreened controls, but who obtain mammograms for themselves outside the study. Both noncompliance and contamination dilute the effect of screening. It is possible to calculate the level of dilution if the rates of noncompliance and contamination are known and it is then necessary to increase the numbers of women in the study to raise its power and obtain a valid result.

Seven RCTs, conducted between the 1960s and 1990s have examined the effect of screening mammography (Forest, 1986; Shapiro et al., 1982; Tabar et al., 2000; Andersson et al., 1988; Frisell et al., 1997; Anon, 1999; Alexander et al., 1999; Miller et al., 2000). For women aged 50 years and over at entry six out of seven showed reduced mortality with screening of between 20–50%. The Canadian national study (Miller et al., 2000) showed increased mortality but its methodology has been criticized (Kopans, 1995).

For women under age 50 the evidence of benefit from screening is less convincing.

Criticism of most of the RCTs (with the exception of the Canadian and Malmo studies) has centred recently around possible bias (Gotzsche & Olsen, 2000). Allegations have been made that randomization was inadequate and that further bias came from postrandomization exclusions and lack of blinding when assessing outcome. Other investigators have counted these as incorrect and unjustifiable criticisms (de Koning, 2000).

What is the evidence that screening works in different age groups?

The effectiveness of screening in reducing breast cancer mortality varies with the age of women screened and I propose to examine the evidence in more detail for different age groups.

Screening in women aged 50–64 years of age

Seven RCTs and five case control studies of screening mammography have been undertaken in this age group (Shapiro et al., 1982; Tabar et al., 2000; Andersson et al., 1988; Frisell, 1997; Anon, 1999; Alexander et al., 1999; Miller et al., 2000; Verbeek et al., 1984; Demmisie, et al. 1998).

As described above an increased mortality in the Canadian national study may be due to the poor quality of mammography and the inadequate randomization process in their study which have been heavily criticized. All other studies show a reduction in mortality for women in this age group offered mammographic screening of between 20 and 50% for RCTs (average 24%) and 56% on average for case control studies.

Demmisie explained the larger reduction in case control studies by the dilution of results of the RCTs due to noncompliance in the study groups and contamination of control groups which occurred to some extent in all RCTs. More recently Tabar et al. (2001) has also reported the effect of the subsequent introduction of service screening in the two counties in Sweden with a persisting reduction in mortality in women invited for screening of 48%. He also reported that those who attended for screening during the Swedish Two Counties trial showed a reduction in mortality of 63% over nonattendees, although this figure may be subject to selection bias. This adds up to strong evidence for the benefit of regular screening on reducing breast cancer mortality in the 50–64 year old age group, both within the setting of trials and that of service screening.

Screening in women over the age of 65

A systematic review of nearly 300 000 women screened and controls in the four Swedish RCTs by Larsson et al. (1996) found the highest mortality reduction of 34% was in the oldest age group, that of women screened aged 60–69. A Dutch study (Van Dijck et al., 1997) of women aged 68–83 comparing mortality in screened versus nonscreened women found a 40% reduction in breast cancer mortality in the study population after 10 years. It appears that screening is acceptable to older women and that screening mammography is at least as effective in women aged 65 and over as in women aged 50–64. There is no currently defined upper age limit at which screening ceases to be effective.

Screening women aged 40–49 years

All seven randomized controlled trials have included women under the age of 50. No randomized controlled trials designed specifically and solely to look at the effect of screening in this age group have yet reported although a UK trial (Moss, 1999) is underway and the results are awaited. Subgroup analysis has been undertaken of the women aged 40–49 included in larger randomized controlled trials and has been reported in the form of meta-analysis and systematic reviews (Feig, 1995; Glasziou and Irwig, 1997).

The results of these subgroup analyses are confusing and range from a relative risk of dying of breast cancer compared to women in the control population which is slightly increased at 1.08 (Frisell, 1997) to a marked reduction at 0.55 (Bjurstam et al., 1997). Some of the differences between different studies may be due to the number of screening views and the screening interval used. An optimistic meta-analysis by Feig gives a 24% risk reduction for regular mammographic screening in women aged 40–49 compared with controls, but Glasziou has calculated an overall absolute gain of four breast cancer deaths averted per 10 000 women screened. The recall rate and benign biopsy rate are both higher than in older women.

Although it appears that there is some reduction in breast cancer mortality due to screening in women aged 40–49 this occurs later and is less than the reduction in women over age 50. It probably reaches significance. It may be dependent on both the use of two views and frequent screening. The costs of screening both in terms of false positive diagnoses and financial costs are higher in this age group.

Why may mammographic screening be less effective in younger women? It has been reported that the sensitivity of mammography for symptomatic cancers reduces with decrease in age (Sibbering et al., 1995) dropping by about 10% per decade down to a sensitivity of 57% for 40 year olds. Reduced sensitivity has been shown with decreasing age and increase in density of the breasts with the greatest reduction for small invasive cancers (Given-Wilson et al., 1997). In addition to cancer being more difficult to diagnose in younger women via mammography, there is also the added problem when evaluating the benefit of mammographic screening that the incidence of breast cancer is lower in this group. It is generally advised that women seeking screening at this age should be made aware of the risks and benefits of screening.

Screening for women under 40 years old

There are few studies of population screening in this age group. Liberman et al. (1993) reviewed the result of screening 5105 women aged 35–39 and reported a 9% recall rate with a less than 0.01% invasive cancer detection rate. Lanninn et al. (1993) reviewed data from the BCDDP and showed a falling sensitivity for both mammography and clinical examination with young age so that under age 40, 36% of cancers were not detectable either clinically or mammographically. This is combined with a relatively low incidence of breast cancer in young women and high incidence of benign disease which contribute to diagnostic difficulties and frequent delay in diagnosis of breast cancer even in the symptomatic setting. In addition, at this young age the risk of cancer induction by radiation from mammography becomes significant. Although the radiation dose in mammography is small (2 mGy per film) sensitivity of breast tissue to cancer induction by radiation increases with reducing age. The risk is less with one per million in the over 50s. It is expressed as a ratio of cancers induced to cancers detected. The calculation of the theoretical risk from available data (Law, 1997) shows cancer induction to detection rates potentially rising greater than 1 in a 100 in under 30s that would outweigh possible benefits of a mass screening in young women.

In conclusion there is no evidence to support population screening of women under 40 who are not at increased risk of breast cancer. The incidence of breast cancer is low, the sensitivity of mammography in this group is low, and the risk of radiation-induced cancer is relatively high.

Organization aspects of screening – the UK model

In order to be successful a screening programme needs to have access to an accurate population register, a failsafe system for invitation and reinvitation,

Table 5.3. Recommendations of the Forrest Committee on breast cancer screening (1986) and current NHSBSP guidelines

- **Target population:** women age 50–64 years by direct invitation, women aged 65 and over may be screened on request. (The NHSBSP has agreed to increase the upper age limit for women invited to 70. There is a multicentre trial of screening women age 40–49 going on under the auspices of the NHSBSP)
- **Interval:** 3 years. (Evaluation of annual versus 3-yearly mammography is ongoing)
- **Number of views:** single medio-lateral oblique view. (Since 1995 two view mammography has been instituted for the prevalent (first) screen, and is about to be introduced also for incident (subsequent) screens)

high-quality mammography and interpretation and facilities for expert assessment and treatment of screen detected lesions. All this needs to be underpinned by strict quality assurance (QA).

Within the UK National Breast Screening Programme (NHSBSP) screening is carried out by 103 local breast screening units. Most are based at multihealth district level and offer screening to target populations of women (aged 50–64) which number between 41 500 women (a Forrest Unit) and 120 000. These units operate under the control of Quality Assurance Reference Centres of which there is one in each region and these are ultimately coordinated by the National Screening Coordinator (Table 5.3).

Breast screening units invite women for screening three yearly from lists taken from health authority computers and checked by the woman's general practitioner. Women will be given an appointment for mammography either at a static or mobile unit. They are not offered clinical examination. Results are sent directly to a woman within two weeks. Over 90% of women screened should receive a negative result. When any possible abnormality has been identified on a woman's mammogram she is recalled to a screening assessment centre. These are staffed by multidisciplinary teams. At an assessment clinic a clinical history will be taken and examination carried out. Further imaging with mammography and ultrasound, as well as needle biopsy, are done as necessary to allow a definitive diagnosis to be reached (Figure 5.3).

Sensitivity and specificity of screening – the performance of the UK NHSBSP

Factors which play a crucial part in the effectiveness of screening are the sensitivity and specificity of the screening test itself. This should be able to detect the majority of cancers (high sensitivity) and reliably exclude people who do not have cancer (high specificity). In the screening programme practical measures of these are the cancer detection rate (particularly the standardized cancer detection ratio (SDR))

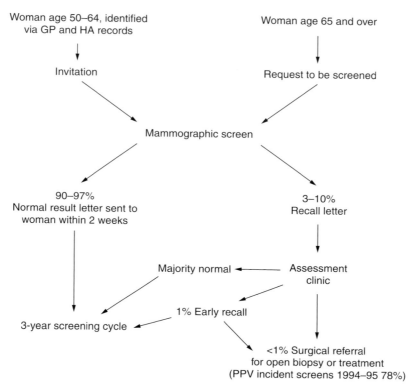

Figure 5.3   Screening process

and the interval cancer rate (sensitivity). For specificity, measures include the recall rate and benign biopsy rate. In the UK programme these measures are contained within the core quality assurance target laid down by the NHSBSP Review (Patnick, 1998) (Table 5.4).

The SDR is a measure of invasive cancer detection corrected for the age of the population screened and the underlying incidence of breast cancer in the population and then compared with the results of the Two Counties study. An SDR of one thus represents a screening performance equivalent to that which would have been achieved by the Two Counties study had it been screening the local British population. This is probably the most accurate measure of sensitivity of the programme for cancer detection. (Blanks et al., 1996).

As can be seen from Table 5.4, the UK screening programme is meeting most of its targets for acceptance and recall rate and small invasive cancer detection rate. If however we look at SDRs within the NHSBSP since its inception, these remained below one for prevalent screens up to the year 1994/95 (national figures varying between 0.74 and 0.96 (personal communication R. Blanks, CSEU). The SDR

Table 5.4. Core quality assurance targets for screening women aged 50–64 in the UK (NHSBSP 1998) and the screening results 1996/97

Objective	Minimum standard 1st screen (target)	Results 96/97 1st screen	Minimum standard further screen (target)	Results 96/97 further screens
To maximize the number of eligible women attending for screening	≥70%	72.5%	≥70%	86.9%
To maximize invasive cancer detection rate per 1000 screened	≥2.7 (3.6)	4.8	≥3.0 (4.0)	3.7%
To maximize small (≥15 mm) invasive cancer detection as a % of invasive cancers detected	50%	53.8%	50%	56.2%
To maximize SDR	≥0.75 (1)	1.17	≥0.75 (1)	0.94
To minimize the numbers recalled for assessment	<10% (7%)	7.6%	<7% (5%)	3.6%
To maximize the number of cancers with a preoperative tissue diagnosis (cytology or core biopsy)	≥70% (90%) (all screens)	62%	≥70% (90%) (all screens)	62%
To minimize benign surgical biopsies/1000 screened	<3.5 (≥1.8)	5.1	<2.0 (≥1.0)	1.3
To minimize the number of interval cancers presenting in the 2 years following a normal screen	<1.2/1000	N/A	<1.2/1000	N/A

SDR = Standardized Cancer Detection Ratio; N/A = Not available.

nationally then rose to 1.1 in 1995/96. This followed the introduction of two-view mammography for prevalent screens coupled with an increase in the recommended optical density of screening films to between 1.4 and 1.8. SDRs for the incident (subsequent) screen remained below 1 (0.85) up to the most recent two years for which figures are available, 1999 and 2000, when they have risen nationally to over 1. This may reflect the fact that the majority of screening programmes were following the NHSBSP guidelines and doing single-view mammography for subsequent screens. The recent improvement corresponds with a shift in most centres from single to double film reading, another method of increasing sensitivity.

Interval cancers are those presenting clinically in the interval between a negative screen and the next screen (standard < 1.2/1000 women screened in the first 24 months after negative screens). The NHSBSP has not published rates of interval cancers nationally but some individual regions have published their interval cancer rates, notably in North Western and East Anglian regions (Woodman et al., 1995; Day et al., 1995). These have shown interval cancer rates in excess of the national targets. South Thames West region has published a comparison of SDRs and interval cancer rates since the inception of breast screening in 1987 (Given-Wilson et al., 1999). The rate, at 1.23 in the first 24 months for the entire region virtually meets the national target. This correlates with an overall SDR of 1 during the same period suggesting that if the detection target for small cancers can be met then the interval cancer target will also be achievable. It appears that this region's success has been partially attributable to the use of two views at all screens and double reading in one of the larger programmes.

The NHSBSP currently operates with a 3-year screening interval. This was based on the Swedish Two County study which used 24 and 36 months (according to age) as the screening interval. Published rates in the UK indicate that at 24 to 36 months after a negative screen the number of women presenting with interval cancers rises to approximately 80% of the expected underlying incidence of breast cancer without screening in the population (Woodman et al., 1995). This may indicate that the screening interval in the UK is too long. It remains under review with an ongoing frequency trial under the auspices of the NHSBSP.

The sensitivity of screening is affected by the number of readers viewing each film. Double reading of films now occurs throughout most of the screening programme (78%) and has also, not surprisingly, been shown to correlate with higher cancer detection rates (Blanks et al., 1998b).

Benefits and adverse effects of breast screening

The major benefit to be gained from the breast screening programme is reduction in breast cancer deaths. The debate around screening centres on the size of this mortality reduction in different groups of women, how it is affected by the method of screening and the costs of achieving it, both human and economic. Breast cancer mortality has fallen rapidly in the UK in the decade 1989–99 by 22% overall and 18% in the USA (Peto et al., 2000). There are a number of contributing factors including improved systemic treatment, cohort effect, the development of specialist breast cancer centres with multidisciplinary teams, greater awareness on the part of women and screening. It is not yet possible to quantify the contribution from each.

As well as a mortality reduction there are also lesser benefits in less radical treatment for women with early tumours and reassurance for women whose test results are negative. One further advantage arising from the presence of the screening service, which is difficult to quantify, is the effect of screening on the symptomatic services. Awareness of screening has been an important catalyst in the development of the multidisciplinary team approach to breast cancer. The expertise developed in screening is now spreading through the symptomatic breast cancer services. There will always be controversy about whether adequate resources are available to meet increasing demands for breast care within both screening and symptomatic breast units where the healthcare budget is finite as in the UK.

Screening generates anxiety in healthy women by making them aware of the possibility of them having cancer unknowingly. For women who are recalled from screening, there is intense short-term anxiety and distress and evidence varies as to whether this is maintained in the months after screening in women not found to have cancer (CRC, 1997). It is difficult to eliminate anxiety when all the women who are involved know that the point of screening is a search for cancer.

Potential harm from low doses (<2 m Gy QA standard) of ionizing radiation used in screening is small and theoretical. At worst the risk of developing breast cancer as a result of undergoing mammography in women over 50 has been calculated as one chance in a million with a latent period of 10 years. This risk reduces with increasing age.

The potential harm from false reassurance for those whose mammograms are negative in the presence of a cancer is extremely difficult to quantify. The literature sent with the screening invitation advises women to seek help for symptoms even though their mammogram may have been negative, emphasizing that mammography does not pick up all cancers. Nevertheless, women who present with an interval cancer within a year or two of a normal screening mammogram, may be angry and wonder whether the screening process has missed their cancer (*Lancet*, 1998).

Screening and subsequent assessment tests are unable to differentiate between cancer and benign disease in all cases. There will be some women who are advised to have surgical biopsies for lesions appearing suspicious at assessment but which subsequently are found to be benign. With greater use of cytology and core biopsy the numbers of such women have been reduced. Numbers tend to be higher at the prevalent (first) screen (1.28 benign biopsies per 1000 women screened, compared with cancer detection 5.9 per 1000 women screened, 1996) than at the incident (subsequent) screen (0.08 benign biopsies per 1000 women screened, compared with 4.3 cancers detected per 1000 women screened, 1996) (Patnick, 1996). These women have had the distress of a possible cancer diagnosis and morbidity from unnecessary surgery for a lesion, which they would have probably been unaware of without screening.

Some screening trials have found a higher incidence of breast cancer in the screened population than the control population with a cumulative excess of 10–21% in the screening population. This suggests that borderline histological lesions may be overdiagnosed. Results from the Swedish Two County Study (Tabar et al., 1992) and the Finnish National Breast Screening Programme (Hakama et al., 1995) suggests that overdiagnosis is limited to the first mammographic examination. Other studies have failed to show overdiagnosis.

Allowing for the mortality reduction of between 20 and 39% in the population offered screening, there will be many women with breast cancer, even those detected on screening, who will still die of their disease. For them screening has not changed their overall prognosis but may bring forward the time of diagnosis thus giving them longer to live with the knowledge of their disease. These women cannot be identified at the time of diagnosis and those who conduct screening know that they will only benefit some women with screen-detected cancers.

Future developments

Challenges facing screening programmes – resources

Screening programmes in many countries will face increasing demands in the coming years due to the baby boom, which occurred following the Second World War and which is now feeding through to the population of women aged 50. This will produce an increase in the workload of most screening programmes. There are already shortages of trained staff to run screening. The major impact so far has been on radiology manpower. There is a widespread shortage of radiologists in most specialities. There is a greater shortage of breast specialist radiologists with 40% of consultant posts unfilled initially in the UK (Field, 1998). Projections for the next few years show that the number of trainee radiologists in the UK is insufficient to cope with rising demand for new posts and to cover retirement vacancies. There are also difficulties in recruiting radiographers for breast screening. It is likely that screening programmes will need to look imaginatively at the use of skill mix. Already in a number of UK centres breast clinicians and radiographers are trained to read film.

Best practice for screening programmes, two views, two readers and extension of age

There are uncertainties over the best number of views for mammography, frequency of mammographic screening and the ideal age group to which a screening programme should be applied. As the UK NHSBSP was set up, trials were also brought into operation to examine each of these questions. The trial of one versus two-view mammography reported in 1995 (Wald et al., 1995) which showed a clear advantage of two-view mammography with an increased cancer detection of 24% and a reduction of 15% in the recall rate. Subsequent to this two-view mammography was introduced for the initial round of screening and SDRs rose nationally. There is now strong evidence that two-view mammography would be equally beneficial at incident screening rounds (Blanks et al., 1998a; Blanks et al., 1998b) and the UK programme is extending to two views at all rounds.

Double reading with two readers viewing each film increases cancer detection by between 5–50%. The benefit gained from a second reader is greater when readers are viewing a single oblique film. Greater benefit is also gained by having a third reader arbitrate after double reading than when using a consensus decision (Blanks et al., 1998a).

The trial of annual versus three-yearly mammography has not yet reported. If a change in the frequency of mammography were to be considered it is more likely that it would be a change to two-yearly rather than annual mammography. This would require a 50% increase in resources throughout the screening programme. This is unlikely to happen in the near future. Organized programmes in most other countries provide screening at two-yearly intervals.

The age limits of the screening programme are under more active consideration. The upper cut-off age of 64 was chosen initially on the grounds that women above the age of 64 would be unlikely to attend for screening rather than any indication that the benefit of screening in this age group was less. Most of the original randomized controlled trials of screening extended up to the age of 70 and showed clear benefit within the 65–70 age group.

The UK programme is extending up to age 70. Sweden recommends inviting women from age 40–70. Meanwhile a randomized controlled trial of screening in the 40–50-year-old age group in the UK has yet to report. This is the only RCT of screening specifically designed to assess the benefit of population screening in this age group (Moss, 1999).

Digital technology and computer aided detection

Current mammography units use screen/film combinations and until recently the resolution of digital radiography has not been sufficient for breast imaging. High resolution digital systems are now available, but there have been technical difficulties with obtaining a field size large enough to take a mammogram rather than imaging a small part of the breast for guiding biopsy or taking magnification views. Commercial full field mammographic digital systems are now in use and it is likely that digital imaging will become more widespread throughout symptomatic and screening mammography. This would then allow PACS (Picture Archiving and Communications Systems) to be extended to breast imaging with potential benefits in film handling, archiving and transmission. It is not yet known whether this will improve the sensitivity of cancer detection. Hand in hand with the development of digital mammography has been work on computer aided detection (CAD). A computer highlights areas of interest such as microcalcifications or areas of stellate distortion on clinical images and indicates the probability of the area being malignant. Such systems have acted as prompts to a radiologist reporting the films rather than providing fully automated reporting. The use of CAD may in the future allow films to be effectively double reported, once by machine and once by a radiologist, despite a shortage of manpower for film reading.

Nonoperative diagnosis

Fine needle aspiration cytology (FNAC), guided either by palpation, ultrasound or stereotaxis is routinely used within screening programmes. There have been difficulties with achieving satisfactory rates of cancers having a preoperative malignant diagnosis (UK 1996/97 results 62%, target 70%) (Patnick, 1998). In addition, cytology cannot reliably distinguish in situ from invasive cancer. There has therefore been a move towards guided core biopy which is capable of providing a more accurate preoperative diagnosis. Many centres are achieving over 90% preoperative malignant diagnosis rates with core biopsy. The availability of a histological diagnosis allows a more definitive discussion of management with a woman prior to surgery and informed counselling. Evaluation is now being undertaken of larger bore guided biopsy needles such as the Mammotome and ABBI breast biopsy systems which allow removal of the majority, or all, of the mammographic abnormality under local anaesthetic and radiological guidance. There are still doubts over the use of these techniques. Not all patients are suitable for them and questions are still unanswered about the accuracy of the histological interpretation of samples obtained this way and the need for obtaining clear margins, wide excision and lymph node staging which may necessitate subsequent operative treatment resulting in a two-stage procedure.

'Family history' screening of younger women

Women who have relatives with breast cancer may be at increased risk of the disease and seek screening at a young age. There are no RCTs aimed at assessing screening in women with a family history. The largest study of screening in such women is a cross-sectional study of nearly 400 000 screened women (Kerlikowske et al., 2000) comparing results in these with and without a first degree relative with breast cancer. This showed results of screening in high-risk women to be similar to those in the general population who are a decade older. A number of smaller cohort studies of women with family histories of breast cancer aged under 50 show similar results of screening to findings in over 50 year olds in larger national and large-scale screening programmes (Tilanus-Linthorst et al., 2000; Moller et al., 1999; Laloo et al., 1998; Kollias et al., 1998). Five-year survival from mammographic screen detected breast cancer in high-risk young women is comparable to that from screen detected cancer in older women (Moller et al., 1999). In most of these studies the average age of participants is 40–50 years. Although there is now evidence that the outcome of screening high-risk women under 50 is similar to RCT data in older women in terms of size and number of cancers detected, evidence for mortality reduction is limited because of the small size of the studies compared with RCTs of population screening. In addition, we know that the sensitivity of mammography is reduced in younger women and may be still less in family history women. Kerlikowske et al. (1996) found reduced sensitivity for cancer detection in women under 50 with a family history compared to those without (68.8 vs. 85.4%). It is also possible that family history women may be more susceptible to cancer induction from radiation. Increased radiation sensitivity is known to be associated with ataxia telangiectasia and there is a suggestion that this may also apply to heterozygotes for the *ATM* gene who have been estimated to make up approximately 0.5–1.5% of the population and may account for up to 8% for all cases of breast cancer (Kastan, 1995).

Despite these drawbacks consensus is emerging that the benefit of screening outweighs the problems in younger women who are at significantly increased risk of cancer. If these are shown to have a lifetime risk greater than twice the average in the population they should be offered screening at a younger age than normal after careful assessment of their level of risk and counselling about benefits and drawbacks of screening (Eccles et al., 2000).

Ongoing research into family history screening is often directed at modalities other than mammography. The use of screening mammography, ultrasound and MRI (magnetic resonance imaging) has been compared in gene carriers and MRI shown to have the highest sensitivity (Kuhl et al., 2000).

Ultrasound for screening

Studies carried out in the 1980s looking at ultrasound for breast screening did not show any benefit (Kopans et al., 1985). In the last 15 years, however, there have been considerable advances in ultrasound technology with the routine introduction of high resolution scanning. The widespread use of ultrasound as an adjunct to mammography in the symptomatic and screening assessment setting has raised the level of radiological expertise with breast ultrasound and there have been a number of reports of impalpable cancers detected solely with ultrasound in women undergoing investigation of lesions elsewhere in the breast. Kolb, Lichy & Newhouse (1998) offered ultrasound screening to women with normal mammograms but dense breasts, and normal physical examination. They ultrasounded 3626 women with a mean age of 54 and increased the numbers of cancers detected solely with imaging by 37% from 30 to 41 tumours in that group. The tumours detected with ultrasound screening were similar in size and stage to mammographically identified impalpable cancers. The cancer detection rate with ultrasound was higher in women who were at high risk because of previous diagnosis, such as breast cancer, but was not increased in women at high risk because of a family history. Nevertheless this was the first large-scale study to indicate that screening ultrasound may be beneficial. Similar detection rates of 3 tumours per 1000 women demonstrated on ultrasound alone were found by Buchberger et al. (1999). As in earlier studies, however, they showed a high false positive rate with 450 out of 6000 women screened undergoing needle or surgical biopsy.

Ultrasound has the benefit as a screening modality that it is harmless, as no ionizing radiation is involved but this may be balanced by a high rate of false positives. Further improvements in ultrasound in the future may make it worthwhile as a screening modality for younger high-risk women with dense breasts.

Magnetic resonance imaging

Contrast enhanced MRI also has the advantage of being free of ionizing radiation. The sensitivity of gadolinium enhanced MRI for detecting breast cancer has been reported at 90–100% (Gilles et al., 1994; Heywang-Kobrunner et al., 1993) but the specificity is much lower varying from 37% to 97% (Kaiser & Reiser, 1992). MRI is expensive, time consuming and invasive compared to other modalities for breast imaging, and these combined with its low specificity make it unsuitable for routine screening. A multicentre study is under way in the UK prospectively comparing enhanced MRI and mammography in younger premenopausal women at high genetic risk of breast cancer (National Multicentre Study, 1997). It is of proven worth in the detection of occult carcinoma in dense breasts and finding multifocal or contralateral carcinomas in the presence of a known cancer. Its value in screening younger women may however be limited by false positive scans due to enhancement with proliferative dysplasias which can resemble both DCIS and invasive ductal carcinoma. (Heywang-Kobrunner, 1995).

Conclusion

Regular mammographic screening for women over 50 can without doubt reduce breast cancer mortality. Screening, however, is a process which carries disadvantages as well as advantages. In order to maximize the benefits of screening it is essential that high quality is maintained in a screening programme. Ten years of having a national screening programme in the UK has allowed areas to be identified where screening could potentially be improved, such as increasing the number of readers. Those working in screening also face other challenges and it is likely that over the next decade more information will become available on other methods of screening and whether they confirm potential benefits particularly in younger women.

REFERENCES

Alexander, F.E., Anderson, T.J., Brown, H.K. et al. (1999). 14 years of follow up from the Edinburgh randomised trial of breast cancer screening. *Lancet*, 353(9168), 1903–8.

Andersson, I., Aspegren, K., Janzon, L. et al. (1988). Mammographic screening & mortality from breast cancer. The Malmo Mammographic Screening Trial. *British Medical Journal*, 297(6654), 943–8.

Anonymous (1999). 16 year mortality from breast cancer in the UK trial of Early Detection of Breast Cancer. *Lancet*, 353(9168), 1909–14.

Bjurstam, N., Bjorneld, L., Duffy, S.W. et al. (1997). The Gothenburg Breast Screening Trial: first results of mortality, incidence, and mode of detection for women ages 30–49 at randomization. *Cancer*, 80, 2091–9.

Blanks, R.G., Day, N.E. & Moss, S.M. (1996). Monitoring the performance of breast screening programmes: use of indirect standardisation in evaluating invasive cancer detection rate. *Journal of Medical Screening*, 3, 79–81.

Blanks, R.G., Given-Wilson, R.M. & Moss, S.M. (1998a). Efficiency of cancer detection deriving routine repeat (incident) mammographic screening: two versus one view mammography. *Journal of Medical Screening*, 5(3), 141–5.

Blanks, R.G., Wallis, M.G. & Moss, S.M. (1998b). A comparison of cancer detection rates achieved by breast cancer screening programmes by number of readers for one and two view mammography: results from the UK National Health Service Breast Screening Programme. *Journal of Medical Screening*, 5(4), 195–201.

Buchberger, W., DeKoekkoek-Doll, P., Springer, P., Obrist, P. & Dunser, M. (1999). Incidental findings on sonography of the breast: clinical significance and diagnostic workup. *American Journal of Roentgenology*, 173, 921–7.

Cancer Research Campaign (1996). *Breast Cancer – UK Factsheet* 6, published by The Cancer Research Campaign.

Cancer Research Campaign (1997). *Breast cancer screening*. UK Factsheet 7.1 Published by The Cancer Research Campaign.

Day, N., McCann, T., Camilleri-Ferrante, C. et al. (1995). Monitoring interval cancers in breast screening programmes: The East Anglian experience. *Journal of Medical Screening*, 2, 180–5.

De Koning, H.J. (2000). Assessment of nationwide cancer-screening programmes. *Lancet*, 355, 80–1.

Demissie, K., Mills, O.F. & Rhoads, G.G. (1998). Empirical comparison of the results of randomised controlled trials and case control studies in evaluating the effectiveness of screening mammography. *Journal of Clinical Epidemiology*, 51(2), 81–91.

Eccles, D.M., Evans, D.G. & Mackay, J. (2000). Guidelines for a genetic risk based approach to advising women with a family history of breast cancer. UK Cancer Family Study Group. *Journal of Medical Genetics*, 37(3), 203–9.

Feig, S.A. (1995). Mammographic screening of women age 40–49 years. Benefit, risk and cost considerations. *Cancer*, 76 (10 suppl.), 2097–106.

Field, S. (1998). Breast Screening Issues. *Royal College of Radiologists Newsletter*, 54, 12–14.

Forrest, A.P.M. (1986). *Breast cancer screening: Report to the Health Ministers of England, Wales, Scotland and Northern Ireland.* London: HMSO.

Frisell, J. & Lidbrink, E. (1997). The Stockholm Mammographic Screening Trial: Risks and benefits in age group 40–49 years. *Journal of the National Cancer Institute. Monographs*, (22), 49–51.

Frissell, J., Lidbrink, E., Hellstrom, L. & Rutguist, L.E. (1997). Follow up after 11 years – update of mortality results in the Stockholm Mammographic Screening Trial. *Breast Cancer Research and Treatment*, 45(3), 263–70.

Gilles, R., Ginnebretiere, J.M., Lucidarme, O. et al. (1994). Non-palpable breast tumours: Diagnosis with contrast-enhanced subtraction dynamic MR imaging. *Radiology*, 191, 625–31.

Given-Wilson, R.M., Blanks, R.G., Moss, S.M. et al. (1999). The evaluation of breast cancer screening – experience from the South Thames (West) Region. *The Breast*, 8, 66–71.

Given-Wilson, R.M., Layer, G., Warren, M. et al. (1997). False negative mammography: causes and consequences. *The Breast*, 6, 361–6.

Glasziou, P. & Irwig, L. (1997). The quality and interpretation of mammographic screening trials for women ages 40–49. *Journal of the National Cancer Institute. Monographs* (22), 73–7.

Gotzsche, P. & Olsen O. (2000). Is screening for breast cancer with mammography justifiable? *Lancet*, 355, 129–34.

Hakama, M., Holli, K., Isola, J. et al. (1995). Agressiveness of screen detected breast cancers. *Lancet*, 345 (8944), 221–4.

Heywang-Kobrunner, S. (1995). *Contrast enhanced MRI of the breast.* 2nd edn., p. 204. Berlin: Springer-Verlag.

Heywang-Kobrunner, S.H., Beck, R., Schmidt, F. et al. (1993). Use of contrast-enhanced MR imaging of the breast for problem cases (abstract). *Radiology*, 189(P), 105.

Kaiser, W.A. & Reiser, M.R. (1992). MR mammography: experience after 650 examinations (Abstract). *Journal of Magnetic Resonance Imaging*, 2(P), 88.

Kastan, M. (1995). Ataxia-Telangiectasia – broad implications for a rare disorder. *The New England Journal of Medicine*, 333(10), 662–3.

Kerlikowske, K., Carney, P.A., Geller, B. et al. (2000). Performance of screening mammography among women with and without a first degree relative with breast cancer. *Annals of Internal Medicine*, 133(11), 855–63.

Kerlikowske, K., Grady, D., Barclay, J. et al. (1996). Effect of age, breast density, and family history on the sensitivity of first screening mammography. *Journal of the American Medical Association*, 276(1), 33–8.

Kollias, J., Sibbering, D.M., Blamey, R.W. et al. (1998). Screening women age less than 50 years with a family history of breast cancer. *European Journal of Cancer*, 34(6), 878–83.

Kopans, D.B. (1995). Mammography screening and the controversy concerning women age 40 to 49. *Radiologic Clinics of North America*, 33(6), 1273–90.

Kopans, D.B., Meyer, J.E. & Lindfors, K.K. (1985). Whole breast ultrasound imaging four year follow up. *Radiology*, 157: 505–7.

Kolb, T.M., Lichy, J. & Newhouse, J.H. (1998). Occult cancer in women with dense breasts: detection with screening US – diagnostic yield and tumour characteristics. *Radiology*, 207, 191–9.

Kukl, L.K., Schmutzler, R.K., Leutner, C.C. et al. (2000). Breast MR Imaging screening in 192 women proved or suspected to be carriers of a breast cancer susceptibility gene: preliminary results. *Radiology*, 215(1), 267–79.

Laloo, F., Boggis, C.R., Evans, D.G. et al. (1998). Screening by mammography, women with a family history of breast cancer. *European Journal of Cancer*, 34(6), 937–40.

Lancet (1998). Editorial. The screening muddle. *Lancet*, 351(9101), 459.

Lanninn, D.R., Harris, R.P., Swanson, F.H. et al. (1993). Difficulties in diagnosis of carcinoma of the breast in patients less than fifty years of age. *Surgery, Gynaecology and Obstetrics*, 177(5), 457–62.

Larsson, L.G., Nystrom, L., Wall, S. et al. (1996). The Swedish Randomised Mammography Scanning Trials: analysis of their effect on the breast cancer related excess mortality. *Journal of Medical Screening*, 3(3), 129–32.

Law, J. (1997). Cancers detected and induced in mammographic screening: new screening schedules and younger women with a family history. *The British Journal of Radiology*, 70, 62–9.

Liberman, L., Dershaw, D.D., Deutch, B.M. et al. (1993). Screening mammography: value in women 35–39 years old. *American Journal of Roentgenology*, 161(1), 53–6.

McIlwaine, G. (1993). Satisfaction with the NHS Breast Screening Programme. Women's views. In *Breast Screening Acceptability, Research and Practice*, ed. J. Austoker, J. Patnick, NHSBSP Publication no. 28, 14–16.

Miller, W.R., Ellis, I.O. & Sainsbury, J.R.C. (1995). Prognostic factors. In: *ABC of Breast Disease*, ed. J.M. Dixon. BMJ Publishing Group.

Miller, A.B., To, T., Baines, C.J. & Wall, C. (2000). Canadian National Breast Screening Study – 2: 13 year results of a randomised trial in women age 50–59 years. *Journal of the National Cancer Institute*, 92(18), 1490–9.

Moller, P., Reis, M.M., Evans, G. et al. (1999). Efficacy of early diagnosis and treatment in women with a family history of breast cancer. European Familial Breast Cancer Collaborative Group. *Disease Markers*, 15(1–3), 179–86.

Moss, S. (1999). A trial to study the effect on breast cancer mortality of annual mammographic screening in women starting at age 40. Trial Steering Group. *Journal of Medical Screening*, 6(3): 144–8.

National Multicentre Study of MRI screening in women at genetic risk of breast cancer (1997). *Lancet http://www. Lancet.*

Patnick, J. (ed.) (1996). *NHS Breast Screening Programme Review 1996*. Published by the NHS Breast Screening Programme.

Patnick, J. (ed.) (1998). *NHS Breast Screening Programme Review 1998*. Published by the NHS Breast Screening Programme.

Peto, R., Boreham, J., Clarke, M. et al. (2000). UK and USA breast cancer deaths down 25% in year 2000 at ages 20–69 years. *Lancet*, 355, 1822.

Shapiro, S. et al. (1982). Fourteen year effect of breast cancer screening on mortality. *Journal of the National Cancer Institute*, 69, 349–55.

Sibbering, D.M., Burrell, H.C., Evans, A.J. et al. (1995). Mammographic sensitivity in women under 50 years presenting symptomatically with breast cancer. *The Breast*, 4, 127–9.

Tabar, L., Chen, H., Duffy, S., Yen, M., Chiang, C., Dean, P. & Smith, R. (2000). A novel method for prediction of long-term outcome of women with T1a, T1b, and 10–14 mm invasive breast cancers: a prospective study. *Lancet*, 355, 429–33.

Tabar, L., Fagerberg, G., Day, N.E. et al. (1992). Breast cancer treatment and natural history: new insights from results of screening. *Lancet*, 339(8790), 412–14.

Tabar, L., Vitak, B., Chen, H.H. et al. (2000a). The Swedish two county trial twenty years later. Updated mortality results & new insights from long-term follow up. *Radiological Clinics of North America*, 38(4), 625–51.

Tabar, L., Vitak, B., Tony, H.H. et al. (2001). Beyond randomised controlled trials: organised mammographic screening substantially reduces breast cancer mortality. *Cancer*, 91(9), 1724–31.

Tilanus-Linthorst, M.M., Bartels, C., Obdeijn, A.I. & Oudkerk, M. (2000b). Earlier detection of breast cancer by surveillance of women at familial risk. *European Journal of Cancer*, 36(4), 514–19.

Van Dijk, J.A., Broeders, M.J. & Verbeek, A.L. (1997). Mammography screening in older women. Is it worthwhile? *Drugs and Ageing*, 10(2), 69–79.

Verbeek, A.L.M. et al. (1984). Reduction of breast cancer mortality through mass screening with modern mammography. *Lancet*, 1, 1222–4.

Wald, N., Chamberlain, J. & Hackshaw, A. (1993). Report of the European Society of Mastology Breast Cancer Screening Evaluation Committee. *The Breast*, 2, 209–16.

Wald, N., Murphy, P., Major, P. et al. (1995). UKCCCR multicentre randomised controlled trial of one and two view mammography in breast cancer screening. *British Medical Journal*, 311, 1189–93.

Wilson, J.M. & Jungner, Y.G. (1968). Principles and practice of mass screening for disease. *Boletin de la Oficina Sanitaria Panamericana*. Pan American Sanitary Bureau, 65:281–393.

Woodman, C.B.J., Threlfall, A., Boggis, C.R.M. et al. (1995). Is the three year breast screening interval too long? Occurrence of interval cancers in NHS breast screening programme's north western region. *British Medical Journal*, 310, 224–6.

6

The management of in situ breast cancer

Zenon Rayter

Bristol Royal Infirmary, Bristol

Introduction

Ductal carcinoma in situ (DCIS) is defined as a proliferation of epithelial cells with cytological features of malignancy within parenchymal structures of the breast and distinguished from invasive carcinoma by the absence of stromal invasion across the basement membrane (National Co-ordinating Committee on Breast Screening Pathology (NCCBSP), 1995). It is conventionally regarded as the principal precursor of breast cancer and is distinct from lobular carcinoma in situ (LCIS), which is now regarded as a high-risk factor for the subsequent development of invasive breast cancer rather than a precursor lesion (Poller & Ellis, 1996).

DCIS of the breast has become an increasingly important pathological entity in the last 15 years with an approximately fourfold increase in incidence in the USA compared with only a modest rise in the incidence of invasive disease (Hankey et al., 1993). This is due mostly to the introduction of screening mammography but may also be due to the increased recognition of DCIS by breast pathologists (Frykberg & Bland, 1994). The incidence of symptomatic DCIS (as opposed to screen-detected DCIS) has not increased significantly and usually presents clinically as a palpable mass, Paget's disease or with nipple discharge and comprises 3–5% of symptomatic cases (Ashikari et al., 1971; Lagios, 1990). In the United Kingdom, there were 1308 cases of DCIS recorded by the National Breast Screening programme for the year 1994/95, accounting for 25.2% of breast cancer cases in the screened population aged 50–64 (Julietta Patnick, personal communication). Recently, however, it has been suggested that DCIS should not be classified as cancer at all and that an entirely new terminology be used to describe the various types of DCIS (Foucar, 1996).

The established view of DCIS as one disease entity is now changing. DCIS is not a homogeneous entity and it seems reasonable to separate DCIS into several disease states. This view is also confirmed by microdissection studies which show loss of heterozygosity (LOH) on chromosomes 16 and 17 in both atypical ductal hyperplasia (ADH) and DCIS (Radford et al., 1993; Lakhani et al., 1995; Stratton et al., 1995), implying that ADH is also part of the spectrum of neoplastic breast disease. However, difficulties may arise in determining the criteria for diagnosis of DCIS compared with ADH, LCIS and microinvasive breast cancer. In addition, some subtypes of DCIS are difficult to recognize and diagnose. Other hotly debated topics include the validity of pathological classification systems for DCIS, as most have not been tested prospectively. Adequacy of pathological excision margins and the use of molecular markers are further areas of uncertainty.

The following summarizes what is known of the epidemiology, pathology and biology of DCIS and reviews its current management.

Epidemiology

A great deal of work has been published on the epidemiology of invasive breast cancer and this has been reviewed recently (McPherson et al., 1994; Hulka & Stark, 1995). The majority of factors related to the epidemiology of breast cancer may be grouped into the following broad headings: age, hormones, genetic factors, sociodemographic factors, diet, lifestyle, biological factors and environmental factors. The relative risks of those factors which are known to be relevant are summarized in Table 6.1. Other factors under suspicion as being important are pesticides, electromagnetic fields and cigarette smoking, but the data on these is conflicting (Hulka & Stark, 1995).

There has been little research on the epidemiology of carcinoma in situ and it has been argued that it is possible that different types of DCIS may have different aetiologies (Millikan et al., 1995). There are several reasons why epidemiological studies of DCIS might give new clues regarding breast cancer risk. First, this may increase the power to detect exposure effects. Secondly, studies of the epidemiology of DCIS would be conducted closer in time to the action of exposures suspected to be causes, as was the case with smoking and colonic polyps (Fielding, 1994). Thirdly, genetic alterations of DCIS are less likely to represent a 'bystander' event such as those which occur in late tumorigenesis.

Some recent data does suggest that there may be subtle differences in epidemiological risk factors in DCIS and LCIS compared with invasive breast cancer. In one study of patients under the age of 45 years, the established risk factors (Table 6.1) for invasive disease also applied to in situ disease but the associations with nulliparity, a previous breast biopsy and body mass index were significantly stronger for in situ disease than for invasive disease, whilst alcohol consumption was associated with an increasing trend in risk for invasive and metastatic disease (Weiss et al., 1996). These observations need to be confirmed by further studies.

Table 6.1. Risk factors for breast cancer

Epidemiological risk factor	High-risk group	Low-risk group
Relative risk > 4.0		
Age	> 50	≤ 30
Geographic area	North America, Northern Europe	Africa, Asia
Positive family history	Two first-degree relatives of young age	No
Previous cancer in one breast	Yes	No
Relative risk 2.1–4.0		
Nodular densities on mammogram (postmenopausal)	> 75% breast volume	No
Positive family history	One first-degree relative	No
Biopsy-confirmed atypical hyperplasia	Yes	No
High-dose radiation to chest	Yes	No
Oophorectomy before age 35	No	Yes
Relative risk 1.1–2.0		
Demographic		
Socioeconomic status	High	Low
Place of residence	Urban	Rural
Race		
Breast cancer > 40 yr	Caucasian	Asian
Breast cancer < 40 yr	Black	Asian
Religion	Jewish	Seventh day Adventist/Mormon
Hormonal		
Age at first full-term pregnancy	> 30 yr	< 20 yr
Age at menarche	< 12 yr	> 14 yr
Age at menopause	> 55 yr	< 45 yr
Obesity (postmenopausal)	Obese	Thin
Parity (postmenopausal)	Nulliparous	Multiparous
Breast feeding	None	Years
Hormonal contraceptives		
Breast cancer < 45 yr	Yes	No
Hormone replacement therapy	Yes	No
Other		
Height	Tall	Short
Previous cancer of colon, ovary or endometrium	Yes	No
Alcohol consumption	Yes	No

Pathology of DCIS

Until recently, DCIS was classified by architectural pattern into comedo, cribriform, micropapillary, solid and mixed subtypes. It is now apparent that the architecture is probably of less importance than was earlier thought and that the nuclear grade, the size of the lesion and the presence or absence of comedo-type necrosis are probably of greater importance (Poller & Ellis, 1996). The European Community Working Group on Breast Screening Pathology have accepted the following guidelines for classification of DCIS into three grades for use in Europe (NCCBSP, 1995).

It has been assumed that lesions of high nuclear grade are more aggressive and there are several series which show an increased incidence of local recurrence after local excision in patients with higher nuclear grade variants of DCIS, those with comedo necrosis and those that are of larger size (*vide infra*). However, subclassification of DCIS into prognostic subtypes has been performed on retrospective series and caution needs to be exercized in the interpretation of these results. It may well be, for example, that lower grade noncomedo DCIS is more difficult to visualize radiographically than comedo DCIS, leading to a falsely low true recurrence rate. Furthermore, the information on margin assessments in some reports is incomplete and the definitions of what constitutes local recurrence varied.

Classification of DCIS (Poller & Ellis, 1996; NCCBSP, 1995)

- High nuclear grade DCIS. Cells have large pleomorphic nuclei and exhibit frequent mitoses. Several growth patterns may be evident, especially solid with comedo-type central necrosis.
- Intermediate grade DCIS. Cells have nuclei with mild to moderate pleomorphism. The growth pattern may be solid, cribriform or micropapillary.
- Low nuclear grade DCIS. Cells have a small and monomorphic appearance. Mitoses are few and necrosis is rare. A cribriform growth pattern is most common although micropapillary growth patterns may also be present within the same lesion.
- Mixed type DCIS. A proportion of cases exhibit features of more than one histological subtype. However, the nuclear grade is usually a more consistent finding throughout even these mixed lesions. In cases where nuclear grade varies, the lesion should be classified on the basis of highest nuclear grade.
- Microinvasive carcinoma. This is defined as a lesion where the dominant lesion is noninvasive but in which there are one or more areas of infiltration, none of which should measure more than 1 mm. These lesions are rare and some authorities suggest these lesions should not be allowed in a classification of DCIS (Royal College of Pathologists, 1990).

- Rare subtypes of DCIS. Tavassoli (1992) has also described six rare subtypes: apocrine; encysted papillary carcinoma in situ; clear cell; signet ring; endocrine; cystic hypersecretory; and male breast DCIS.

An alternative classification has been proposed by Silverstein et al. (1995a) which also groups DCIS into three categories defined by the presence or absence of high nuclear grade and comedo-type necrosis. Thus, group 1 is characterized as non-high-grade DCIS without comedo-type necrosis. Group 2 is non-high-grade DCIS with comedo-type necrosis and group 3 is high-grade DCIS with or without comedo-type necrosis. The utility of this classification is claimed to be valid by the differing prognostic outcomes of these subtypes. Thus small cell micropapillary cribriform DCIS is claimed to have a relatively low invasive potential (Rosen et al., 1980; Page et al., 1982; Lagios, 1990; Silverstein et al., 1995a) and rarely progresses or recurs, whereas comedo and other large cell types are said to be associated with a poorer prognosis, larger lesion size and have a significantly higher incidence of recurrence, suggesting a more aggressive biological behaviour (Lagios et al., 1982; Page et al., 1982; Schnitt et al., 1988; Schwartz et al., 1989; Baird et al., 1990; Moore, 1991; Pierce et al., 1992; Schwartz et al., 1992; Simpson et al., 1992; Silverstein et al., 1995a). The major problem with the subclassification of DCIS into lesions giving prognostic categories is that the subclassification of these lesions has been derived from retrospective studies and has not been tested prospectively. Finally, the micropapillary form of DCIS is generally regarded as being multifocal and therefore should always be treated by mastectomy (Bellamy et al., 1993). This would, therefore, not allow the confirmation that this is a low-grade lesion in studies involving breast-conserving surgery.

Natural history of DCIS

There is surprisingly little known about the natural history of DCIS as little prospective data is available. The critical question is whether DCIS progresses to invasive cancer. Historically DCIS has been treated very successfully by mastectomy with almost 100% cure, making the frequency with which invasive recurrence occurred almost impossible to assess. Furthermore, the natural history of mammographically detected DCIS is likely to be quite different to that of symptomatic DCIS, which usually presents with a mass, nipple discharge or Paget's disease. This makes the results of older studies not necessarily applicable to screen-detected DCIS.

It is now known that DCIS arises within the terminal duct lobular units (TDLU) of the breast (Wellings et al., 1975; Holland et al., 1990; Faverly et al., 1994), although the size of the ducts suggest that extralobular ducts are also involved in

DCIS (Rosen & Oberman, 1993). The current belief is that DCIS originates in the terminal ducts and acini of the breast, grows and expands these ducts until at some stage in its natural history it becomes invasive and penetrates the basement membrane. One method of discerning the natural history of DCIS has been to determine its frequency in autopsies of patients dying from an unrelated condition. In one autopsy series from Denmark, the incidence of asymptomatic DCIS was 15% (Anderson et al., 1985), indicating that DCIS may remain occult and clinically unimportant for a long time. In contrast, three other autopsy studies demonstrated DCIS much less frequently (Alpeers & Wellings, 1985; Bartow et al., 1987; Nielsen et al., 1987). These studies are in marked contrast to an incidence of 40% found in the breast when an invasive cancer was present and an incidence of 60% in the contralateral breast of patients undergoing bilateral mastectomy for unilateral invasive cancer (Alpeers & Wellings, 1985).

Holland et al., using a variety of techniques including three-dimensional reconstruction and serial subgross pathology, have mapped out the distribution of DCIS and have shown that the majority if not all cases of DCIS exist as one lesion (Holland et al., 1990; Faverly et al., 1992; Faverly et al., 1994). The fact that only some 66% of DCIS lesions occur within a quadrant of the breast is irrelevant, as a breast quadrant is a descriptive account of the breast tissue encompassed by a 90° arc and is not an anatomically distinct unit. These observations imply that DCIS is unifocal in origin despite the observation that it is sometimes discontinuous (previously interpreted as implying multifocality). The view that DCIS is a single clonal process has been further supported recently by the work of Noguchi et al. who have shown the monoclonal origin of DCIS and atypical ductal hyperplasia using the polymerase chain reaction (Noguchi et al., 1994), and by recent work which has shown loss of heterozygosity at the same chromosome locus in all 12 cases of DCIS studied (Stratton et al., 1995).

It is unknown what proportion of DCIS lesions will become malignant but some clues regarding this can be gleaned from the following studies. Two retrospective studies of patients who had undergone excision biopsy for lesions considered benign at the time but on subsequent review were found to have DCIS have suggested that these patients are at greater risk of developing invasive cancer. The incidence of subsequent ipsilateral invasive cancer in these studies was between 25% and 30% (Rosen et al., 1980; Page et al., 1982). In most cases the invasive disease occurred at the site of the previously excised DCIS with a mean time to detection of the invasive cancers of 6.1 to 9.7 years. These studies lacked important information on adequacy of the excision margin and also represented the more benign spectrum of DCIS changes. Two prospective studies have reported recurrence rates of 13% (5 of 38 patients; Arnesson et al., 1989) and 17% (5 of 28 patients; Carpenter et al., 1989). A worrying feature was that 3 of these 10 patients presented with a recurrence which was invasive after follow-up of between 3 and 5 years.

These tentative data suggest that some but not all cases of DCIS will progress to invasive cancer and that this process may take many years to become evident. Some retrospective studies have suggested that known poor prognostic factors in invasive breast cancer may be indicators of subsequent recurrence of DCIS when these are present in the lesion but none of these have yet been tested prospectively.

Molecular biology of DCIS

Interphase cytogenetics

A wide variety of genetic changes have been described in invasive cancer, DCIS and ADH (reviewed by Poller & Ellis, 1996). A recent fluorescent in situ hybridization (FISH) study (Micale et al., 1994) described true gains of chromosome 1 in 34% of nuclei in one case of DCIS, with true gains of chromosomes 17 and 18 using pericentrometric probes for chromosomes 1, 16, 17 and 18. Other workers have also found loss of heterozygosity associated with pure DCIS (Radford et al., 1993) and DCIS associated with invasive cancer (Stratton et al., 1995) on chromosomes 16 and 17 in up to 50% of cases. These allelic imbalances may be due to loss of one allele in neoplastic cells or an increase in copy number of the other allele. There are no large studies of the familial breast cancer gene *BRCA1* in DCIS which is also located on chrosome 17 (17q12–q21), but a small study has shown loss of heterozygosity in the region of the *BRCA1* gene in 10–20% of informative cases of DCIS studied (Futreal et al., 1994), implying, as in invasive cancer, a limited role for this gene in sporadic DCIS. These observations at present have no clinical utility.

Oncogenes and steroid receptors

Different subtypes of DCIS vary in the frequency with which they express the proto-oncogene c-*erb*B-2(HER2/*neu*). This is an oncogene that is overexpressed in 15–25% of invasive breast cancers and is associated with a poorer prognosis and decreased response to endocrine therapy and chemotherapy (Ramachandra et al., 1990; Barnes et al., 1992; Gusterson et al., 1992; Wright et al., 1992). Overexpression of c-*erb*B-2 has been found in 50–60% of all DCIS lesions (Allred et al., 1992; Barnes et al., 1992), and in 77–90% of the comedo subtype, being significantly associated with large cell type and increased proliferative activity as measured by thymidine labelling index and S-phase fraction (Barnes et al., 1992). Another study (Allred et al., 1992) has shown that the frequency of c-*erb*B-2 overexpression in DCIS associated with invasive cancer was approximately 30%, half that seen in pure DCIS. These observations suggest that c-*erb*B-2 may be important in breast cancer initiation but not in progression. Another interpretation is that invasive breast cancers which do not overexpress c-*erb*B-2 do not arise from a significant in situ phase.

The expression of the protein product of the mutated tumour suppressor gene p53 has also been investigated in DCIS. In one study, 33% of DCIS cases expressed the mutated p53 protein product, a similar proportion to that of invasive cancer (Poller et al., 1992). Significant associations of p53 expression were lack of oestrogen receptor (ER) expression, high tumour grade, c-*erb*B-2 and epidermal growth factor receptor overexpression (Poller et al., 1993a), all factors associated with a lack of response to hormone therapy.

The expression of ER in DCIS has been much more variable and inconsistent. Two studies found an incidence of ER-positive DCIS of 60% (Malafa et al., 1990; Chandhuri et al., 1993), a similar proportion to that found in invasive breast cancer (Rayter, 1991). However, in a larger study of 151 cases of DCIS from Nottingham, only 31.8% of cases were ER-positive (Poller et al., 1993b). This was significantly associated with noncomedo architecture, small cell size, higher S-phase fraction and lack of c-*erb*B-2 overexpression. This study is much more consistent with the observed inverse relationship of ER to c-*erb*B-2 seen in invasive breast cancer (Rayter, 1991) and more consistent with those studies which have shown a high incidence of c-*erb*B-2 overexpression in DCIS (Allred et al., 1992; Barnes et al., 1992). There have been few studies of progesterone receptor in DCIS and frequencies of positivity vary from 31% to 73% (Poller & Ellis, 1996). The significance of steroid receptors regarding treatment of DCIS will be further discussed.

A wide variety of oncogene and growth factor changes in DCIS have been discovered (for review, see Poller & Ellis, 1996) and although very interesting, they require prospective evaluation before it is known whether they will have any therapeutic implications.

Diagnosis of DCIS

DCIS is diagnosed by mammography in the vast majority of cases, in over 80% because of microcalcification (Stomper et al., 1989; Evans et al., 1994). A minority of cases may present with mammographic abnormalities without microcalcification, most commonly as ill-defined and spiculate masses. Symptomatic cases may present with nipple discharge (Fung et al., 1990), Paget's disease or a palpable mass and these comprise only 2% of cases. In 6% of cases, mammographically detected DCIS is found incidentally (Stomper et al., 1989).

A preoperative cellular diagnosis of malignancy can be achieved by stereotactic fine needle aspiration (FNA) cytology if, as in the majority of cases, the lesion is impalpable. However, FNA cytology cannot distinguish between DCIS and invasive malignancy. It may also be difficult to reliably differentiate between DCIS and ADH (Lilleng & Hagmar, 1992; Sneige & Staerkel, 1994). The results of FNA cytology should be used as part of the 'triple assessment', combining cytology with mammographic and clinical findings. Experience has shown that the positive predictive value of this triple assessment in the diagnosis of screen-detected DCIS falls short of that achieved for screen-detected or symptomatic invasive breast cancer. This is partly due to difficulties in obtaining enough cellular material for cytology to be diagnostic and partly due to the uncertainty of whether the sample is representative of the whole lesion.

Because of these difficulties, some groups have advocated the use of stereotactic core biopsy techniques to obtain a preoperative *histological* diagnosis. Several studies have now been published comparing the histology of core biopsies of non-palpable breast lesions with the final histology of the same lesion subsequently surgically excised using the fine wire guided biopsy technique. Excellent correlations of the order of 90% have been achieved by several groups (Caines et al., 1994; Gisvold et al., 1994; Liberman et al., 1994). The accuracy of this technique for a diagnosis of invasive cancer can be increased to 97% if as many as six core biopsies of the lesion are taken (Liberman et al., 1994). However, the diagnostic accuracy of this technique is unreliable in excluding malignancy if the histology of the core biopsy shows benign features with atypical findings (Jackman et al., 1994).

The role of stereotactic core biopsy of impalpable mammographic lesions has been reviewed recently by Morrow (1995). Arguments in favour of this technique are that it is safe and has a low (0.2%) complication rate. Because as many as half of mammographically detected lesions which are excised prove to be benign, stereotactic core biopsy may have the potential to spare patients with benign lesions an open surgical biopsy. Proponents of this technique also point out that fine wire guided biopsy also has a failure rate although this is less than 1% in specialized units, a figure much lower than the misdiagnosis rate of stereotactic core biopsy. It is also argued that if stereotactic core biopsy spares patients with benign lesions from an open surgical biopsy, it will prove to be a cost-effective method of evaluating lesions of low mammographic suspicion.

However, there are arguments against the widespread introduction of stereotactic core biopsy. The accuracy of the procedure varies with the type of mammographic lesion, the technique being more reliable in the evaluation of a mass lesion compared with microcalcification. The reproducibility of the technique remains uncertain and the ability of the core biopsy to determine definitive surgical therapy remains to be evaluated prospectively. Finally, the cost-effectiveness of the technique also requires careful evaluation, as do quality assurance standards (Morrow, 1995). Nevertheless, stereotactic core biopsy does seem a technique of great potential, although it will have to be demonstrated that the missed cancer detection rate is similar to that of fine wire localization biopsy before it is widely introduced.

The standard technique used for diagnosis of mammographically detected abnormalities which subsequently prove to be DCIS is by fine wire localization biopsy. In this technique, the mammographic abnormality is localized with a fine wire (a variety are available) stereotactically. The patient is subsequently transferred to the operating theatre and, under a general anaesthetic, the wire is used as a guide to excise the area of breast tissue under investigation. Following removal, orientation sutures or clips are placed on the surgical specimen and this is X-rayed with the wire still in situ to confirm that the suspicious lesion has been removed before it is sent for pathological evaluation. The majority of authors report miss rates of non-palpable lesions to be 1–5% (Homer et al., 1992; Morrow, 1995). However, the best results achieve a miss rate of only 0.2% (Kopans, 1993; Morrow, 1995).

Frozen section examination of impalpable lesions suspected of being DCIS is not recommended in the UK (NCCBSP, 1995) for the following reasons. Margins of excision cannot be adequately assessed on frozen section examination, thorough sampling of lesions cannot be properly performed to exclude foci of micro-invasion or frank invasive disease and the pathological grade of DCIS or invasive breast cancer cannot be assessed on frozen sections (NCCBSP, 1995). In the USA, frozen section diagnosis seems to be used much more frequently and some centres have published a frozen section accuracy of 97.7% (Ferreiro et al., 1995).

Treatment of DCIS

Historical perspective

Simple mastectomy used to be the standard treatment of symptomatic DCIS in view of the perceived hazards of multifocality and evolution into invasive carcinoma (Lewis & Geschikter, 1938; Rosen et al., 1979; Rosen et al., 1980; Von Rueden & Wilson, 1984; Schu et al., 1986; Lagios, 1990; Swain, 1992; Frykberg & Bland, 1993). The results of mastectomy in this setting are well established and are excellent (Smart et al., 1978). The combined data from 1061 women who underwent mastectomy for DCIS reported in 14 published studies with follow-up ranging from 2 to more than 15 years shows an overall local recurrence rate of only 0.75% (Fowble, 1989), and an overall cancer-related mortality of only 1.7% (Frykberg et al., 1991; Frykberg & Bland, 1993, 1994). However, local recurrence rates vary widely from 0% to 10% (Carter & Smith, 1977; Rosner et al., 1980; Lagios et al., 1982; Fisher et al., 1986; Carpenter et al., 1989; Lagios, 1990).

In view of the trend towards breast-conserving surgery for invasive breast

Table 6.2. Results of treatment of DCIS by wide local excision alone

Author	Year	Type of study	No. of patients	Mean FU (months)	No. of recurrences Total n (%)	Invasive n (%)
Arnesson	1989	Retrospective	38	60	5 (13)	2 (40)
Baird	1990	Retrospective	30	39	4 (13)	1 (25)
Carpenter	1989	Retrospective	28	38	5 (18)	1 (20)
Cataliotti	1992	Retrospective	46	105	5 (11)	5 (100)
Fisher	1986	Prospective	22	39	5 (23)	2 (40)
Fisher	1991	Prospective	21	83	9 (43)	5 (55)
Fisher	1993	Prospective	391	43	64(16)	32(50)
Gallagher	1989	Retrospective	13	100	5 (38)	3 (60)
Lagios	1989	Retrospective	79	44	8 (10)	4 (50)
Page	1982	Retrospective	25	192	7 (28)	7 (100)
Price	1990	Retrospective	35	108	22(63)	12(55)
Reynolds	1993	Retrospective	16	34	3 (19)	1 (33)
Ringberg	1991	Retrospective	21	84	3 (14)	3 (100)
Sanchez	1992	Retrospective	18	108	4 (22)	3 (75)
Schwartz	1992	Retrospective	72	49	11(15)	3 (27)
Silverstein	1992	Pros/Randomized	26	63	2 (8)	1 (50)
Silverstein	1996	Retrospective	195	79 (median)	32 (16)	14 (44)
Temple	1989	Retrospective	17	72	2 (12)	2 (100)
Vrouenraets	1991	Retrospective	14	73	5 (36)	1 (20)
Total			1107		201 (18)	102 (51)

% invasive recurrences expressed as % total recurrences.

cancer with results which are comparable to those of mastectomy in randomized prospective studies (Fisher et al., 1985, 1989; Veronesi et al., 1990), it seems appropriate that breast-conserving treatment should be applied to DCIS. Table 6.2 shows the results of a number of such studies, mostly retrospective, in which patients with DCIS were treated by wide local excision alone (Page et al., 1982; Fisher et al., 1986, 1991, 1993; Arnesson et al., 1989; Carpenter et al., 1989; Gallagher et al., 1989; Lagios et al., 1989; Temple et al., 1989; Baird et al., 1990; Ringberg et al., 1991; Vrouenraets et al., 1991; Cataliotti et al., 1992; Sanchez Forgach et al., 1992; Schwartz et al., 1992; Silverstein et al., 1992; Reynolds et al., 1993). With a mean follow-up of 38 to 192 months, local recurrence rates varied from 10% to 63%, although the average for all patients was 18.5%. Approximately half (52%) recurred as potentially incurable invasive disease (Table 6.2). It is evident from these studies that the incidence of local recurrence was greatest for palpable DCIS larger than 20 mm, as has been shown by other workers (Lagios et al., 1982, 1989) and in cases in which a pathological margin of excision was uncertain. Most local recurrences were located in the immediate vicinity of the original biopsy site, suggesting inadequate excision as the cause of the local recurrence rather than any intrinsic biological behaviour of DCIS.

The above studies are interesting but suffer from being retrospective, have widely different follow-up data, and mix palpable DCIS with screen-detected DCIS. However, three prospective studies of wide local excision without radiotherapy confirm the above findings of an unacceptable high rate of local recurrence with this form of therapy over a relatively short length of follow-up (Fisher et al., 1986, 1991, 1993). Those studies which have reported the lowest rates of local recurrence have been those in which the DCIS was found incidentally in biopsies for benign breast disease and in which the size of the lesion was <10 mm (Patchefsky et al., 1989; Schwartz et al., 1989, 1992). Thus one study employing wide excision alone for DCIS reported a local recurrence rate of 15.3% over a mean follow-up period of 49 months (Schwartz et al., 1989). All local recurrences exclusively occurred in cases of comedo DCIS, an association noted by other workers (Fisher et al., 1991, 1993).

A number of studies, again mostly retrospective, have also reported the results of treatment of DCIS by wide local excision with the addition of radiotherapy (Table 6.3; Fisher et al., 1986, 1991, 1993; Zafrani et al., 1986; Kurtz et al., 1989; Baird et al., 1990; Hafty et al., 1990; McCormick et al., 1990; Stotter et al., 1990; Bornstein et al., 1991; Recht et al., 1991; Ringberg et al., 1991; Vrouenraets et al., 1991; Silverstein et al., 1992; Solin et al., 1993). These have demonstrated very good results over follow-up intervals of up to 92 months. The addition of radiotherapy reduces local recurrence within the breast to an average of 9%, although 45% of these recur as invasive cancer (Table 6.3). Cancer-related mortality in these patients has been very low, averaging only approximately 1% (Zafrani et al., 1986; Kurtz et al., 1989; Stotter et al., 1990). The largest study of local excision and radiotherapy for DCIS was the B-17 protocol of the NSABP which randomized 818 women with purely noninvasive DCIS to undergo either wide excision alone or wide excision with postoperative breast irradiation (Fisher et al., 1993). After a mean follow-up of 43 months, the addition of radiotherapy significantly reduced the incidence of local breast recurrence by 58.8% and reduced the rate of ipsilateral recurrence of invasive cancer by 77%. The uncertainties of the potential value of radiotherapy in reducing *early* recurrence of noninvasive and invasive cancer have, however, not been eliminated by this study as margin status was not accurately assessed in many specimens and it was not possible to define a group of patients who might not benefit from adjuvant

Table 6.3. Results of treatment of DCIS by local excision and breast radiotherapy

Author	Year	No. of patients	Median FU (months)	No. of recurrences Total n (%)	Invasive n (%)
Baird	1990	8	39[a]	2 (25)	1 (50)
Bornstein	1991	38	81	8 (21)	5 (62.5)
Cataliotti	1992	34	105	3 (9)	3 (100)
Fisher	1986	29	39[a]	2 (7)	1 (50)
Fisher	1991	27	83	2 (7)	1 (50)
Fisher	1993	399	43[a]	28 (7)	8 (29)
Haffty	1990	60	43	4 (7)	1 (25)
Kurtz	1989	43	61	3 (7)	3 (100)
McCormick	1990	54	36	10 (10)	5 (50)
Recht	1991	193	76	21 (11)	10 (48)
Silverstein	1992	103	63	10 (10)	5 (50)
Silverstein	1996	138	79	23 (17)	12 (52)
Solin	1993	172	84	16 (9)	7 (44)
Stotter	1990	42	92	4 (9)	4 (100)
Vrouenraets	1991	28	73[a]	1 (4)	1 (100)
Zafrani	1986	55	55	3 (5.5)	1 (33)
Total		1415		140(10)	68 (49)

[a]

radiotherapy. It should also be emphasized that follow-up is still relatively short and it is possible that the effect of radiotherapy is to delay the appearance of local recurrence rather than prevent its occurrence. A further criticism of this study is that the extent of the margin of excision was unclear. Although it has been demonstrated in a retrospective study that breast-conserving surgery and radiotherapy for DCIS is associated with a reduced survival compared with mastectomy (Silverstein et al., 1995b), the safety of breast conservation needs to be tested prospectively by a randomized trial.

Breast-conserving surgery

What can be learned from the above studies regarding which patients can be treated by breast-conserving surgery? Some guidance regarding patient selection can be obtained from the current UK DCIS trial protocol. This trial was designed to compare the effectiveness of complete local excision (CLE) alone with CLE followed by radiotherapy to the residual ipsilateral breast tissue with or without tamoxifen, 20 mg/day for 5 years, in reducing the incidence of subsequent invasive carcinoma of the breast. A subsidiary aim is to compare, within the treatment arms of the trial, the incidences of subsequent DCIS in the ipsilateral breast distant from the original lesion and in the contralateral breast. The trial has a 2 × 2 factorial design as follows:

CLE ALONE   CLE + TAMOXIFEN

CLE + RADIOTHERAPY   CLE + RADIOTHERAPY + TAMOXIFEN

Entry criteria include patients with unilateral or bilateral DCIS which is cosmetically suited to breast conservation, which has been detected as a result of attendance at a screening centre, which is without evidence of invasion and which has been completely excised as determined by free margins on histological examination. Other patients suitable for entry into the trial are patients with similarly defined DCIS lesions in whom the diagnosis of DCIS has been made as a result of mammograms taken following referral to a diagnostic clinic. Clearly, the major determinant of a patient's suitability for this trial (besides informed consent) is the suitability of the DCIS lesion to be treated by breast-conserving surgery. To this extent, one can apply the same criteria as is applicable to invasive breast cancer; that is, size of the lesion compared to size of the breast, absence of multifocal/multicentric disease and a site in the breast sufficiently away from the nipple-areolar complex (NAC) which allows the nipple to be safely retained. Other factors which need to be taken into consideration are the relationship of size of the lesion to the likelihood of multicentricity, multifocality and axillary metastases.

It is useful to consider the definitions of multifocality and multicentricity in the therapeutic setting. Multicentric tumours are defined as separate tumours arising in the breast epithelium independently, whereas multifocal tumours are defined as metastatic deposits from a single primary neoplasm (Noguchi et al., 1994). Most workers now agree that the majority of cases of DCIS are unifocal and that multifocality may be due to the observation that the growth of DCIS may be discontinuous in up to half of all cases. Thus 'gaps' may occur between areas of DCIS within the same ductal tree. Most lesions (80%) revealed gaps which were less than 5 mm and only 10% of DCIS lesions exhibited gaps of > 10 mm. This has been correlated with the histological subtype of DCIS, and gaps are more frequently found in well-differentiated lesions than in moderately or poorly differentiated lesions (Holland et al., 1992). This is extremely important when consideration is given to what constitutes a clear margin, as it is obvious that even a clear margin of > 10 mm (often quoted as a reasonable definition of a clear margin, Sibbering et al., 1995) may leave behind DCIS in up to 10% of DCIS lesions even though the disease is really unifocal.

There is also the consideration of size of the DCIS lesion and its relationship to occult invasion (microinvasion). It has been shown that the frequency of microinvasion in DCIS is related to the extent of DCIS. Thus, lesions < 25 mm are very unlikely to exhibit areas of microinvasion, but 46% of lesions larger than 25 mm show areas of microinvasion and this rises to 70% for lesions larger than 50 mm (Lagios et al., 1982). Although the overall incidence of lymph node metastasis in DCIS is only 0–2% (Silverstein et al., 1987), this incidence rises with the presence of microinvasion and this in turn is related to the size of the lesion (Lagios et al., 1982). Finally, consideration needs to be given to the frequency with which the nipple or nipple-areolar complex are involved if breast-conserving surgery is contemplated. One French study suggested that spread to the NAC occurred in the majority of cases (Recht et al., 1994). This discrepancy from most other pathological studies, as well as from clinical experience in which tumour recurrence in the NAC is rare even when local excision alone has been employed, may be explained by differences in the size of the lesions studied in different series. Thus, involvement of the NAC is likely to be frequent only for larger (30–50 mm) lesions. Therefore, special attention to the NAC is only warranted in patients with frank Paget's disease and lesions in the subareolar region (Recht et al., 1994).

With these considerations in mind, which patients can be treated by breast-conserving surgery? The vast majority of such patients will have asymptomatic, mammographically detected lesions. It must be stressed that careful preoperative evaluation with the radiologist is required to assess the extent of the lesion. It is well documented that the pathological extent of poorly differentiated DCIS correlates well with the radiological extent of the lesion but that the mammographic extent of well-differentiated lesions substantially underestimates their pathological extent. However, when routine mammograms are supplemented by magnification views, they detect many more calcifications than can be detected by routine mammograms and this substantially reduces the discrepancy between radiological and pathological size of the lesion. A preoperative diagnosis of malignancy may be obtained by stereotactic cytology and this may be histologically confirmed by stereotactic core biopsy. If the size of the lesion (usually < 40 mm), size of the breast and the site of the lesion within the breast suggest that a breast-conserving procedure can be employed, then the lesion can be excised using the fine wire guided localization technique with the aim of completely removing the lesion with a surrounding rim of 'normal' breast tissue. One method of excision suggested is to remove a cylinder of breast tissue extending from the skin to the pectoral fascia with the aim of obtaining a minimum 10 mm clear margin around the lesion (Sibbering et al., 1995). The edges of the specimen should be marked in three planes with either orientation sutures or clips to aid identification of the orientation of the margins.

Specimen radiography is then performed which allows an assessment of completeness of excision and may allow a judgement at the time of surgery, whether a further excision need be performed. The major limitation of this assessment of completeness of excision is that most centres obtain only one radiographic view and this only allows the assessment of two rather than three dimensions. An alternative method of radiographic assessment is 'tetrahedron' radiography. This method involves placing the excised breast specimen in a tetrahedron and obtaining radiographs in four planes. A preliminary assessment of this technique in the laboratory has demonstrated its superiority over conventional specimen radiography in its detection of microcalcification near a surgical excision margin (Kulka et al., 1995). This method of assessment needs to be tested at the time of surgical excision before its role in the management of lesions with microcalcification can be defined.

The most important component in the assessment of completeness of excision is meticulous pathological examination of the surgical specimen which requires close collaboration between surgeon, radiologist and pathologist. The margins of excision should be inked and then extensively sampled. The lesion should be typed and completeness of excision assessed so that the minimum clear margin can be ascertained. Although there is consensus that this should be performed, there is still no clear consensus on what constitutes a clear margin. This has been defined previously as anything from as little as 1 mm (Silverstein et al., 1995a) to 10 mm (Sibbering et al., 1995). In studies which have looked at the presence of residual tumour in further excision specimens (whether local excisions or mastectomy specimens) after a 'clear' margin has been achieved histologically, the incidence of residual tumour associated with clear margins of 1 mm was 45% (Recht et al., 1994). It appears from retrospective studies that the smaller the margin of clearance the higher the incidence of subsequent local recurrence (Silverstein et al., 1996) of DCIS and invasive breast cancer. Thus in one study in which a clear margin was defined as 1 mm, 13.5% of patients treated by excision and radiotherapy developed local recurrence after a median follow-up of 95 months (Silverstein et al., 1995b). In another study which looked at the role of wide excision (sector resection) of DCIS without the addition of radiotherapy, the risk of local recurrence was 38% if tumour extended histologically to within 5 mm of the resection margin compared to only 6% when the width of the microscopically clear margin was greater than 5 mm (Arnesson et al., 1989). In a recent study from Nottingham, a policy of ensuring a minimum clear margin of 10 mm after wide excision alone for DCIS of 40 mm or less in size has shown excellent short-term results, with no local recurrences in 48 patients after 42 months follow-up. The largest and most recent study to have been published which related local recurrence to margin width is that by Silverstein et al. (1999).

In this study, margin width was assessed by ocular micrometry on 469 specimens of DCIS from patients who had been treated with breast-conserving therapy with or without postoperative radiotherapy. The estimated probability of recurrence at 8 years was only 0.04 among 133 patients who had a margin width of 10 mm or more in every direction. These patients did not seem to benefit from adjuvant radiotherapy. There was also no statistically significant benefit from radiotherapy in those patients in whom a definite clear margin of 1–10 mm was present. The only subgroup who benefited from radiotherapy was those patients in whom margin widths were < 1 mm. It can be seen from these studies and from studies which have looked at completeness of excision of an extensive intraduct component associated with invasive breast cancer (Holland et al., 1990), that completeness of excision is desirable and may have a bearing on rates of local recurrence. The size of the clear margin may also influence the necessity for radiotherapy after surgery. It is also likely that the extent of the clear margin required to minimize the risk of local recurrence may also vary with the histological subtype of DCIS.

What is the role of re-excision of breast tissue if a positive margin exists after breast-conserving surgery? It has become apparent that excision of all microscopic foci of DCIS is paramount in reducing the risk of local recurrence and re-excision is recommended if tumour is present at a margin of the original excision specimen. If the original DCIS lesion was < 40 mm, then it may still be possible to re-excise breast tissue, achieve a clear margin (however this is defined) and preserve the breast. However, in general, lesions > 40 mm do not lend themselves to preservation of the breast, although the EORTC 10853 trial is currently enrolling patients with lesions up to 49 mm in size. Mastectomy may therefore be the only surgical option available when further excision is required for unicentric disease and is the treatment of choice for widespread multifocal or multicentric disease. In practice, some 50% of patients with screen-detected asymptomatic DCIS are unsuitable for breast-conserving surgery and should be treated by mastectomy. Because this has such a high cure rate and avoids the need for postoperative radiotherapy, these patients are ideally suited to immediate breast reconstruction which should be offered routinely to all patients.

Role of radiotherapy

The data presented from retrospective studies and prospective clinical trials which have compared breast-conserving surgery with surgery and radiotherapy suggest that early recurrence is at least delayed and at best reduced in the preserved breast by the addition of radiotherapy. However, even in the prospective clinical trials, these studies did not set the minimum clear margin which was acceptable for withholding radiotherapy and it is possible that a wider margin of excision may reduce the need to add postoperative radiotherapy to the preserved breast. There is still some debate as to whether histological subtype (Recht et al., 1994) or high nuclear grade (Holland et al., 1992) are important factors in early recurrence of DCIS. Recently, a prognostic index has been derived based on tumour size, margin width and pathological classification in determining the likelihood of local recurrence in patients who had been treated by breast-conserving surgery with or without radiotherapy (Silverstein et al., 1996). This suggested that patients with low scores (3, 4) could safely be treated by surgery alone, patients with intermediate scores (5–7) gained a 17% benefit in terms of reduction of local recurrence with the addition of radiotherapy and patients with high scores (8, 9) had such a high rate of local recurrence (60% at 8 years) that they should be treated by mastectomy. The major problem with this study is that it requires to be tested prospectively before it can be universally applied.

Role of adjuvant medical therapy

There is only one reported trial evaluating the addition of adjuvant systemic therapy to local treatment. In the NSABP B-24 trial (Fisher et al., 1999), 1804 women with DCIS (including those whose resected sample margins were involved by tumour) were randomly assigned to local excision, radiotherapy and placebo or to local excision, radiotherapy and tamoxifen (20 mg/day for 5 years). Median follow-up was 74 months. Women in the tamoxifen group had fewer breast cancer events at 5 years than those on placebo (8.2% vs. 13.4%, $p = 0.0009$). The cumulative incidence of ipsilateral invasive breast cancer at 5 years in the tamoxifen group was 2.1% vs. 4.2% in the placebo group and the corresponding rates for contralateral breast cancer were 1.8 vs. 2.3% respectively. Close scrutiny of the results for recurrence of DCIS showed no statistically significant difference in the two groups. This study was disappointing in that it allowed entry into the study of patients whose specimens had involved margins. Furthermore, the recurrence rate seems high considering 80% of tumours were 1 cm or less in diameter. Recurrence was commoner in patients with involved margins compared with patients whose specimens had clear margins but, nevertheless, invasive recurrence was reduced even in margin-positive patients. This is the first study which suggests a role for adjuvant endocrine therapy of patients with DCIS treated by local excision and radiotherapy.

The United Kingdom DCIS study is also studying the effect of adjuvant tamoxifen in patients undergoing breast-conserving treatment (see p. 139), but as yet no results are available. A proportion of DCIS lesions are ER positive and adjuvant tamoxifen in patients with ER-positive lesions may be beneficial, especially if occult residual ER-positive disease is present elsewhere in the preserved breast or in the contralateral breast. However, if all the DCIS has been completely excised and no occult tumour exists, then it is likely that the importance of adjuvant tamoxifen will be in the likelihood that a second cancer in the contralateral breast may be delayed or even prevented, even in those patients who initially have ER-negative lesions (Cuzick & Baum, 1985; Baum et al., 1992).

The role of adjuvant endocrine therapy in completely excised DCIS with a clear margin in patients who do not receive radiotherapy is still unknown, and there is still no study published on randomizing patients with completely excised DCIS on the basis of the ER status of the tumour.

Role of axillary surgery

The incidence of positive axillary nodes in patients with DCIS is only 0–2% (Silverstein et al., 1987) and therefore there is very little place for axillary surgery in the management of patients with DCIS. The fact that occasionally metastases to the axillary nodes has occurred probably represents inadequate sampling of the breast tissue or failure to detect microinvasion or frank invasive tumour. The incidence of microinvasion increases with increasing size of the DCIS lesion (Lagios et al., 1982) and therefore only patients with relatively large (>50 mm) lesions will be at risk of axillary lymph node deposits. There is no consensus on which patients should (if at all) undergo axillary surgery. Clearly, patients with lesions which are pure DCIS should not undergo axillary surgery to harvest lymph nodes. The difficulty arises when a patient with extensive DCIS exhibits microinvasion in the breast. If a mastectomy is required to adequately excise all of the lesion, then there is a reasonable argument for an axillary sampling procedure which in our opinion should not be more than a level 1 dissection (taking all the axillary lymph nodes below the level of pectoralis minor) as a complete axillary clearance would not be justified. If a breast-conserving procedure has been employed and microinvasion has been identified within the DCIS lesion, then a decision on whether postoperative irradiation is required will need to be made and the lower axilla can then be included in the radiotherapy field. Patients with microinvasion are not suitable for the UK DCIS trial and therefore randomization to an arm with no radiotherapy will not apply. There are uncertainties with these approaches as no trials of breast-conserving therapies in patients with DCIS with microinvasion have been published.

Follow-up

Some authorities recommend a postoperative mammogram of the preserved breast in patients with DCIS who have undergone breast-conserving therapy (Recht et al., 1994) to try and ensure that all of the lesion has been excised, although there is no consensus on this subject. Other unknown factors are how often to screen the affected breast and the contralateral breast. Whether DCIS increases the risk of a contralateral DCIS lesion occurring to the same degree as that of invasive cancer is as yet unknown.

Future studies

It can be seen from the above discussions that a great variety of uncertainties regarding treatment exist. Immediate priorities should include standardization of the pathological classification of DCIS, the prospective evaluation of different subcategories of pathology as predictors of local recurrence, the effect of a clear tumour margin on local recurrence, the size of the clear margin and its relationship to pathological type on the likelihood of developing local recurrence, and the prospective use of prognostic markers in identifying patients with such a low risk of recurrence that postoperative radiotherapy in patients treated by breast-conserving surgery is not required. From a clinical point of view, a randomized prospective trial needs to be performed to compare breast-conserving techniques with mastectomy. The difficulty with a study of this type is the lack of certainty in identifying patients in whom this approach is justifiable especially with the current trend for breast preservation for invasive breast cancer. It is hoped that the current UK DCIS trial will provide some answers regarding the use of adjuvant tamoxifen in patients with completely excised DCIS.

Studies on the biological nature of DCIS are clearly also important and in the future may lead to a greater understanding of the relationship of DCIS to invasive cancer and may have a role in identifying patients suitable for breast-conserving therapy. These biological markers will then need to be tested prospectively. Finally, further study is required to look at ways of improving preoperative diagnosis and especially novel methods of imaging of the breast such as magnetic resonance imaging and high frequency ultrasound scanning.

Conclusion

DCIS can be regarded as a heterogeneous group of conditions whose optimal therapy for different pathological subtypes is under intense investigation. Previously thought to be rare and the sole province of the surgeon, it will be increasingly encountered by nonsurgical oncologists. Current research regarding treatment will increasingly become multidisciplinary in nature and research on the biology and genetics of these lesions will hopefully shed further light on the relationship of DCIS to invasive breast cancer.

REFERENCES

Allred, D.C., Clark, G.M., Molina, R. et al. (1992). Overexpression of *HER-2/neu* and its relationship with other prognostic factors. Change during progression of in situ to invasive breast cancer. *Human Pathology*, 23, 974–9.

Alpeers, C.E. & Wellings, S.R. (1985). The prevalence of carcinoma in situ in normal and cancer-associated breasts. *Human Pathology*, 16, 796–807.

Anderson, J., Nielsen, M. & Christiansen, L. (1985). New aspects of the natural history of in situ and invasive carcinoma in the female breast: results from autopsy investigations. *Verhandlungen der Deutschen Gesellschaft fur Pathologie*, 69, 88–95.

Arnesson, L.G., Smeds, S., Fagerberg, G. et al. (1989). Follow-up of two treatment modalities for ductal carcinoma in situ of the breast. *British Journal of Surgery*, 76, 672–5.

Ashikari, R. Hajdu, S.E. & Robbins, G.F. (1971). Intraductal carcinoma of the breast (1960–1969). *Cancer*, 28, 1182–7.

Baird, R.M., Worth, A. & Hislop, G. (1990). Recurrence after lumpectomy for comedo-type intraductal carcinoma of the breast. *American Journal of Surgery*, 159, 479–81.

Barnes, D.M., Bartkova, J., Camplejohn, R.S. et al. (1992). Overexpression of the *c-erbB2* oncoprotein: Why does this occur more frequently in ductal carcinoma in situ than in invasive mammary carcinoma and is this of prognostic significance? *European Journal of Cancer*, 28, 644–8.

Bartow, S.A., Pathak, D.R., Black, W.C. et al. (1987). Prevalence of benign, atypical and malignant breast lesions in populations at different risk of breast cancer: a forensic autopsy study. *Cancer*, 60, 2751–60.

Baum, M., Houghton, J. & Riley, D. (1992). Results of the cancer research campaign adjuvant trial for perioperative cyclophosphamide and long-term tamoxifen in early breast cancer reported at the tenth year of follow-up. *Acta Oncologica*, 31, 251–7.

Bellamy, C.O.C., McDonald, C., Salter, D.M. et al. (1993). Noninvasive ductal carcinoma of the breast: The relevance of histologic categorization. *Human Pathology*, 24, 16–23.

Bornstein, B.A., Recht, A., Connolly, J.L. et al. (1991). Results of treating ductal carcinoma in situ of the breast with conservative surgery and radiation therapy. *Cancer*, 67, 7–13.

Caines, J.S., McPhee, M.D., Konok, G.P. et al. (1994). Stereotaxic needle core biopsy of breast lesions using a regular mammographic table with an adaptable stereotaxic device. *American Journal of Radiology*, 163, 317–21.

Carpenter, R., Boulter, P.S., Cooke, T. et al. (1989). Management of screen detected ductal carcinoma in situ of the female breast. *British Journal of Surgery*, 76, 564–7.

Carter D. & Smith, R.R. (1977). Carcinoma in situ of the breast. *Cancer*, 40, 1189–93.

Cataliotti, L., Distante, V., Ciatto, S. et al. (1992). Intraductal breast cancer: a review of 183 consecutive cases. *European Journal of Cancer*, 28A, 917–20.

Chandhuri, B., Crist, K.A., Mucci, S. et al. (1993). Distribution of estrogen receptor in ductal carcinoma in situ of the breast. *Surgery*, 113, 134–7.

Cuzick, J. & Baum, M. (1985). Tamoxifen and contralateral breast cancer. *Lancet*, ii, 282.

Evans, A., Pinder, S., Wilson, R. et al. (1994). Ductal carcinoma in situ of the breast. Correlations between mammographic findings and pathological findings. *American Journal of Roentgenology*, 162, 1307–11.

Faverly, D., Holland, R. & Burgers, L. (1992). An original stereomicroscopic analysis of the mammary glandular tree. *Virchows Archives A. Pathological Anatomy*, 421, 115–19.

Faverly, D.R.G., Burgers, L., Bult, P. et al. (1994). Three dimensional imaging of mammary ductal carcinoma in situ: clinical implications. *Seminars in Diagnostic Pathology*, 11, 193–8.

Ferreiro, J.A., Gisvold, J.J. & Bostwick, D.G. (1995). Accuracy of frozen section diagnosis of mammographically directed breast biopsies. Results of 1,490 consecutive cases. *American Journal of Surgical Pathology*, 19(11), 1267–71.

Fielding, J. (1994). Preventing colon cancer: yet another reason not to smoke. *Journal of the National Cancer Institute*, 86, 162–4.

Fisher, B., Bauer, M., Margolese R. et al. (1985). Five year results of a randomised clinical trial comparing total mastectomy and segmental mastectomy with or without radiation in the treatment of breast cancer. *New England Journal of Medicine*, 312, 665–73.

Fisher, E.R., Sass, R., Fisher, B. et al. (1986). Pathologic findings from the National Surgical Adjuvant Breast Project (protocol 6). 1. Intraductal carcinoma (DCIS). *Cancer*, 57, 197–208.

Fisher, B., Redmond, C., Poisson, R. et al. (1989). Eight year results of a randomised trial comparing total mastectomy and lumpectomy with or without irradiation in the treatment of breast cancer. *New England Journal of Medicine*, 320, 822–8.

Fisher, E.R., Leeming, R., Anderson, S. et al. (1991). Conservative management of intraductal carcinoma (DCIS) of the breast. Collaborating NSABP investigators. *Journal of Surgical Oncology*, 47, 139–47.

Fisher, B., Constantino, J., Redmond C. et al. (1993). Lumpectomy compared with lumpectomy and radiation therapy for the treatment of intraductal breast cancer. *New England Journal of Medicine*, 328, 1581–6.

Fisher, B., Dignam, J., Wolmark, N. et al. (1999). Tamoxifen in treatment of intraductal breast cancer: National Surgical Adjuvant Breast and Bowel Project B-24 randomised controlled trial. *Lancet*, 353, 1993–2000.

Foucar, E. (1996). Carcinoma in situ of the breast: have pathologists run amok? *Lancet*, 347, 707–8.

Fowble, B.L. (1989). Intraductal noninvasive breast cancer: a comparison of three local treatments. *Oncology*, 3, 51–69.

Frykberg, E.R. & Bland, K.I. (1993). In situ breast carcinoma. *Advances in Surgery*, 26, 29–72.

Frykberg, E.R. & Bland, K.I. (1994). Overview of the biology and management of ductal carcinoma in situ of the breast. *Cancer*, 74, 350–61.

Frykberg, E.R., Ames, F.C. & Bland, K.I. (1991). Current concepts for management of early (in situ and occult invasive) breast carcinoma. In: *The breast: comprehensive management of benign and malignant diseases*, ed. K.I. Bland & E.M. Copeland, pp. 731–51. Philadelphia: Saunders.

Fung, A., Rayter, Z., Fisher, C. et al. (1990). Preoperative cytology and mammography in patients with single duct nipple discharge treated by surgery. *British Journal of Surgery*, 77, 1211–12.

Futreal, P.A., Liu, Q., Eidens, D.S. et al. (1994). BRCA 1 mutations in primary breast and ovarian carcinomas. *Science*, 266, 120–2.

Gallagher, W.J., Koerner, F.C. & Wood, W.C. (1989). Treatment of intraductal carcinoma with limited surgery: long term follow up. *Journal of Clinical Oncology*, 7, 376–80.

Gisvold, J.J., Goellner, J.R., Grant, C.S. et al. (1994). Breast biopsy: A comparative study of stereotaxically guided core and excisional techniques. *American Journal of Radiology*, 162, 815–20.

Gusterson, B.A., Gelber, R.D., Goldhirsch, A. et al. (1992). Prognostic importance of *c-erbB2* expression in breast cancer. *Journal of Clinical Oncology*, 10, 1049–56.

Haffty, B.G., Peschel, R.E., Papadopoulos, D. et al. (1990). Radiation therapy for ductal carcinoma in situ of the breast. *Connecticut Medicine*, 54, 482–4.

Hankey, B.F., Brinton, L.A., Kessler, L.G. et al. (1993). Breast Cancer. In *SEER Cancer Statistics Review 1973–1990*, ed. Miller, B.A., Ries, L.A.G., Hankey, B.F., Kosary, C.L., Harras A., Devesa, S.S. & Edwards, B.J., pp. IV.1–IV.4. Washington DC: US National Cancer Institute NIH Publication No. 93–2789.

Holland, R., Connolly J.L., Gelman, R. et al. (1990). The presence of an extensive intraductal component following a limited excision correlates with prominent residual disease in the remainder of the breast. *Journal of Clinical Oncology*, 8, 113–18.

Holland, R., Hendriks, J.H., Vebeek A.L.M. et al. (1992). Extent, distribution and mammographic/histologic correlations of breast ductal carcinoma in situ. *Lancet*, 335, 519–22.

Homer, M.J., Smith, T.J. & Safaii, H. (1992). Pre-biopsy needle localization: methods, problems and expected results. *Radiological Clinics of North America*, 30, 139–53.

Hulka, B.S. & Stark, A.T. (1995). Breast cancer: cause and prevention. *Lancet*, 346, 883–7.

Jackman, R.J., Nowels, K.W., Shepard, M.J. et al. (1994). Stereotaxic large-core needle biopsy of 450 nonpalpable breast lesions with surgical correlation in lesions with cancer or atypical hyperplasia. *Radiology*, 193, 91–5.

Kopans, D.B. (1993). Review of stereotaxic large-core needle biopsy and surgical biopsy results in nonpalpable breast lesions. *Radiology*, 189, 665–6.

Kulka, J., Davies, J.D., Sharp, S. et al. (1995). Tetrahedron radiography of the microcalcifications of comedo ductal carcinoma in situ: three-dimensional assessment of surgical excision. *The Breast*, 4, 117–21.

Kurtz, J.M., Jacqenier, J., Torhorst, J. et al. (1989). Conservation therapy for breast cancers other than infiltrating ductal carcinoma. *Cancer*, 63, 1630–5.

Lagios, M.D. (1990). Duct carcinoma in situ. *Surgical Clinics of North America*, 70, 853–71.

Lagios, M.D., Westdhal, P.R. Margolin, F.R. et al. (1982). Duct carcinoma in situ: relationship of extent of noninvasive disease to the frequency of occult invasion, multicentricity, lymph node metastases and short term treatment failures. *Cancer*, 50, 1309–14.

Lagios, M.D., Margolin, F.R., Westdhal, P.R. et al. (1989). Mammographically detected duct carcinoma in situ: frequency of local recurrence following tylectomy and prognostic effect of nuclear grade on local recurrence. *Cancer*, 63, 618–214.

Lakhani, S.R., Collins, N., Stratton, M.R. et al. (1995). Atypical ductal hyperplasia of the breast: clonal proliferation with loss of heterozygosity on chromosomes 16q and 17p. *Journal of Clinical Pathology*, 48, 611–15.

Lewis, D. & Geschikter, C.F. (1938). Comedo carcinoma of the breast. *Archives of Surgery*, 36, 225–44.

Liberman, L., Dershaw, D.D., Rosen, P.P. et al. (1994). Stereotaxic 14-guage breast biopsy: How many core biopsy specimens are needed? *Radiology*, 192, 793–5.

Lilleng, R. & Hagmar, B. (1992). The comedo subtype of intraductal carcinoma. Cytologic characteristics. *Acta Cytologica*, 36, 731–41.

Malafa, M., Chandhuri, B., Thornford, N.R. et al. (1990). Estrogen receptors in ductal carcinoma in situ of the breast. *American Surgeon*, 56, 436–9.

McCormick, B., Rosen, P.P., Kinne, D.W. et al. (1990). Duct carcinoma in situ of the breast: does conservation surgery and radiotherapy provide acceptable local control? (abstract). *International Journal of Radiation Oncology, Biology, Physics*, 19 (Suppl. 1), 132.

McPherson, K. Steel, C.M. & Dixon, J.M. (1994). ABC of breast diseases. Breast cancer-epidemiology, risk factors and genetics. *British Medical Journal*, 309, 1003–6.

Micale, M.A., Visscher, D.W., Guilino, S.E. et al. (1994). Chromosomal aneuploidy in proliferative breast disease. *Human Pathology*, 25, 29–35.

Millikan, R., Dressler, L., Geradts, M.D. et al. (1995). The need for epidemiological studies of in-situ carcinoma of the breast. *Breast Cancer Research and Treatment*, 35, 65–77.

Moore, M.M. (1991). Treatment of ductal carcinoma in situ of the breast. *Seminars in Surgical Oncology*, 7, 267–70.

Morrow, M. (1995). When can stereotactic core biopsy replace excisional biopsy? A clinical perspective. *Breast Cancer Research and Treatment*, 36, 1–9.

National Co-ordinating Committee on Breast Screening Pathology (NCCBSP). (1995). Pathology reporting in breast cancer screening: Guidelines for Pathologists.

Nielsen, M., Thomsen, J.L., Primdahl, S. et al. (1987). Breast cancer and atypia among young and middle aged women: a study of 110 medicolegal autopsies. *British Journal of Cancer*, 56, 814–19.

Noguchi, S., Motomura, K., Inaji, H. et al. (1994). Clonal analysis of predominantly intraductal carcinoma and precancerous lesions of the breast by means of the polymerase chain reaction. *Cancer Research*, 54, 1849–53.

Page, D.L., Dupont, W.D., Rogers, L.W. et al. (1982). Intraductal carcinoma of the breast. Follow up after biopsy only. *Cancer*, 49, 751–8.

Patchefsky, A.S., Schwartz, G.F., Finklestein, S.D. et al. (1989). Heterogeneity of intraductal carcinoma of the breast. *Cancer*, 63, 731–41.

Pierce, S.M., Schnitt, S.J. & Harris, J.R. (1992). What to do about mammographically detected ductal carcinoma in situ. *Cancer*, 70, 2576–8.

Poller, D.N & Ellis, I.O. (1996). Ductal carcinoma in situ (DCIS) of the breast. In: *Progress in Pathology 2*, 47–85.

Poller, D.N., Hutchings, C.E., Galea, M. et al. (1992). p53 protein expression in human breast carcinoma: relationship to expression of epidermal growth factor receptor, *c-erbB2* overexpression and oestrogen receptor. *British Journal of Cancer*, 66, 583–8.

Poller, D.N., Roberts, E.C., Bell, J.A. et al. (1993a). p53 protein expression in mammary ductal carcinoma in situ: relationship to immunohistochemical expression of oestrogen receptor and *c-erbB2* protein. *Human Pathology*, 24, 463–8.

Poller, D.N., Snead, D.R.J., Roberts, E.C. et al. (1993b). Oestrogen receptor expression in ductal carcinoma in situ of the breast: relationship to flow cytometric analysis of DNA and expression of the *c-erbB2* oncoprotein. *British Journal of Cancer*, 68, 156–61.

Price, P., Sinnett, H.D., Gusterson, B. et al. (1990). Duct carcinoma in situ: predictors of local recurrence and progression in patients treated by surgery alone. *British Journal of Cancer*, 61, 869–72.

Radford, D.M., Fair, K., Thompson, A.M. et al. (1993). Allelic loss on a chromosome 17 in ductal carcinoma in situ of the breast. *Cancer Research*, 53, 2947–50.

Ramachandra, S., Machin, L., Ashley, S. et al. (1990). Immunohistochemical distribution of *c-erbB2* in in situ breast carcinoma – a detailed morphological analysis. *Journal of Pathology*, 161, 7–14.

Rayter, Z. (1991). Steroid receptors in breast cancer. *British Journal of Surgery*, 78, 528–35.

Recht, A., Solin, L.J., Kurtz, J.M. et al. (1991). Conservative surgery and radiotherapy (cs and rt) for ductal carcinoma in situ (DCIS) (meeting abstract). *Proceedings of the Annual Meeting of the American Society of Clinical Oncology*, 10, A62.

Recht, A., van Dongen, J.A., Fentiman, I.S. et al. (1994). Third meeting of the DCIS working party of the EORTC. (Fondazione Cini, Isola S. Giorgio, Venezia, 28 February, 1994). *European Journal of Cancer*, 30A, 1895–901.

Reynolds, J.V., Sweeney, J.P., Nolan, N. et al. (1993). Management of ductal carcinoma in situ of the breast. *Irish Journal of Medical Science*, 162, 45–8.

Ringberg, A., Andersson, I., Aspegren, K. et al. (1991). Breast carcinoma in situ in 167 women-incidence, mode of presentation, therapy and follow up. *European Journal of Surgical Oncology*, 17, 466–76.

Rosen, P.P. & Oberman, H.A. (1993). Intraepithelial (pre-invasive or in-situ carcinoma). In: *Tumours of the mammary gland*. Washington DC: Armed Forces Institute of Pathology, p. 119.

Rosen, P.P., Senie, R., Schottenfield, D. et al. (1979). Noninvasive breast carcinoma: frequency of invasion and implications for treatment. *Annals of Surgery*, 189, 377–82.

Rosen, P.P., Braun, D.W. Jr. & Kinne, D.E. (1980). The clinical significance of preinvasive breast carcinoma. *Cancer*, 46, 919–25.

Rosner, D., Bedwani, R.N., Vana J. et al. (1980). Noninvasive breast cancer: result of a national survey by the American College of Surgeons. *American Surgeon*, 192, 139–47.

Royal College of Pathologists Working Group. (1990). Pathology reporting of breast cancer screening. NHS Breast Screening Programme.

Sanchez Forgach, E., Mamounas, E.P., Penetrante, R. et al. (1992). Ductal carcinoma in situ (dcis): clinical presentation and long term results (meeting abstract). *Proceedings of the Annual Meeting of the American Society of Clinical Oncology*, 11, A169.

Schnitt, S.J., Silen, W., Sadowski, N.L. et al. (1988). Ductal carcinoma in situ (intraductal carcinoma) of the breast. *New England Journal of Medicine*, 318, 893–903.

Schu, M.E., Nemoto, T., Penetrante, R.B. et al. (1986). Intraductal carcinoma: analysis of presentation, pathologic findings and outcome of disease. *Archives of Surgery*, 121, 1303–7.

Schwartz, G.F., Patchefsky, A.S., Finkelstein, S.D. et al. (1989). Nonpalpable in situ ductal carcinoma of the breast. Predictors of multicentricity and microinvasion and implications for treatment. *Archives of Surgery*, 124, 29–32.

Schwartz, G.F, Finkel, G.C, Garcia, J.C. et al. (1992). Subclinical ductal carcinoma in situ: treatment by local excision and surveillance alone. *Cancer*, 70, 2468–74.

Sibbering, D.M., Obuszko, Z., Ellis, I.O. et al. (1995). Radiotherapy may be unnecessary after adequate wide local excision of ductal carcinoma in situ.(abstract). *The Breast*, 4, A60, 244.

Silverstein, M.J., Rosser, R.J., Gierson, E.D. et al. (1987). Axillary lymph node dissection for intraductal breast carcinoma – is it indicated? *Cancer*, 59, 1819–24.

Silverstein, M.J., Cohlan, B.F., Gierson, E.D. et al. (1992). Duct carcinoma in situ: 227 cases without micrinvasion. *European Journal of Cancer*, 28, 630–4.

Silverstein, M.J., Poller, D.N., Waisman, J.R. et al. (1995a). Prognostic classification of breast ductal carcinoma in situ. *Lancet*, 354, 1154–7.

Silverstein, M.J., Barth, A., Poller, D.N. et al. (1995b). Ten-year results comparing mastectomy to excision and radiation therapy for ductal carcinoma in situ of the breast. *European Journal of Cancer*, 31A, 1425–7.

Silverstein, M.J., Lagios, M.D., Craig, P.M. et al. (1996). A prognostic index for ductal carcinoma in situ of the breast. *Cancer*, 77, 2267–74.

Silverstein, M.J., Lagios, M.D., Groshen, S. et al. (1999). The influence of margin width on local control of ductal carcinoma in situ of the breast. *New England Journal of Medicine*, 340, 1455–61.

Simpson, T., Thirlby, R.C. & Dail, D.H. (1992). Surgical treatment of ductal carcinoma in situ of the breast; 10- to 20-year follow up. *Archives of Surgery*, 127, 468–72.

Smart C.R., Myers M.H. & Gloeckler, M.A. (1978). Implications of SEER data on breast cancer management. *Cancer*, 41, 787–9.

Sneige, N. & Staerkel, G.A. (1994). Fine needle aspiration cytology of ductal hyperplasia with and without atypia and ductal carcinoma in situ. *Human Pathology*, 25, 485–92.

Solin, L.J., Yeh, I.-T., Kurtz, J.M. et al. (1993). Ductal carcinoma in situ (intraductal carcinoma) of the breast treated with breast-conserving surgery and definitive irradiation. *Cancer*, 71, 2532–42.

Stotter, A.T., McNeese, M., Oswald, M.J. et al. (1990). The role of limited surgery with irradiation in primary tratment of ductal in situ breast cancer. *International Journal of Radiation Oncology, Biology and Physics*, 18, 283–7.

Stomper, P.C., Connolly, J.L., Meyer, J.E. et al. (1989). Clinically occult ductal carcinoma in situ detected with mammography: analysis of 100 cases with radiologic-pathologic correlation. *Radiology*, 172, 235–41.

Stratton, M.R., Collins, N, Lakhani, S.R. et al. (1995). Loss of heterozygosity in ductal carcinoma in situ of the breast. *Journal of Pathology*, 175, 195–201.

Swain, S.M. (1992). Ductal carcinoma in situ. *Cancer Investigation*, 10, 443–54.

Tavassoli, F.A. (1992). *Pathology of the breast.* Norwalk, Connecticut: Appleton & Lange.

Temple, W.J., Jenkins, M., Alexander, F. et al. (1989). Natural history of in situ breast cancer in a defined population. *Annals of Surgery*, 210, 653–7.

Veronesi, U., Banfi A. & Savadori, B. (1990). Breast conservation is the treatment of choice in small breast cancers: long term results of a randomised trial. *European Journal of Cancer*, 26, 668–70.

Vrouenraets, B.C., Peterse, J.L. & van Dongen, J.A. (1991). Breast-conserving therapy of ductal carcinoma in situ: frequency of local recurrence after wide excision with and without additional radiotherapy; a retrospective study of 42 cases. *Netherlands Journal of Surgery*, 43, 51–5.

Von Rueden, D.G. & Wilson, R.E. (1984). Intraductal carcinoma of the breast. *Surgery, Gynecology and Obstetrics*, 158, 105–11.

Weiss, H.A., Brinton, L.A., Brogan, D. et al. (1996). Epidemiology of *in situ* and invasive breast cancer in women aged under 45. *British Journal of Cancer*, 73, 1298–305.

Wellings, S.R., Jensen, M.H. & Marcum, R.G. (1975). An atlas of subgross pathology of the human breast with special reference to possible precancerous lesions. *Journal of the National Cancer Institute*, 55, 231–73.

Wright, C., Nicholson, S., Angus, B. et al. (1992). Relationship between *c-erbB2* protein product expression and response to endocrine therapy in advanced breast cancer. *British Journal of Cancer*, 65, 118–21.

Zafrani, B., Fourquet, A., Vilcoq, J.R. et al. (1986). Conservative management of intraductal breast carcinoma with tumorectomy and radiation therapy. *Cancer*, 57, 1299–301.

7

Adjuvant systemic therapy

T.R.J. Evans

CRC Department of Medical Oncology, University of Glasgow

The rationale for systemic adjuvant therapy

Up until approximately 25 years ago, it was considered that breast cancer metastases developed according to the anatomical and mechanistic principles first proposed by Halstead (1907). Metastases spread in a predictable fashion from the breast to the regional lymph nodes and subsequently to distant sites. Consequently, the aim of early breast cancer treatment was extensive surgery to remove local and regional disease. However, the Halstead principles were subsequently challenged by laboratory findings, biological hypotheses and clinical observations which have formed the rationale for systemic adjuvant chemotherapy. There is no orderly pattern of cancer cell dissemination, and the blood stream is of considerable importance as a route of dissemination (Fisher & Fisher, 1966), and so regional lymph nodes are of prognostic rather than anatomical significance. The high recurrence rate, especially during the first three years after a Halstead radical and extended radical mastectomy, suggest that micrometastases, which are not clinically detectable, are present at the time of surgery for the primary tumour and are unaffected by local treatment (Valagussa et al., 1978). Several studies have evaluated breast-conserving surgery alone or with radiotherapy (Fisher et al., 1991; Veronesi et al., 1993; Liljegren et al., 1994). A higher local recurrence rate among women who underwent lumpectomy did not adversely affect survival. Moreover, six randomized trials have demonstrated that the survival of patients treated with a breast-conserving operation (either lumpectomy, wide excision or quadrantectomy) plus radiotherapy is equivalent to that of patients treated with mastectomy (Fisher et al., 1989a; Sarrazin et al., 1989; Veronesi et al., 1990; Blichert-Toft et al., 1992; Van Dongen et al., 1992; Jacobson et al., 1995).

Operable breast cancer is therefore considered to be a systemic disease at presentation such that therapy directed at the primary tumour fails to affect these micrometastases. There is convincing evidence that systemic adjuvant therapy both alters the natural history of breast cancer and improves survival of certain patient subsets.

Adjuvant chemotherapy

The Goldie–Coldman hypothesis, formulated in 1979, suggests that a given tumour will contain resistant clones when a patient is newly diagnosed (Goldie & Coldman, 1979). Consequently, resistance could be a problem even with small tumour burdens (such as micrometastases). Furthermore, the tumour models established in rodents by Skipper and colleagues suggest that the cytotoxic effects of cancer drugs follow log-kill kinetics, that is, the absolute cell kill is proportional, regardless of tumour burden (Skipper et al., 1950, 1964; Skipper, 1978). In practice, however, human tumours follow Gompertzian rather than exponential growth kinetics. That is, the growth fraction of the tumour is not constant but decreases exponentially with time. Consequently, when the tumour is clinically undetectable, as in the adjuvant setting, its growth fraction would be at its largest, and although the numerical reduction in cell number is small, the fractional cell kill from chemotherapy would be higher than in more extensive disease. On the basis of these kinetic models, combination chemotherapy has proven to be more effective than single agent chemotherapy in the management of advanced disease and also in adjuvant therapy.

The first randomized trials based on modern concepts of adjuvant chemotherapy were performed in patients with positive axillary lymph nodes. The first National Surgical Adjuvant Breast Project (NSABP) study used single-agent chemotherapy with melphalan or L-phenylalanine mustard (Fisher et al., 1975a) and the National Cancer Institute of Italy used cyclophosphamide, methotrexate and 5-fluorouracil (CMF) (Bonadonna et al., 1975). The results of 20 years of follow-up of the Milan adjuvant CMF trial are now available (Bonadonna et al., 1995). A total of 391 node-positive patients under the age of 75 years who had undergone a radical mastectomy were randomly assigned to receive no chemotherapy or CMF chemotherapy for 12 monthly cycles. At the 20-year analysis both relapse-free and overall survival remained significantly better in patients treated with surgery plus adjuvant chemotherapy than in patients treated with surgery alone. In the control group the median time to relapse was 40 months, as compared with 83 months in the CMF group; the median lengths of overall survival were 104 and 137 months respectively. Most recurrences occurred within the first 3 years after radical mastectomy. The median survival after the diagnosis of relapse was 36 months in the control group compared with 32 months in the CMF group; 18 years after relapse and after receiving a variety of salvage treatments (Valagussa et al., 1989), 4% of the women in the control group were alive with disease compared with 5% of the women in the CMF group. Salvage therapy had the same palliative effect regardless of whether the patient had received chemotherapy, which further re-enforces the fact that the difference in overall survival was due to the adjuvant treatment and not to salvage therapy. Overall, the benefit translated into a 34% reduction in the relative risk of relapse and a 26% reduction in the relative risk of death. In all subgroups of patients, based on menopausal status, tumour size or the number of involved nodes, a significant benefit from adjuvant CMF was seen except in postmenopausal women and patients with four to ten positive nodes. However, the difference in efficacy of the regimen between premenopausal and postmenopausal women may be due to the low dose of chemotherapy that the postmenopausal patients received, either by protocol design, or protocol violations, particularly the lack of compliance for oral cyclophosphamide (Bonadonna & Valagussa, 1981). Furthermore, the Cancer and Leukaemia Group B (CALG B) study showed that both premenopausal and postmenopausal women, when given regimens involving high or moderate doses of cyclophosphamide, doxorubicin, and fluorouracil, had significantly better disease-free and overall survival from those given regimens involving low doses (Wood et al., 1994). This underlines the importance of avoiding reduced doses of chemotherapy if maximal benefit is to be achieved. Furthermore, there may be some additional benefit to early initiation of adjuvant chemotherapy at least in premenopausal node-positive oestrogen receptor (ER)-negative women in whom there is a significant advantage in the 10-year disease-free survival (60% vs. 34%) if chemotherapy is initiated within 20 days of surgery as compared with 21 to 86 days after surgery (Colleoni et al., 2000). Subsequent studies have attempted to determine if standard CMF is the optimal regimen for adjuvant therapy. The second adjuvant CMF programme evaluated the efficacy of 6 cycles versus 12 cycles of combination chemotherapy. After 14 years, the relapse-free and total survival rates were equal in the two treatment groups (Bonadonna, 1992).

The standard CMF adjuvant schedule contains oral cyclophosphamide. Whether the addition of prednisolone improves treatment outcome remains controversial. Furthermore, in an attempt to improve patient compliance, regimens which include intravenous cyclophosphamide have been evaluated. Although the intravenous administration on days 1 and 8 of all three drugs provides a greater dose intensity, a recent trial of intravenous cyclophosphamide as part of a CMF regimen at three-weekly intervals in women with one to three positive nodes gave similar results to those achieved with standard CMF at 5 years (Moliterni et al., 1991). Other effective chemotherapy combinations have also been extensively used as adjuvant therapy, and include FA(adriamycin)C, AC and CA (Harris et al., 1993).

Table 7.1. Some of the combination chemotherapy regimens used adjuvantly for breast cancer

Regimen	Dose (mg/m^2)	Route	Days of treatment	Cycle frequency
CMF				
Cyclophosphamide	600	i.v.	1	3 weekly
Methotrexate	40	i.v.	1	
5-fluorouracil	600	i.v.	1	
CMF				
Cyclophosphamide	100	p.o.	1–14	4 weekly
Methotrexate	40	i.v.	1 and 8	
5-fluorouracil	600	i.v.	1 and 8	
CA				
Cyclophosphamide	200	p.o.	3–6	3–4 weekly
Doxorubicin	40	i.v.	1	
AC				
Doxorubicin	60	i.v.	1	3 weekly
Cyclophosphamide	600	i.v.	1	
FAC				
5-fluorouracil	500	i.v.	1 and 8	4 weekly
Doxorubicin	50	i.v.	1	
Cyclophosphamide	500	i.v.	1	

Node-negative patients

Initially it was considered that histologically node-negative breast cancer was an invariably 'curable' disease. However, on review of the 10-year follow-up data of radical mastectomy in large surgical series, it was apparent that the relapse-free survival in this group of patients was 70–75% (Valagussa et al., 1978; Fisher et al., 1975b). Furthermore, as in the case with node-positive patients, approximately 50% of recurrences became apparent in the first 3 years after locoregional treatment, once again suggesting the presence of occult distant micrometastases (Henderson et al., 1990).

As a result, the role of adjuvant chemotherapy in node-negative patients has been investigated by several groups (Fisher et al., 1989a; Mansour et al., 1990; Bonadonna, 1992; Zambetti et al., 1992). Although there were some variables in the designs of these studies, all gave comparable results at 5-year follow up, with an at least 30% reduction in annual odds of recurrence. Indeed, this improvement was still apparent at 8-year follow up in the Milan study (Bonadonna, 1992), and was equally valid for both premenopausal and postmenopausal women.

However, as at least 70% of node-negative women are unlikely to relapse on observation alone, it is difficult to justify routine adjuvant chemotherapy in all node-negative women. It is possible to identify patients with a low ($< 15\%$) risk of recurrence: these include patients with tumours less than 1 cm in diameter, grade I differentiation on histology, positive, oestrogen receptor (ER) and progesterone receptor (PR) and absence of vascular invasion. Conversely, patients with tumours ≥ 2 cm in diameter, negative steroid receptors, presence of vascular invasion and grade II–III histology, have a greater than 30% risk of recurrence and therefore are advised to receive adjuvant chemotherapy. For those with intermediate risk (tumours 1–2 cm in diameter, ER-positive, grade I–II), adjuvant chemotherapy should be discussed with the individual patient and individual risks and toxicity discussed.

An overview of the randomized trials of adjuvant chemotherapy in early breast cancer has been reported (Early Breast Cancer Trialists Collaborative Group, 1998a). This meta-analysis reports on information gathered in 1995 on each woman in any randomized trial beginning before 1990 and involved treatment groups that differed only with respect to the chemotherapy regimens that were being compared. Thus, 18 000 women in 47 trials of prolonged combination chemotherapy versus no chemotherapy were analysed, with about 6000 women in 11 trials of longer versus shorter chemotherapy, and about 6000 women in 11 trials of anthracycline-containing regimens versus CMF.

Combination chemotherapy gave a significant reduction in odds of recurrence both among women aged under 50 years (35% reduction; $p < 0.00001$) and among those aged 50–69 (20% reduction; $p < 0.00001$). Similarly, there was also a significant reduction in mortality for women aged < 50 years (27% reduction; $p < 0.00001$) and for women aged 50–69 years (11% reduction; $p < 0.0001$). The reductions in recurrence were most apparent during the first 5 years of follow-up, whereas the survival differences grew throughout the first 10 years.

The proportional reductions in risk were similar for women with node-positive and node-negative disease. The proportional mortality reduction observed for women aged under 50 at randomization would change a 10-year survival of 71% to 78% for those with node-negative disease (absolute benefit of 7%) and of 42% to 53% for those with node-positive disease (absolute benefit of 11%). The small proportional mortality reduction observed in women aged 50–69 would similarly translate into smaller absolute benefits in survival. Thus for those with node-negative disease the 10-year survival would be increased from 67% to 69% (absolute gain of 2%), and from 46% to 49% (absolute gain of 3%) for patients with node-positive disease. The age-specific benefits of adjuvant chemotherapy were independent of menopausal status at presentation, ER status, and independent of whether adjuvant endocrine therapy had been used. Furthermore, there was a reduction of approximately one-fifth in the occurrence of contralateral breast cancer, and no apparent increase in deaths from causes other than breast cancer. Moreover, the randomized comparisons of longer versus shorter durations of adjuvant chemotherapy did not indicate any survival advantage with the use of more than 3–6 months of chemotherapy.

This overview analysis, and the St Gallen Consensus Panel (Goldhirsch et al., 1998a) has identified patient subsets who should benefit from chemotherapy. While adjuvant chemotherapy is beneficial for patients <70 years with node-positive and node-negative disease, the absolute benefit decreases with advancing age. For patients with low-risk node-negative disease, the toxicity of therapy outweighs the relatively small benefit achieved. Although we can define a group of patients in whom a satisfactory significant relapse-free and overall survival benefit occurs, a significant proportion of these patients receive chemotherapy from which they do not benefit, highlighting the importance of improving prediction of clinical benefit.

The place of anthracyclines

An equally contentious issue is whether all women receiving chemotherapy should receive an anthracycline. The most effective single-agent drug in the treatment of advanced breast cancer is the anthracycline doxorubicin (Bonadonna et al., 1970). Anthracycline-containing regimens of combination chemotherapy result in a consistently higher response rate in patients with locally advanced or disseminated breast cancer compared with regimens that do not. However, this has not resulted in a superior duration of response or overall survival. Initial nonrandomized studies did not demonstrate a clear superiority for doxorubicin-containing regimens over CMF or CMFP (Buzdar et al., 1990; Dalton et al., 1987). However, after it became clear that adjuvant chemotherapy could be limited to about 6 months, several randomized trials with anthracycline-containing regimens were performed in Europe and the USA (Bonadonna et al., 1985; Bondadonna, 1989; Fisher et al., 1989a, 1989b; Buzzoni et al., 1991; Moliterni et al., 1991; Shapiro et al., 1991). In an initial NSABP study doxorubicin (30 mg/m^2) was administered every 3 weeks in combination with PF (5-fluorouracil and prednisolone). However, there was only a marginal advantage at 5 years compared with patients given PF alone and similar outcome if adjuvant tamoxifen was added to both drug combinations (Fisher et al., 1989b). However, the dose of doxorubicin used in this study was low. In a subsequent NSABP trial (B-15), 2194 node-positive patients with tamoxifen nonresponsive tumours were randomized to one of three treatment arms: doxorubicin (60 mg/m^2) plus cyclophosphamide (600 mg/m^2) every 3 weeks for 4 cycles (AC regimen); AC followed 6 months later by 3 monthly cycles of modified intravenous CMF; or standard CMF for 6 monthly cycles. Results at 3 years did not show any significant difference in outcome among the three arms with relapse-free survival rates of 62% (AC), 68% (AC + CMF) and 63% (CMF) (Fisher et al., 1990a). Moreover, at the Dana-Farber Cancer Institute, 15 and 30 weeks of a three-weekly AC regimen consisting of doxorubicin (45 mg/m^2) and cyclophosphamide (500 mg/m^2) were compared in node-positive women, and resulted in comparable disease-free survival in both groups at 8-year analysis (Shapiro et al., 1991).

Data from trials at the Milan Cancer Institute have suggested that the use of an anthracycline can improve outcome (Bonadonna, 1992; Buzzoni et al., 1991; Moliterni et al., 1991). Patients with one to three positive nodes were randomized to receive either 12 courses of intravenous CMF at three-weekly intervals or to receive 8 courses of intravenous CMF followed by 4 courses of doxorubicin (75 mg/m^2) at 3-weekly intervals. Comparable relapse-free survival rates were noted at the 5-year analysis, with no clear superiority for the anthracycline containing regimen. However, for patients with more than three positive nodes, a superior relapse-free survival rate (61%) was observed in patients who received sequential administration of four courses of doxorubicin followed by eight courses of CMF compared with alternating administration of the same drug regimens (relapse-free survival rate of 38%). This superiority was noted both for pre and postmenopausal women, and was still maintained at the 6-year analysis. It is likely that the use of doxorubicin and this scheduling account for these superior results.

A French study has also confirmed the superiority of an adriamycin-containing regimen in premenopausal women with any node-positive disease after 16 years follow up (Misset et al., 1996) in terms of both disease-free and overall survival. Similar results have been reported for FEC in comparison with CMF (Coombes et al., 1996). Furthermore, the CALG B 8541 study has suggested that an increased intensity of adriamycin dose confers further benefit in node-positive women (Budman et al., 1998).

The overview meta-analysis (EBCTCG, 1998a) suggested that anthracycline-containing regimens yielded a further 12% proportional reduction in recurrence compared to standard CMF regimens, with a marginally significant further 11% proportional reduction in mortality with the anthracycline-containing regimens. This translates into a small, but real, absolute benefit of 3.2% improvement in relapse free survival and a 2.7% improvement in overall survival at 5 years. Although a benefit has been observed in high-risk node-negative women (Hutchins et al., 1998) as well as in node-positive women, there will be many subgroups of patients with relatively low risk for whom toxicity might outweigh the small absolute benefit.

Numerous trials involving adjuvant taxane therapy have been initiated, although only one has been reported (CALG B 9344), and this in abstract form only with a short median follow-up (Henderson et al., 1998). Early analysis suggests a significant reduction in relapse free and overall survival for the addition of four cycles of adjuvant paclitaxel in addition to anthracyclines. However, this is an early analysis in patients with four or more positive lymph nodes, and it remains to be seen if there is an absolute benefit and whether it can be extrapolated into meaningful clinical benefit in other patient subgroups.

Poor risk patients and dose intensification

High-dose adjuvant chemotherapy

Retrospective data from the Milan CMF studies has shown that outcome at 5 and 10 years is related to the use of full doses of drugs (Bonadonna & Valagussa, 1981; Bonadonna et al., 1985). Furthermore, Hryniuk and colleagues showed a highly significant relationship between projected dose intensity and the 3-year relapse free survival in both premenopausal and postmenopausal women with either less than three or more than three axillary nodes involved by tumour (Hryniuk et al., 1987). In patients with advanced disease, higher doses of CMF are superior to lower doses of CMF (Tannock et al., 1986; Engelsman et al., 1991). However, the most convincing clinical data to support the hypothesis of a dose-response relationship in breast cancer are from the use of high-dose chemotherapy with autologous bone marrow transplantation in patients with metastatic breast cancer. In one such study approximately 40% of such patients achieved objective response, with approximately 25% achieving temporary complete remissions (Eder et al., 1986). Historically, the toxicity associated with this form of therapy has been substantial. However, advances in the field of haematopoietic support, by using peripheral blood stem cell pooling and growth factor support, have substantially reduced the morbidity and mortality associated with high-dose chemotherapy. It should theoretically be more effective to use dose-intensive chemotherapy in minimal disease states, such as in high-dose adjuvant therapy for high-risk patients. Currently the role of high-dose chemotherapy as adjuvant therapy in breast cancer is being further evaluated in comparison to conventional dose chemotherapy in randomized clinical trials, and is discussed more fully in Chapter 12a of this book.

Toxicity

Side-effects of adjuvant chemotherapy, both in conventional and high-dose regimens, is still a major concern. The toxicity of adjuvant chemotherapy varies with the particular drug regimens employed and the dose intensity. All regimens potentially cause nausea and vomiting, but the development of more effective antiemetic regimens, particularly including the serotonin-3 receptor antagonists, has considerably reduced the frequency of what is considered by patients to be among the worst side-effects of chemotherapy. Marked alopecia (i.e. needing to wear a wig) occurs in less than 10% of patients receiving CMF, but is observed almost universally in patients who receive an anthracycline containing regimen. Weight gain (average of 3–4 kg) has been observed in at least half the women during adjuvant chemotherapy, irrespective of menopausal status and also unrelated to whether drug-induced amenorrhoea occurs in premenopausal women. Thromboembolic phenomena are relatively uncommon complications of adjuvant chemotherapy alone, occurring in approximately 0.5% of cases of CMF therapy, although the incidence of this complication is considerably increased on addition of prednisolone (1.5%) or prednisolone plus tamoxifen (3.5%) to chemotherapy (Tormey et al., 1986).

Other significant acute toxicities include myelosuppression and thrombocytopenia, which occur in fewer than approximately 10% of patients who receive CMF (Harris et al., 1993), although toxic deaths occur in fewer than 0.5% of patients (Harris et al., 1993). Persistent neutropenia (with or without sepsis) may necessitate dose reductions and delays; lowering the dose below 85% has been shown to compromise survival. The use of growth factors to maintain the dose and reduce delays is currently under investigation.

The major delayed toxicity of adjuvant chemotherapy is irreversible amenorrhoea, which occurs after treatment with regimens containing alkylating agents such as cyclophosphamide. The incidence of amenorrhoea is clearly age related, occurring in approximately 40% of women who receive adjuvant chemotherapy under the age of 40, compared with an incidence of 95% in women over the age of 40 years. Furthermore, reversibility of amenorrhoea is also age related – 40% of women younger than 40 years of age who develop amenorrhoea will subsequently regain menses. However, it remains unclear whether the development of amenorrhoea confers any outcome benefit following adjuvant chemotherapy. Both the NSABP and Milan trials did not show any advantage in terms of disease-free interval or overall survival in patients who developed amenorrhoea compared with those who did not (Fisher et al., 1979; Bonadonna et al., 1981). Furthermore, in the Milan study, premenopausal women who relapsed were equally likely to respond to subsequent ovarian ablation irrespective of whether they had developed prior amenorrhoea (Bonadonna et al., 1981). In contrast, however, Bianco et al.

observed a significant correlation between drug-induced amenorrhoea and treatment outcome (Bianco et al., 1991) and Goldhirsch et al. reported a marginally significant improvement in the 4-year relapse-free survival rate in women with drug induced amenorrhoea (68%) in comparison with women without amenorrhoea (61%) (Goldhirsch et al., 1990). Similarly, amenorrhoea induced by adjuvant chemotherapy was associated with a significantly better disease-free survival ($p = 0.09$) in women treated in IBCSG Trial VI (Pagani et al., 1998). Consequently, an endocrine effect due to cytotoxic chemotherapy cannot be excluded.

The major late toxicity of adjuvant chemotherapy is the development of secondary neoplasms. There may be a slightly increased risk of myeloproliferative disease in patients treated with melphalan containing regimens, but leukaemia occurring after CMF has only been reported occasionally (Fisher et al., 1985; Valagussa et al., 1987). Although there does not appear to be an increased incidence of subsequent solid tumours after adjuvant chemotherapy, longer follow-up is required before this possibility can be excluded (Valagussa et al., 1987; Arriagada & Rutqvist, 1991). Cardiotoxicity is a well-established side-effect of anthracyclines which can occur more than one year after drug exposure. Furthermore, subclinical cardiotoxicity of adjuvant therapy might manifest itself only several decades after treatment. Indeed, subclinical cardiac damage has been documented following adjuvant dose-escalated FEC chemotherapy (Erselcan et al., 2000). Consequently, longer follow-up of the studies with anthracycline-containing regimens of adjuvant taxanes, and high-dose therapy, is necessary to exclude long-term toxicity, including cardiac disease, in these patients.

Adjuvant endocrine therapy

Ovarian ablation

One third of patients with breast cancer have hormone-dependent tumours (Henderson & Canellos, 1980). Animal studies and clinical trials of antioestrogens and inhibitors of oestrogen biosynthesis have confirmed that oestrogens are the most important hormones involved in supporting growth of hormone-dependent breast cancers (Segaloff, 1978; Kirschner, 1979). Initially, ovarian ablation was used as an adjuvant endocrine manipulation and several randomized studies including several prospective randomized studies have shown improvement in recurrence-free and overall survival rates in premenopausal women (Pritchard, 1987; Gibson & Jordan, 1990; Stewart, 1991; Goldhirsch & Valagussa, 1991). In the Toronto study, patients aged 45 years or older were randomized into one of three groups: radiation-induced ovarian ablation; radiation-induced ovarian ablation followed by 5 years of prednisolone (7.5 mg daily); or no adjuvant systemic therapy. Postmenopausal patients showed no survival gain from either of the adjuvant regimens. Patients who were premenopausal and who were treated with a combination of prednisolone and ovarian ablation had a significantly increased survival rate at 10 years compared with the patients who were given no adjuvant systemic therapy (Meakin et al., 1983).

The Early Breast Cancer Trialists' Collaborative Group (EBCTCG) has reported a meta-analysis of 12 randomized studies begun before 1990 that assess the effects of ovarian ablation by irradiation or surgery in over 2000 women younger than 50 years of age, most of whom are presumed to be premenopausal (EBCTCG, 1996). As the hormone receptor status for these patients was unavailable, it is likely that both ER-positive and ER-negative patients would have been included. Furthermore, as the benefit of ovarian ablation is likely to be limited largely to patients with ER-positive tumours, these trials may well underestimate the effects of ovarian ablation in appropriate patients.

The meta-analysis confirms that after 15 years follow-up, there is a significantly improved relapse-free survival (45% vs. 39%; $p = 0.0007$) and overall survival (52.4% vs. 46.1%; $p = 0.001$) for patients randomized to receive ovarian ablation. Subgroup analyses are unreliable because of small numbers, but the benefit seemed to be significant for women with both node-positive and node-negative cancers. Conversely, no significant improvement in relapse-free survival and overall survival was observed with ovarian ablation in approximately 1300 women of greater than 50 years of age included in this analysis. Most of these would presumably be peri or postmenopausal, confirming that the benefit of ovarian ablation is limited to premenopausal women.

Several large trials are in progress or have been completed evaluating the use of LHRH analogues with or without tamoxifen and/or chemotherapy in premenopausal women (Davidson et al., 1999; Jakesz et al., 1999; Rutqvist, 1999). Preliminary data are only available in abstracts at present and longer follow-up is required to determine the potential benefit of this approach.

Adjuvant tamoxifen

Most frequently, however, adjuvant endocrine therapy has focused on the use of the antioestrogen tamoxifen. Tamoxifen competitively inhibits the high affinity binding of oestradiol to specific oestrogen receptors and attenuates the biological effects of the natural hormone (Jordan, 1984). The tamoxifen receptor complex is not entirely biologically inert, however, and can induce a variety of biological responses including complete blockade of oestrogen action as well as minimizing the effects of oestradiol (Furr & Jordan, 1984). Furthermore, tamoxifen has additional effects through growth factor mechanisms, including the induction of an increase in secretion of transforming growth factor β (TGFβ) by ER-positive cells, which in turn may inhibit growth of adjacent cells (Knabbe et al., 1987). Moreover, tamoxifen may act as a biological response modifier through enhancing natural killer cell activity in patients with early breast cancer (Berry et al., 1987). Consequently tamoxifen may exert an antitumour effect even in tumours with a predominantly ER-negative cellular component. The function of the ER, and the biological mechanisms of tamoxifen and other antioestrogens, have been extensively reviewed (Chander et al., 1993).

In 1977, the Nolvadex Adjuvant Trial Organization designed an adjuvant trial with randomization to tamoxifen or to a no-treatment control arm. In a series of 1151 patients with either node-positive or node-negative breast cancer, the 5 and 10-year results provided evidence that overall survival was moderately, but significantly, improved with the use of adjuvant tamoxifen (Baum et al., 1990). Subsequently, numerous research groups have carried out many trials, although with a diversity of approaches. Many of the European groups have compared tamoxifen with untreated controls in patients unselected according to ER status. Many other groups have chosen to compare adjuvant chemotherapy with adjuvant chemotherapy plus long-term tamoxifen with all patients selected for tamoxifen according to ER status. Moreover, selection of menopausal and nodal groups has further complicated the picture. Most of the trials include postmenopausal women with predominantly node-positive disease. However, the NATO, Scottish and CRC trials have looked at tamoxifen as single-agent adjuvant therapy in premenopausal women for node-positive patients, for node-negative patients, and for both node-positive and node-negative patients respectively (Baum et al., 1983; Scottish Cancer Trials Office, 1987; CRC Adjuvant Breast Trial Working Party, 1988). Other complicating variables amongst these trials include the duration of tamoxifen (ranging from 1 to 5 years) and the dose of tamoxifen – most trials have used 20 mg/day although some have evaluated 30 mg or 40 mg/day. In an attempt to overcome these variables, an overview of adjuvant trials has been performed (Early Breast Cancer Trialists' Collaborative Group, 1998b).

This updated meta-analysis was performed in 1995 and includes results from 37 000 women in 55 trials, comprising about 87% of the world-wide evidence. Compared with previous such overviews, this approximately doubles the amount of evidence from trials of about 5 years of tamoxifen and, taking all trials together, on events occurring more than 5 years after randomization.

The overall effects of tamoxifen appeared to be small in almost 8000 women who had a low, or zero, level of the ER protein in their primary tumour. Consequently, subsequent analyses of recurrence and total mortality were restricted to the remaining women with ER-positive tumours ($n = 18\,000$), or unknown ER status ($n = 12\,000$, of which an estimated 8000 should have been ER positive). For trials of 1, 2 and about 5 years of adjuvant tamoxifen, the proportional recurrence reductions for these 30 000 women during about 10 years of follow-up were 21%, 29% and 47% respectively, with a highly significant trend towards a greater effect with longer treatment ($p < 0.00001$). The corresponding mortality reductions for these groups were 12%, 17% and 24%, respectively, with again a significant test for trend ($p = 0.003$). The absolute improvement in recurrence was greater during the first 5 years, whereas the improvement in survival grew steadily larger throughout the first 10 years. The proportional mortality reductions were similar for women with node-positive and node-negative disease, but the absolute mortality reductions were greater in node-positive women. In the trials of about 5 years of adjuvant tamoxifen the absolute improvements in 10-year survival were 10.9% for node-positive women (61.4% vs. 50.5% survival; $p < 0.00001$) and 5.6% for node-negative (78.9% vs. 73.3% survival; $p < 0.00001$) women. These benefits appeared to be largely irrespective of age, menopausal status, tamoxifen dose (usually 20 mg/day) and of whether chemotherapy had also been given. In terms of other outcomes among all women studied (i.e. including those with 'ER-poor' tumours), the proportional reductions in contralateral primary breast cancers were 13%, 26%, and 47% for 1, 2 and 5 years of adjuvant tamoxifen respectively. These findings led the St Gallen Consensus Panel to consider tamoxifen as part of adjuvant therapy for virtually all women with ER-positive breast cancer, but to recommend against its use in women in ER-negative breast cancer outside of a clinical trial (Goldhirsh et al., 1998a).

Duration of tamoxifen

The EBCTCG meta-analysis also provides strong evidence for the use of at least 5 years of tamoxifen therapy, particularly for women under the age of 50 years. Trials of longer tamoxifen administration were not included in this meta-analysis, but several trials have attempted to define the optimal duration of adjuvant therapy.

A randomized trial of 2 or 5 years of adjuvant tamoxifen (20 mg/day) in 2937 patients showed no difference in overall survival between the two groups, but there was a statistically significant delay in the time to relapse for patients receiving the longer treatment (Current Trials Working Party of the Cancer Research Campaign Breast Cancer Trials Group, 1996). However, the median follow-up in this study was only 2 years at this preliminary analysis and there was also flexibility in allowing adjuvant chemotherapy in this study. Three individual trials have failed to demonstrate further benefit with use of tamoxifen beyond 5 years (Fisher et al., 1996; Stewart et al., 1996; Tormey et al., 1996). Because the trials together encompass approximately 1700 women, most of whom were node negative, the value of longer tamoxifen duration is still somewhat uncertain (Peto, 1996). For this reason, further trials are ongoing to determine the optimal duration of adjuvant tamoxifen (aTTOM, ATLAS). However, given our current state of knowledge, it is reasonable to discontinue tamoxifen at 5 years in standard practice.

Side-effects of tamoxifen

Generally, tamoxifen is well tolerated and less than 3% of patients need to discontinue treatment as a result (Litherland & Jackson, 1988). The side-effects which occur most frequently include gastrointestinal upset, weight gain, hot flushes and menstrual disturbance in premenopausal women. There does not appear to be any adverse effect on bone mineral density in either premenopausal or postmenopausal women who have been treated with tamoxifen (Wolter et al., 1988; Fentiman et al., 1989; Powles et al., 1989); indeed, an increase in bone mass has been reported in tamoxifen-treated patients compared with those receiving a placebo. Thromboembolism has been reported in some studies on the use of adjuvant tamoxifen. In the NSABP-B14 and Eastern Cooperative Oncology Group (ECOG) trials there was a statistically significant increase in thromboembolic events in patients receiving tamoxifen compared to those receiving either placebo or chemotherapy alone (Healey et al. 1987; Fisher et al. 1989c). Other studies, however, have shown no such association (Goldhirsch, 1984; Ingle et al., 1988). Most of the concern surrounding the adverse effects of long-term tamoxifen administration has focused on the increased risks of endometrial cancer. The cumulative frequency of infiltrating endometrial cancer in women receiving adjuvant tamoxifen is 0.5% compared with 0.1% in the control group (Nayfield et al., 1991). However, when the Stockholm Trial (Fornander et al., 1989) (in which higher doses of tamoxifen were used) is excluded there is a twofold increase in risk of endometrial cancer, which is similar to the increased risk associated with postmenopausal oestrogen replacement therapy. The most recent meta-analysis (EBCTCG, 1998b) placed the incidence of endometrial cancer as approximately doubled in trials of 1 or 2 years of tamoxifen and approximately quadrupled in trials of 5 years of tamoxifen (although the number of cases was small and these ratios were not significantly different from each other). The absolute decrease in contralateral breast cancer was about twice as large as the absolute increase in the incidence of endometrial cancer. Clearly, the favourable side-effect profile of tamoxifen justifies its use in an adjuvant setting.

Adjuvant aromatase inhibitors

In addition to ovarian ablation and tamoxifen, the aromatase inhibitor amino-glutethamide, given for 2 years with hydrocortisone, has also been evaluated as adjuvant endocrine therapy in comparison with placebo in a randomized, double blind trial in postmenopausal women (Coombes et al., 1987). An early analysis indicated that aminoglutethamide and hydrocortisone caused a similar delay in relapse to that reported for adjuvant tamoxifen. Furthermore, there are large ongoing trials evaluating the combination of tamoxifen with the aromatase inhibitor arimidex in adjuvant therapy versus either agent used alone (ATAC Study). Other aromatase inhibitors including exemestane and letrozole are also under evaluation as adjuvant therapy within clinical trials given at 2–3 years and after 5 years of tamoxifen respectively in postmenopausal women with ER-positive or ER-unknown breast cancer. The exemestane study compares a further 2–3 years of exemestane (total 5 years) with continuing tamoxifen whereas the letrozole study involves 5 years of letrozole compared with placebo.

Newer antioestrogens, including toremifene (Holli, 1998) are being evaluated in clinical trials and it is anticipated that pure antioestrogens such as faslodex may be suitable candidates for adjuvant studies in the future.

Combined chemotherapy and endocrine therapy

Breast cancer is a biologically heterogenous tumour and it is likely to consist of various populations of cells with a range of sensitivities to cytotoxic and hormonal agents. Given the beneficial results achieved using adjuvant chemotherapy and adjuvant tamoxifen, it would seem reasonable to evaluate the use of a combination of chemotherapy and hormonal therapy in ER-positive tumours to determine if these treatment modalities have any additive or synergistic effect when given as adjuvant therapy. The EBCTCG meta-analysis suggested that tamoxifen adds significant benefit regardless of whether chemotherapy is used; the chemotherapy meta-analysis suggested that the reverse is also true. Several studies have attempted to determine if combined therapy provides a clinically meaningful advantage to the patient.

An initial NSABP study (Fisher et al., 1986) evaluated chemoendocrine therapy (L-phenylalanine, 5-fluorouracil and tamoxifen) versus chemotherapy alone. A total of 1891 women with positive axillary lymph nodes were randomized in this study. At 5 years there was a significant prolongation of disease-free survival ($p = 0.002$) associated with chemoendocrine therapy for all patients, but not of overall survival. The benefit was almost entirely restricted to patients greater than 50 years of age with 4, or more, positive axillary lymph nodes. In this group there was a 66% greater chance of remaining disease free when combined modality treatment was administered ($p < 0.001$) and there was also a significant survival benefit ($p = 0.02$). In addition to the patient's age and nodal status, the advantage derived from combined modality therapy was associated with the ER and PR status of the tumour. Conversely, there was no significant advantage for the addition of tamoxifen to combination chemotherapy (cyclophosphamide, 5-fluorouracil, prednisolone) in the Mayo Clinic Study (Ingle et al., 1988), nor in the Eastern Cooperative Oncology Group Study (Tormey et al., 1990). In contrast, the addition of tamoxifen to adjuvant chemotherapy with doxorubicin and ftorafur confers significantly higher 5-year disease-free rate and overall survival, with the same apparent benefit for ER-negative and premenopausal women as for the ER-positive and postmenopausal subgroups (Uchino et al., 1994).

The use of combined chemotherapy and endocrine therapy has also been addressed by the International (Ludwig) Breast Cancer Study Group who have reported their 15-year follow-up data (Castiglione-Gertsch et al., 1994). In premenopausal women with one to three positive axillary lymph nodes the addition of low-dose continuous prednisolone to a CMF combination did not give any advantage for either disease-free survival or overall survival. In premenopausal women with four or more positive nodes there was an improved outcome in ER-positive tumours when surgical oophorectomy was used in addition to CMF/prednisolone alone (disease-free survival 23% vs. 15%, $p = 0.13$; overall survival 41%, $p = 0.12$). For postmenopausal women under 65 years old, combined chemoendocrine therapy (1 year of CMF/prednisolone and tamoxifen) improved both disease-free survival and overall survival compared with endocrine therapy alone (prednisolone and tamoxifen) or no adjuvant treatment (disease free survival 35% vs. 25% vs. 14%, $p < 0.0001$; overall survival 48% vs. 36% vs. 32%, $p = 0.01$). Moreover, the addition of chemotherapy to tamoxifen has resulted in superior treatment outcome compared with adjuvant tamoxifen alone in postmenopausal patients with ER-positive tumours in other trials (Fisher et al., 1990b; Pearson et al., 1989). In addition, the IBCSG have retrospectively analysed four adjuvant trials performed between 1978 and 1993 and demonstrated that premenopausal women over 35 years had a significantly worse disease-free survival if they had ER-positive tumours compared with women with ER-negative tumours, and concluded that chemotherapy alone was insufficient for women in this age group with ER-positive tumours (Aebi et al., 2000). On the basis of these, and other more recent trials, the St Gallen Consensus Panel made recommendations for different clinical scenarios (Goldhirsch et al., 1998a).

Premenopausal women with node-positive, receptor-positive breast cancer

Although none of the above initial trials of combined chemoendocrine therapy demonstrated any appreciable benefit in this situation, many of these trials had short periods of tamoxifen therapy. More recent studies that have used 5 years of tamoxifen have demonstrated a clear reduction in recurrence rates with combined modality treatments (Tormey et al., 1992; Davidson et al., 1999). Consequently, the St Gallen Consensus Panel regarded chemotherapy plus tamoxifen as standard for these women (Goldhirsch et al., 1998a).

Postmenopausal women with node-positive, receptor-positive breast cancer

In addition to the studies of Fisher and Pearson outlined above, a statistical advantage of combined chemoendocrine adjuvant therapy has also been demonstrated in two other studies (International Breast Cancer Study Group, 1997; Albain et al., 1997). This benefit is most pronounced in the younger postmenopausal women and in women with lymph node burden. Moreover, the improved therapeutic outcome with chemoendocrine therapy in this patient population may well be related to the chemotherapy regimen used. Chemotherapy regimens such as the 'classical' CMF provide an advantage in combination with tamoxifen but no such additional benefit was observed when the modified CMF regimens, e.g. three-weekly i.v. CMF regimen, was used (Goldhirsch et al., 1998b).

Tamoxifen and chemotherapy for node-negative, receptor-positive breast cancer

The NSABP-B20 randomized 2306 women to either adjuvant tamoxifen alone, or CMF plus tamoxifen, or methotrexate, 5-FU plus tamoxifen. There was a significant improvement in both disease-free survival and overall survival with chemoendocrine therapy compared to tamoxifen alone, irrespective of tumour size and ER status (Fisher et al., 1997). However, the greatest benefit was observed for younger patients and those with larger tumours. The St Gallen Consensus Panel considered that women with node-negative, receptor-positive breast cancer of >2 cm were candidates for chemoendocrine therapy and that tamoxifen with or without chemotherapy should be considered for women whose tumour measured 1–2 cm. Women with tumours <1 cm do not routinely require chemotherapy.

Concurrent versus sequential chemohormonal therapy

In vitro studies have demonstrated that endocrine therapies may decrease the cytotoxic effect of chemotherapy drugs by altering tumour cell kinetics (Osborne et al., 1989). At only 4 years follow-up, there is no apparent difference in disease outcome for postmenopausal women with node-positive, ER-positive breast cancer randomized to CAF followed by 5 years of tamoxifen or CAF with concurrent tamoxifen for 5 years (Albain et al., 1997). Further follow-up is necessary to confirm this finding, although a higher rate of thromboembolic events has been reported with combined therapy, and consequently many clinicians choose the sequential approach pending the final analysis of this study.

Future prospects

Despite the improvements in disease-free survival, overall survival and mortality with the current recommended adjuvant therapy regimens, many issues remain unresolved. Further clinical trials are needed to address these issues, and many of these are currently in progress. These include the place of high-dose chemotherapy with appropriate haematopoietic support, the optimal chemotherapy regimen for patients with four or more positive axillary lymph nodes, the role of ovarian ablation in addition to chemotherapy and/or tamoxifen in premenopausal women, the optimal chemoendocrine combination, and the identification of subsets of node-negative patients who would benefit from adjuvant chemotherapy and/or endocrine therapy. There is already an emphasis, within clinical trials, for evaluating newer chemotherapy agents (e.g. taxanes) and newer endocrine agents (e.g. aromatase inhibitors) as adjuvant therapy. The use of new technologies such as high-density cDNA arrays to measure thousands of genes simultaneously on a single tumour specimen has the potential to increase our understanding of putative prognostic factors in early breast cancer, and of potential predictive factors, when designing adjuvant therapies. This is likely to be particularly relevant with the introduction of novel biologic therapies such as anti-HER-2 monoclonal antibodies and antiangiogenesis agents into systemic adjuvant therapy strategies. Indeed adjuvant trials incorporating Herceptin within therapy schedules are planned both in Europe and in the USA with the primary endpoint being disease-free survival although overall survival and cardiotoxicity will be other significant secondary endpoints. It is anticipated that these trials will also contribute to resolving the on-going controversies surrounding the predictive value of HER-2 status for treatment outcome.

REFERENCES

Aebi, S., Gelber, S., Castiglione-Gertsch, M. et al. (2000). Is chemotherapy alone adequate for young women with oestrogen-receptor positive breast cancer? *Lancet*, 355, 1869–74.

Albain, K., Green, S., Osborne, K. et al. (1997). Tamoxifen (T) versus cylophosphamide, adriamycin, and 5-FU plus either concurrent or sequential T in postmenopausal receptor (A), node(+), breast cancer: A Southwest Oncology Group phase II Intergroup trial (SWOG-8814 INT-0100). *Proceedings of the American Society of Clinical Oncology*, 16, 128a, Abstract 450.

Arriagada, R. & Rutqvist, L.E. (1991). Adjuvant chemotherapy in early breast cancer and incidence of new primary malignancies. *Lancet*, 338, 535–8.

Baum, M., Brinkley, D.M., Dossett, J.A. et al. (1983). Controlled trial of tamoxifen as adjuvant agent in managment of early breast cancer. *Lancet*, i, 257–61.

Baum, M., Ebbs, S. & Brooks, M. (1990). Biological fall out from trials of adjuvant tamoxifen in early breast cancer. In *Adjuvant therapy of cancer*, VI. Ed. S.E. Salman, Philadelphia: W.B. Saunders, pp. 269–74.

Berry, J., Green, B.J. & Matheson, D.S. (1987). Modulation of natural killer cell activity by tamoxifen in stage I postmenopausal breast cancer. *European Journal of Cancer and Clinical Oncology*, 23, 517–20.

Bianco, A.R., Del Mastro, L., Gullo, C. et al. (1991). Prognostic role of amenorrhoea induced by adjuvant chemotherapy in premenopausal patients with early breast cancer. *British Journal of Cancer*, 63, 799–803.

Blichert-Toft, M., Rose, C., Anderson, J.A. et al. (1992). Danish randomised trial comparing breast conservation therapy with mastectomy: six years of life-table analysis. *Monographs of the National Cancer Institute*, 11, 19–25.

Bonadonna, G. (1989). Conceptual and practical advances in the management of breast cancer. Karnofsky Memorial Lecture. *Journal of Clinical Oncology*, 7, 1380–97.

Bonadonna, G. (1992). Evolving concepts in the systemic adjuvant treatment of breast cancer. *Cancer Research*, 52, 2127–37.

Bonadonna, G. & Valagussa, P. (1981). Dose-response effect of adjuvant chemotherapy in breast cancer. *New England Journal of Medicine*, 304, 10–15.

Bonadonna, G., Monfardini, S., Delena, M. et al. (1970). Phase I and preliminary phase II evaluation of adriamycin (NSC-123127). *Cancer Research*, 30, 2572–82.

Bonadonna, G., Brusamolino, E., Valagussa, P. et al. (1975). Combination chemotherapy as an adjuvant treatment in inoperable breast cancer. *New England Journal of Medicine*, 294, 405–10.

Bonadonna, G., Valagussa, P. & De Palo, G. (1981). The results of adjuvant chemotherapy are predominantly caused by the hormonal changes such therapy induces. Opposed. (1981). In *Medical Oncology, Controversies in cancer treatment*, ed. M.B. Van Scoy-Mosler, Boston: G.K. Hall, 100–9, 112–15.

Bonadonna, G., Valagussa, P., Rossi, A. et al. (1985). Ten-year results with CMF-based adjuvant chemotherapy in resectable breast cancer. *Breast Cancer Research and Treatment*, 5, 95–115.

Bonadonna, G., Valagussa, P., Moliterni, A. et al. (1995). Adjuvant cyclophosphamide, methotrexate and fluorouracil in node-positive breast cancer. *New England Journal of Medicine*, 332, 901–6.

Budman, D.R., Berry, D.A., Cirrincione, C.T. et al. (1998). Dose and dose intensity as determinants of outcome in the adjuvant treatment of breast cancer. The Cancer and Leukaemia Group B. *Journal of the National Cancer Institute*, 90, 1205–11.

Buzdar, A.U., Hortobagyi, G.N. & Kau, S.W. (1990). Doxorubicin-containing adjuvant therapy for patients with stage II breast cancer. M.D. Anderson Cancer Center Experience. In *Adjuvant therapy of cancer*, VI. Ed. S.E. Salman, Philadelphia: W.B. Saunders, pp. 210–15.

Buzzoni, R., Bonadonna, G., Valagussa, P. et al. (1991). Adjuvant chemotherapy with doxorubicin plus cyclophosphamide, methotrexate and fluorouracil in the treatment of resectable breast cancer with more than three positive axillary nodes. *Journal of Clinical Oncology*, 9, 2134–40.

Castiglione-Gertsch, M., Johnsen, C., Goldhirsch, A. et al. (1994). The International (Ludwig) Breast Cancer Study Group Trials I–IV: 15 years follow-up. *Annals Oncology*, 5, 717–24.

Chander, S.K., Sahota, S.S., Evans, T.R.J. et al. (1993). The biological evaluation of novel anti-oestrogens for the treatment of breast cancer. *Critical Reviews in Oncology Hematolology*, 15, 243–69.

Colleoni, M., Bonetti, M., Coates, A.S. et al. (2000). Early start of adjuvant chemotherapy may improve treatment outcome for premenopausal breast cancer patients with tumours not expressing estrogen receptors. *Journal of Clinical Oncology*, 18, 584–90.

Coombes, R.C., Powles, T.J., Easton, D. et al. (1987). Adjuvant aminoglutethamide therapy for postmenopausal patients with primary breast cancer. *Cancer Research*, 47, 2496–9.

Coombes, R.C., Bliss, J.M., Wils, J. et al. (1996). Adjuvant cyclophosphamide, methotrexate and fluorouracil versus fluorouracil, epirubicin and cyclophosphamide chemotherapy in premenopausal women with axillary node-positive operable breast cancer: results of a randomised trial. The International Collaborative Cancer Group. *Journal of Clinical Oncology*, 14, 35–45.

CRC Adjuvant Breast Trial Working Party (1988). Preliminary analysis: cyclophosphamide and tamoxifen as adjuvant therapies in the management of breast cancer. *British Journal of Cancer*, 57, 604–7.

Current Trials Working Party of the Cancer Research Campaign Breast Cancer Trials Group (1996). Preliminary results from the cancer research campaign trial evaluating tamoxifen duration in women aged fifty years or older with breast cancer. *Journal of the National Cancer Institute*, 88, 1834–9.

Dalton, W., Brooks, R. & Jones S. (1987). Breast cancer adjuvant therapy trials at Arizona Cancer Center using adriamycin and cyclophosphamide. In: *Adjuvant Therapy of Cancer* V. Ed. S.E. Salman, Philadelphia: Grune and Stratton, pp. 263–9.

Davidson, N., O'Neill, A., Vukov, A. et al. (1999). Effect of chemohormonal therapy in premenopausal, node(+), receptor(+) breast cancer: an Eastern Cooperative Oncology Group Phase III Intergroup Trial (E5188, INT-0101). *Proceedings of the American Society of Clinical Oncology*, 18, Abstract 249.

Early Breast Cancer Trialists' Collaborative Group (1996). Ovarian ablation in early breast cancer: overview of the randomised trials. *Lancet*, 348, 1189–96.

Early Breast Cancer Trialists' Collaborative Group (1998a). Polychemotherapy for early breast cancer: an overview of the randomised trials. *Lancet*, 352, 930–42.

Early Breast Cancer Trialists' Collaborative Group (1998b). Tamoxifen for early breast cancer: an overview of the randomised trials. *Lancet*, 351, 1451–67.

Eder, J.P., Antman, K., Peters, W.P. et al. (1986). High dose combination alkylating agents chemotherapy with autologous bone marrow support for metastatic breast cancer. *Journal of Clinical Oncology*, 4, 1592–7.

Engelsman, E., Klijn, J.C.M., Rubens, R.D. et al. (1991). 'Classical' CMF versus a 3-weekly intravenous CMF schedule in postmenopausal patients with advanced breast cancer. An EORTC Breast Cancer Cooperative Group phase III trial (10808). *European Journal of Cancer*, 27, 966–70.

Erselcan, T., Kairemo, K.J.A., Wiklund, T.A. et al. (2000). Subclinical cardiotoxicity following adjuvant dose-escalated FEC, high-dose chemotherapy, or CMF in breast cancer. *British Journal of Cancer*, 82, 777–81.

Fentiman, I.S., Caleffi, M., Rodin, A. et al. (1989). Bone mineral content of women receiving tamoxifen for mastalgia. *British Journal of Cancer*, 60, 262–4.

Fisher, B. & Fisher, E.R. (1966). The interrelationship or hematogenous and lymphatic tumor cell dissemination. *Surgery, Gynaecology and Obstetrics*, 122, 791–8.

Fisher, B., Carbone, P., Economou, S.G. et al. (1975a). L-Phenylalanine mustard (L-PAM) in the management of primary breast cancer: a report of early findings. *New England Journal of Medicine*, 292, 117–22.

Fisher, B., Slack, N., Katrych, D. et al. (1975b). Ten-year follow-up results of patients with carcinoma of the breast in a co-operative clinical trial evaluating surgical adjuvant chemotherapy. *Surgery Gynecology Obstetrics*, 240, 528–34.

Fisher, B., Sherman, B., Rockette, H. et al. (1979). L-Phenylalanine mustard (L-PAM) in the management of premenopausal patients with primary breast cancer: lack of association of disease-free survival with depression of ovarian function. *Cancer*, 44, 857–7.

Fisher, B., Rockette, H., Fisher, E.R. et al. (1985). Leukaemia in breast cancer patients following adjuvant chemotherapy or postoperative therapy: the NSABP experience. *Journal of Clinical Oncology*, 3, 1640–58.

Fisher, B., Redmond, C., Brown, A. et al. (1986). Adjuvant chemotherapy with and without tamoxifen in the treatment of primary breast cancer: 5-year results from the NSABP trial. *Journal of Clinical Oncology*, 4, 459–71.

Fisher, B., Redmond, C., Poisson, R. et al. (1989a). Eight-year results of a randomised trial comparing total mastectomy and lumpectomy with or without irradiation in the treatment of breast cancer. *New England Journal of Medicine*, 320, 822–8.

Fisher B., Redmond, C., Wickerham, D.L. et al. (1989b). Doxorubicin-containing regimens for the treatment of stage II breast cancer. The National Surgical Adjuvant Breast and Bowel Project experience. *Journal of Clinical Oncology*, 7, 572–82.

Fisher, B., Brown, A.M., Dinitrov, N.V. et al. (1990a). Two months of doxorubicin-cyclophsophamide with and without interval reintroduction therapy compared with 6 months of cyclophosphamide, methotrexate and fluorouracil in positive node breast cancer patients with tamoxifen nonresponsive tumour: results from the National Surgical Adjuvant Breast and Bowel Project B-15. *Journal of Clinical Oncology*, 8, 1493–6.

Fisher, B., Redmond, C., Legault-Poisson, S. et al. (1990b). Postoperative chemotherapy and tamoxifen compared with tamoxifen alone in the treatment of postive-node breast cancer aged 50 years and older with tumors responsive to tamoxifen: results from the National Surgical Adjuvant Breast and Bowel Project B-16. *Journal of Clinical Oncology*, 8, 1005–18.

Fisher, B., Constantino, J., Redmond, C. et al. (1989c). A randomised clinical trial evaluating tamoxifen in the treatment of patients with node-negative breast cancer who have oestrogen-receptor positive tumours. *New England Journal of Medicine*, 320, 479–84.

Fisher, B., Anderson, S., Fisher, E.R. et al. (1991). Significance of ipsilateral breast tumour recurrences after lumpectomy. *Lancet*, 338, 327–31.

Fisher, B., Dignam, J., Bryant, J. et al. (1996). The worth of five versus more than five years of tamoxifen therapy for breast cancer patients with negative lymph nodes and estrogen receptor-positive tumors. *Journal of the National Cancer Institute*, 88, 1529–42.

Fisher, B., Dignam, J., Wolmark, N. et al. (1997). Tamoxifen and chemotherapy for lymph node-negative, estrogen receptor-positive breast cancer. *Journal of the National Cancer Institute*, 89, 1673–82.

Fornander, T., Rutqvist, L.E., Cedermark, B. et al. (1989). Adjuvant tamoxifen in early breast cancer: occurrence of new primary cancers. *Lancet*, 1, 117–20.

Furr, B.J.A. & Jordan, V.C. (1984). The pharmacology and clinical uses of tamoxifen. *Pharmacology Therapeutics*, 25, 127–205.

Gibson, D.F.C. & Jordan, V.C. (1990). Adjuvant antioestrogen therapy for breast cancer: past, present, and future. *Surgical Clinics of North America*, 70, 1103–13.

Goldhirsch, A. (1984). Adjuvant therapy for postmenopausal women with operable breast cancer. Part I – a randomised trial of chemoendocrine versus endocrine therapy versus mastectomy alone. *Adjuvant Therapy of Cancer,* IV, 379–91.

Goldhirsch, A. & Valagussa, P. (1991). Old and new trends in the adjuvant treatment of early breast cancer. *Annals of Oncology (Editorial),* 2, 320–2.

Goldhirsch, A., Gelber, R.D. & Castiglione, M. (1990). The magnitude of endocrine effects of adjuvant chemotherapy for premenopausal breast cancer patients. *Annals of Oncology,* 1, 183–8.

Goldhirsch, A., Glick, J.H., Gelber, R.D. et al. (1998a). Meeting highlights: international consensus panel on the treatment of primary breast cancer. *Journal of the National Cancer Institute,* 90, 1601–8.

Goldhirsch, A., Coates, A.S., Colleoni, M. et al. (1998b). Adjuvant chemoendocrine therapy in postmenopausal breast cancer: cyclophosphamide, methotrexate and fluorouracil dose and schedule may make a difference. International Breast Cancer Study Group. *Journal of Clinical Oncology,* 16, 1358–62.

Goldie, J.H. & Coldman, A.J. (1979). A mathematical model for relating the drug sensitivity of tumours to the spontaneous mutation rate. *Cancer Treatment Reports,* 63, 1727–33.

Halstead, W.S (1907). The results of radical operations for the cure of carcinoma of the breast. *Annals of Surgery,* 46, 1–19.

Harris, J.R., Morrow, M. & Bonadonna, G. (1993). Cancer of the breast. In: *Principles and Practice of Oncology.* eds. DeVita Jr, V.T., Hellman, S., Rosenberg, S.A., Lippincott, J.B. Philadelphia, 1264–332.

Healey, B., Tormey, D.C., Gray, K. et al. (1987). Arterial and venous thrombotic events in ECOG adjuvant breast cancer trials. *Proceedings of the American Society of Clinical Oncology,* 6, 54, Abstract 208.

Henderson, I.C. & Canellos, G.P. (1980). Cancer of the breast: the past decade (Part 1). *New England Journal of Medicine,* 302, 17–30.

Henderson, I.C., Hayes, D.F., Parker, L.M. et al. (1990). Adjuvant systemic therapy for patients with node-negative tumours. *Cancer,* 65, 2132–47.

Henderson, I.C., Berry D., Demetri, G. et al. (1998). Improved disease-free (DFS) and overall survival (OS) from the addition of sequential paclitaxel (T) but not from the escalation of doxorubicin (A) dose level in the adjuvant chemotherapy of patients with node-positive primary breast cancer. *Proceedings of the American Society of Clinical Oncology,* 17, 101a, Abstract 390.

Holli, K. (1998). Adjuvant trials of toremifene vs tamoxifen: the European experience. *Oncology,* 12, 23–7.

Hryniuk, W.M., Bonadonna, G. & Valagussa, P. (1987). The effect of dose intensity in adjuvant chemotherapy. In: *Adjuvant Therapy of Cancer V.* Philadelphia: ed. Salman, S.E., Grune and Stratton, 13–23.

Hutchins, L., Green, S., Ravidin, P. et al. (1998). CMF versus CAF with and without tamoxifen in high-risk node-negative breast cancer patients and a natural history follow-up study in low-risk node-negative patients: first results of Intergroup trial INT 0102. *Proceedings of the American Society of Clinical Oncology,* 17, 1a, Abstract 2.

Ingle, J.N., Everson, L.E., Wieand, S. et al. (1988). Randomised trial of observation versus adjuvant therapy with cyclophosphamide, fluorouracil, prednisolone with or without tamoxifen following mastectomy in postmenopausal women with node-positive breast cancer. *Journal of Clinical Oncology*, 6, 1388–96.

International Breast Cancer Study Group (1997). Effectiveness of adjuvant chemotherapy in combination with tamoxifen for node-positive postmenopausal breast cancer patients. *Journal of Clinical Oncology*, 15, 1385–94.

Jacobson, J.A., Danforth, D.N., Cowan, K.H. et al. (1995). Ten-year results of a comparison of conservation with mastectomy in the treatment of stage I and II breast cancer. *New England Journal of Medicine*, 332, 907–11.

Jakesz, R., Haurmaninger, H., Samonigg, H. et al. (1999). Comparison of adjuvant therapy with tamoxifen and goserelin vs CMF in premenopausal stage I and II hormone-responsive breast cancer patients: four-year results of Austrian Breast Cancer Study Group (ADCSG) Trial 5. *Proceedings of the American Society of Clinical Oncology*, 18, Abstract 250.

Jordan, V.C. (1984). Biochemical pharmacology of anti-oestrogen action. *Pharmacology Reviews*, 36, 245–76.

Kirshner, M.A. (1979). The role of hormones in the development of human breast cancer. In *Breast Cancer 3: Advances in Research and Treatment, current topics*. Ed. W.L. McGuire. Plenum Press: New York, pp. 199–226.

Knabbe, C., Lippman, M.E., Wakefield, L.M. et al. (1987). Evidence that transforming growth factor is a hormonally regulated negative growth factor β in human breast cancer cells. *Cell*, 48, 417–28.

Liljegren, G., Holmberg, L., Adami, H.O. et al. (1994). Sector resection with or without postoperative radiotherapy for stage I breast cancer: five year results of a randomised trial. *Journal of the National Cancer Institute*, 86, 717–22.

Litherland, S. & Jackson, I.M. (1988). Anti-oestrogens in the management of hormone dependent cancer. *Cancer Treatment Reports*, 15, 183–94.

Mansour, E.G., Ejday, L., Shatila, A.H. (1990). Adjuvant therapy in node-negative breast cancer: is it necessary for all patients? An Intergroup study. In: *Adjuvant therapy of Cancer VI*. Ed. S.E. Salman, Philadephia: Saunders, W.B., pp. 174–89.

Meakin, J.W., Allt, W.E.C., Beale, F.A. et al. (1983). Ovarian irradiation and prednisone following surgery and radiotherapy for carcinoma of the breast. *Breast Cancer Research Treatment*, 3 (Suppl. 1), 45–8.

Misset, J.L., diPalma, M., Delgado, M. et al. (1996). Adjuvant treatment of node-positive cancer with cyclophosphamide, doxorubicin, fluorouracil and vincristine versus cyclophosphamide, methotrexate and fluorouracil: final report after a 16 year median follow-up duration. *Journal of Clinical Oncology*, 14, 1136–45.

Moliterni, A., Bonadonna, G., Valagussa, P. et al. (1991). Cyclophosphamide, methotrexate and fluorouracil with and without doxorubicin in the adjuvant treatment of resectable breast cancer with one to three positive axillary nodes. *Journal of Clinical Oncology*, 9, 1124–30.

Nayfield, S.G., Karp, J.E., Ford, L.G. et al. (1991). Potential role of tamoxifen in prevention of breast cancer. *Journal of the National Cancer Institute*, 83, 1450–9.

Osborne, C.K., Kilten, L. & Arteaga, C.L. (1989). Antagonism of chemotherapy-induced cytotoxicity for human breast cancer cells by antioestrogens. *Journal of Clinical Oncology*, 7, 710–17.

Pagani, O., O'Neill, A., Castiglione, M. et al. (1998). Prognostic impact of amenorrhoea after adjuvant chemotherapy in premenopausal breast cancer patients with axillary node involvement: results of The International Breast Cancer Study Group (IBCSG) Trial VI. *European Journal of Cancer*, 34, 632–40.

Pearson, O.H., Hubay, C.A., Gordon, N.H. et al. (1989). Endocrine versus endocrine plus five-drug chemotherapy in postmenopausal women with stage II oestrogen-receptor positive breast cancer. *Cancer*, 64, 1819–23.

Peto, R. (1996). Five years of tamoxifen, or more? *Journal of the National Cancer Institute*, 88, 1791–3.

Powles, T.J., Hardy, J.R., Ashley, S.E. et al. (1989). A pilot trial to evaluate the acute toxicity and feasibility of tamoxifen for prevention of breast cancer. *British Journal of Cancer*, 60, 126–31.

Pritchard, K.L. (1987). Current status of adjuvant endocrine therapy for resectable breast cancer. *Seminars in Oncology*, 14, 23–33.

Rutqvist, L.E. (1999). Zoladex and tamoxifen as adjuvant therapy in premenopausal breast cancer: a randomised trial by the Cancer Research Campaign (CRC) Breast Cancer Trials Group, the Stockholm Breast Cancer Study Group, the South-East Sweden Breast Cancer Group, and the Gruppo Interdisciplinare Valutazione Interventi in Oncologia (GIVIO). *Proceedings of the American Society of Clinical Oncology*, 18, Abstract 251.

Sarrazin, D., Le, M.G., Arriagada, R. et al. (1989). Ten-year results of a randomised trial comparing a conservative treatment to mastectomy in early breast cancer. *Radiotherapy Oncology*, 14, 177–84.

Scottish Cancer Trials Office (1987). Adjuvant tamoxifen in the management of operable breast cancer. The Scottish Trial. *Lancet*, ii, 171–5.

Segaloff, A. (1978). Hormones and mammary carcinogenesis. In: *Advances in Research and Treatment: experimental biology*. Ed. W.L. McGuire. Plenum Press: New York, pp. 1–22.

Shapiro, C.L., Henderson, I.C. & Gelman, R.S. (1991). A randomised trial of 15 vs 30 weeks of adjuvant chemotherapy in high risk breast cancer patients: results after a median follow up of 9.1 years. *Proceedings of the American Society of Clinical Oncology*, Abstract, 10, 44 (50).

Skipper, H.E. (1978). Reasons for success and failure in treatment of murine leukaemias with the drugs now employed in treating human leukaemias. In *Cancer Chemotherapy*, vol. 1. Ann Arbor, MI: University Microfilms International, 1–166.

Skipper, H.E., Schabel, F.M. Jr. & Mellet, L.B. (1950). Implications of biochemical, cytotoxic, pharmacologic, and toxicologic relationships in the design of optimal therapeutic schedules. *Cancer Chemotherapy Reports*, 54, 431–50.

Skipper, H.E., Schabel, F.M. Jr. & Wilcox, W.S. (1964). Experimental evaluation of potential anticancer agents: XII: on the criteria and kinetics associated with 'curability' of experimental leukaemias. *Cancer Chemotherapy Reports*, 35, 1–111.

Stewart, H.J. (1991). Adjuvant endocrine therapy for operable breast cancer. *Bulletins in Cancer*, 78, 379–84.

Stewart, H.J., Forrest, A.P., Everington, D. et al. (1996). Randomised comparison of 5 years of adjuvant tamoxifen with continuous therapy for operable breast cancer: The Scottish Cancer Trials Breast Group. *British Journal of Cancer*, 74, 297–9.

Tannock, I.F., Boyd, N.F., De Boer, G. et al. (1986). A randomised trial of two dose levels of cyclophosphamide, methotrexate and 5-fluorouracil chemotherapy for patients with metastatic breast cancer. *Journal of Clinical Oncology*, 6, 1377–87.

Tormey, D.C., Gray, R., Taylor, S.G. et al. (1986). Postoperative chemotherapy and chemohormonal therapy in women with node-positive breast cancer. *National Cancer Institute Monographs*, 1, 75–80.

Tormey, D.C., Gray, R., Gilchrist, K. et al. (1990). Adjuvant chemohormonal therapy with cyclophosphamide, methotrexate, 5-fluorouracil, and prednisolone (CMFP) or CMFP plus tamoxifen compared with CMF for premenopausal breast cancer patients: an Eastern Cooperative Oncology Group Trial. *Cancer*, 65, 200–6.

Tormey, D.C., Gray, R., Abeloff, M.D. et al. (1992). Adjuvant therapy with a doxorubicin regimen and long-term tamoxifen in premenopausal breast cancer patients: an Eastern Cooperative Oncology Group Trial. *Journal of Clinical Oncology*, 10, 1848–56.

Tormey, D.C., Gray, R., Falkson, H.C. (1996). Postchemotherapy adjuvant tamoxifen therapy beyond five years in patients with lymph node-positive breast cancer. *Journal of the National Cancer Institute*, 88, 1818–33.

Uchino, J., Samejima, N., Tanabe, T. et al. (1994). Positive effect of tamoxifen as part of adjuvant chemo-endocrine therapy for breast cancer. *British Journal of Cancer*, 69, 767–71.

Valagussa, P., Bonadonna, G., Veronesi, U. (1978). Patterns of relapse and survival following radical mastectomy: analysis of 716 consecutive patients. *Cancer*, 41, 1170–8.

Valagussa, P., Tancini, G. & Bonadonna, G. (1987). Second malignancies after CMF for resectable breast cancer. *Journal of Clinical Oncology*, 5, 1138–42.

Valagussa, P., Brambilla, C., Zambetti, M. et al. (1989). Salvage treatments in relapsing resectable breast cancer. *Recent Results in Cancer Research*, 115, 69–76.

Van Dongen, J.A., Bartelink, H., Fentiman, I.S. et al. (1992). Randomised clinical trial to assess the value of breast-conserving therapy in stage I and II breast cancer: EORTC 10801 trial. *Monographics of the National Cancer Institute*, 11, 15–18.

Veronesi, U., Banfi, A., Salvadori, B. et al. (1990). Breast conservation is the treatment of choice in small breast cancer: long-term results of a randomised trial. *European Journal of Cancer*, 26, 668–70.

Veronesi, U., Luini, A., Del Vecchio, M. et al. (1993). Radiotherapy after breast-preserving surgery in women with localized cancer of the breast. *New England Journal of Medicine*, 328, 1587–91.

Wolter, J., Ryan, W.G., Subbaiah, P.V. et al. (1988). Apparent beneficial effects of tamoxifen on serum lipoprotein subfractions and bone mineral content in patients with breast cancer. *Proceedings of the American Society of Clinical Oncology*, 7, 10 Abstract 14.

Wood, W.C., Budman, D.R., Korzun, A.H. et al. (1994). Dose and dose intensity of adjuvant chemotherapy for stage II, node-positive breast carcinoma. *New England Journal of Medicine*, 330, 1253–9.

Zambetti, M., Bonadonna, G., Valagussa, P. et al. (1992). Adjuvant CMF for node-negative and estrogen receptor-negative breast cancer patients. *Journal of the National Cancer Institute*, 11, 77–83.

8

Adjuvant radiotherapy in the management of breast cancer

Gillian Ross[a], David Landau[b] and Andrew Tutt[a]

[a]Institute of Cancer Research, London
[b]The Royal Marsden Hospital, London

Introduction

Adjuvant radiotherapy (RT) has an established role in the reduction of risk of locoregional breast cancer recurrence, both postmastectomy and after breast-conserving surgery (BCS). Importantly, results of recent clinical trials also suggest that locoregional RT may impact on overall survival, adding to the benefits accruing to systemic adjuvant therapy. This chapter will review the evidence base for current recommendations for adjuvant RT, highlight areas of ongoing research activity and indicate directions for future treatment optimization.

Radiotherapy and breast conservation

The aims of breast-conservation therapy using tumorectomy and adjuvant radiotherapy are to ensure survival equivalent to mastectomy, whilst optimizing the cosmetic outcome and minimizing risks of disease recurrence in the conserved breast. Since the 1970s, there have been six prospective randomized trials in which breast-conserving surgery has been compared with mastectomy. These studies have confirmed the efficacy of BC + RT with respect to survival (Table 8.1). Differing surgical and RT techniques lead to varying rates of recurrence in the breast from 4% to 20% at 10 years. Importantly, despite undergoing a more radical surgical procedure, associated with significant rates of psychosexual morbidity, it was observed that mastectomy still conferred a risk of local recurrence of 2–9%.

As a result of these randomized studies, and many retrospective large single-centre studies of BCT and RT, this approach has become the standard of care for women who wish to opt for BCT. Efforts have since focused on refining and improving the therapeutic ratio by examining and modifying factors contributing

Table 8.1. Local recurrence rates in randomized trials comparing conservative surgery and radiotherapy with mastectomy

Trial	Follow-up (years)	Local recurrence (%) Mastectomy	BCS + RT	Type of BCS	Reference
Gustave-Roussy	10	9	7	2 cm margin	Sarrazin et al, 1989
Milan	10	2	4	quadrantectomy	Veronesi et al., 1990a
NSABP B-06	8	8	10	lumpectomy	Fisher et al., 1989
NCI	8	6	20	gross excision	Lichter et al., 1992
EORTC	8	9	13	1 cm margin	Van Dongen et al., 1992
Danish Breast Group	6	4	3	wide excision	Blichert-Toft et al., 1992

to risk of local recurrence, and late effects such as cosmesis, and treatment-related complications.

Risk factors for recurrence following breast-conserving surgery

The ability to conserve a woman's breast can be expected to have significant effects on quality of life but for most women these benefits must not be gained at the expense of a reduced expectation of survival or an unacceptably increased risk of local recurrence. As a result of prospective trials comparing breast-conservation strategies with mastectomy, breast cancer clinicians can provide much information to guide women in this decision.

The local recurrence rates observed in both randomized and retrospective studies range from 8% to 20% at 10 years. However, some of the longest follow-up has been obtained in retrospective studies. Kurtz et al. (1989) have documented an actuarial incidence of recurrence increasing from 7% at 5 years, to 14% at 10 years, rising to 20% at 20 years. The study group comprised 1593 women with stage I or II breast cancer, completely excised; 79% of the recurrences were in the vicinity of the tumour bed, but with increasing time interval, an increasing percentage of recurrences were located elsewhere in the breast. A majority of recurrences after 10 years were considered new tumours. Locoregional control was 88% at 5 years after salvage mastectomy and 64% after breast-conserving salvage procedures.

Factors which influence local recurrence include: patient factors, e.g. age; tumour factors, such as an extensive intraduct component, lymphovascular invasion, and grade III histology; and finally, treatment factors, including resection margins, intensity of radiotherapy and adjuvant systemic treatment. Although tumour size and lymph node positivity are the most important predictive factors for overall survival, neither has been shown to impact on local failure in the breast (Clarke et al., 1985; Halverson et al., 1993), although this may be difficult to resolve due to competing risks of systemic failure in the case of node positivity.

Pathological studies of the extent of microscopic invasive and in situ carcinoma which surrounds the macroscopic tumour in mastectomy specimens indicate that microscopic tumour extends some distance from the gross tumour. In T1 and T2 invasive cancers microscopic extension may be present more than 2 cm from the tumour in more than 40% of patients (Holland et al., 1985; Ohtake et al., 1995). This accords with the 42% probability of breast recurrence seen in the lumpectomy without RT arm of NSABP B-06 (Fisher et al., 1989; Fisher et al., 1995). The principles behind modern BCS/RT are the surgical removal of sufficient breast tissue such that the residual microscopic tumour burden is sufficiently low to be sterilized by moderate dose adjuvant RT. In all epithelial malignancies the total radiation dose required to control disease increases as tumour clonogen bulk increases. At the high-radiation doses required to sterilize macroscopic disease or even large quantities of microscopic disease there is very little therapeutic ratio in favour of tumour control over normal tissue damage. This leads to unacceptable late radiation effects in the breast and underlying chest wall. The 12% probability of ipsilateral breast recurrence in the adjuvant RT arm compared to 8% in the mastectomy arm of NSABP B-06 suggests that moderate-dose RT can achieve acceptable local control when the margins of excision are microscopically free of tumour cells (Fisher et al., 1989; Fisher et al., 1995).

Modern randomized controlled comparisons of BCS/RT and adjuvant RT with mastectomy indicate that breast preservation is not associated with any detriment to overall survival. However, local recurrence within the treated breast (3–20%) is more common than chest wall recurrence after mastectomy (4–9%) (Blichert-Toft et al., 1988; Fisher et al., 1989; Sarrazin et al., 1989; Veronesi et al., 1990; Straus et al., 1992; van Dongen et al., 1992; Fisher et al., 1995).

Natural history of and risk factors for local recurrence

The natural history of local recurrence is protracted with recurrence risks of 1–2% per year over at least 10 years following BCS/RT with most recurrences occurring within the index quadrant (Fourquet et al., 1989; Kurtz et al., 1989). In contrast, postmastectomy recurrence tends to occur within 3 years of surgery.

The selection of patients for a BCS/RT strategy should take into account factors known to increase the risk of breast recurrence. Young patient age (< 35–40 years) has been found to be a risk factor by several authors (Kurtz et al., 1988; Fourquet et al., 1989; Boyages et al., 1990; Kurtz et al., 1990a) and although youth correlates with the presence of adverse histopathological factors (Kurtz et al., 1990b) it independently signifies increased risk (Fourquet et al., 1989). Retrospective analyses indicate that patients younger than 35 years also have an increased risk of recurrence despite mastectomy (Donegan et al., 1966; Matthews et al., 1988). The prospective trials of BCS/RT versus mastectomy do not show any survival advantage for mastectomy in the subgroup of young patients. Youth is therefore not considered a contraindication to BCS/RT and adjuvant RT.

Tumour multifocality, high tumour grade, vascular invasion, the presence of an extensive intraduct component (EIC) and the inadequacy of the surgical margins of excision have been shown also to be risk factors for breast recurrence on multivariate analyses (Davis et al., 1986; Osteen et al., 1987; Smitt et al., 1995; Touboul et al., 1999; van Tienhoven et al., 1999). The presence of EIC correlates with the most extensive infiltration of intraduct carcinoma into breast tissue surrounding a macroscopic tumour (Ohtake et al., 1995). The increased risk of local recurrence associated with EIC is lost in a multivariate analysis controlled for the presence of a tumour-free margin of excision (Fourquet et al., 1989; Solin et al., 1991; Anscher et al., 1993; Borger et al., 1994; Gage et al., 1996). This suggests that the presence of EIC in the tumour, and a microscopically involved surgical margin, indicate a surrounding tumour bulk, which is less likely to be eradicated by moderate dose RT. If the excision margins are clear of tumour the significance of EIC is lost. This is presumably because the surrounding tumour burden is now sufficiently low to be sterilized by adjuvant RT.

The importance of local recurrence

Postmastectomy breast reconstruction has narrowed the cosmetic advantage of BCS/RT over mastectomy. This smaller advantage may not be considered to be sufficient by some women to risk the increase in local recurrence, which occurs if BCS/RT is undertaken in the presence of these risk factors. Whereas risk factors such as youth and tumour pathological features are beyond the control of clinicians, the adequacy of tumour excision may not be. It should be remembered that the standard management of a breast recurrence following adjuvant RT is mastectomy. Therefore, if prevention of local recurrence can be achieved by re-excision of the margin there may be considerable cosmetic advantage over the treatment of a subsequent recurrence by mastectomy.

The effect of breast recurrence on overall survival is controversial. The apparent lack of detriment to survival of BCS/RT, despite an increased risk of ipsilateral breast recurrence, argues against any detrimental effect of local recurrence on survival (Fisher et al., 1989; Sarrazin et al., 1989; Veronesi et al., 1990a; Blichert-Toft et al., 1992; Straus et al., 1992; van Dongen et al., 1992; Fisher et al., 1995). More recently, the effect of prevention of local or regional recurrence on survival has been demonstrated in the 15-year follow-up results of two trials of postmastectomy RT (Overgaard et al., 1997; Ragaz et al., 1997). They highlight the very long follow-up required to see differences in survival attributable to metastasis from local recurrence. This is especially the case in the context of BCS/RT as local recurrence is later than that occurring postmastectomy and risk of recurrence continues for at least 10 years following treatment (Fourquet et al., 1989; Kurtz et al., 1989). The NSABP B-06 trial has shown that patients with local recurrence following BCS without RT have an increased risk of metastatic disease (Fisher et al., 1995). Touboul et al. have found isolated and local recurrence to be an independent risk factor for metastatic disease with a relative risk (RR) of 9.9 (95% CI: 5.5–18) after a mean follow-up of 7 years (Touboul et al., 1999). It can be argued that these results may simply represent the effect of lead-time bias as those with local recurrence may have early metastatic disease detected when they are restaged. However, others argue that it is intuitive that local recurrence may lead to metastasis and thus compromise survival. The observed increases in distant metastasis associated with high rates of local recurrence may precede reductions in overall survival as observed in trials with 15-year follow-up (Hellman, 1997). Despite the controversy it seems sensible to minimize the risk of local recurrence associated with breast conservation if this can be achieved with good cosmetic outcome. If not, one should consider mastectomy and breast reconstruction in those whose risk factors indicate a risk of local recurrence unacceptable to the individual patient.

The balance between optimal local control and cosmesis

It has been shown in the Milan II trial that the risk of breast recurrence is inversely related to the volume of breast tissue resected. Quadrantectomy is associated with a risk of local recurrence of 5.3% and lumpectomy 13.3%, despite both being followed by RT. Microscopic involvement of the surgical margin by tumour occurred in 3% of the quadrantectomy group and 16% of the lumpectomy group. Cosmesis is significantly worse following quadrantectomy (Veronesi et al., 1990b). Others have confirmed this finding (Van Limbergen et al., 1989). There is thus a difficult balance between minimizing the volume of breast tissue removed in order to maintain a good cosmetic result and removing sufficient microscopic disease to allow maintenance of the radiation dose below that which leads to unacceptable late radiation damage which itself compromises cosmesis (Wazer et al., 1992).

Several important questions are thus raised when guiding a woman in making this choice. What are the risks of local recurrence contingent upon the differing microscopic status of the surgical excision margin? Can an increased dose of RT eradicate any increased risk of local recurrence without so adversely affecting breast cosmesis or the chest wall that mastectomy and breast reconstruction may be preferable to that patient? Does adjuvant systemic therapy reduce an increased risk of local recurrence associated with adverse margin status? Can re-excision reduce the risk of local recurrence?

The information in the literature is confounded by the heterogeneity of pathological margin assessment techniques, definitions of margin involvement, re-excision practices, breast radiation doses and the adequacy of length of follow-up required to detect recurrence following breast conservation. It should be noted that studies make no distinction between invasive tumour and the carcinoma in situ component when describing the surgical margin of excision.

Margin status and local recurrence risk

A number of authors have reported increased risk of breast recurrence following BCS/RT and RT associated with microscopic involvement of the final surgical margin, with actuarial recurrence rates of 2–5% for margin-negative groups and

16–21% for margin-positive groups (Kurtz et al., 1990b; Anscher et al., 1993; Borger et al., 1994; Spivack et al., 1994; Gage et al., 1996). More recent publications have suggested that although diffuse involvement of the margin is associated with an increased recurrence rate, focal involvement of the margin is not associated with increased risk of recurrence (Smitt et al., 1995; DiBiase et al., 1998; Peterson et al., 1999), at least not in the absence of EIC (Gage et al., 1996). The presence of more diffuse margin involvement and an EIC-positive tumour is associated with risk of breast recurrence as high as 40% (Gage et al., 1996). Other investigators have concluded that microscopic involvement of the surgical margin does not increase recurrence risk (Clarke et al., 1985; Schmidt-Ullrich et al., 1989; Solin et al., 1991).

Discussion of some of these individual reports is informative. Schmidt-Ullrich et al. (1989) found no increased risk of local recurrence associated with a positive surgical margin, with no patient in their series of 108 women suffering a local recurrence. However, they conservatively define a positive margin as tumour within 2 mm of the inked margin rather than the NSABP definition of malignant cells at the margin. Furthermore, all patients who had 'positive' resectable margins (i.e. not adjacent to the chest wall) were subsequently re-excised such that only seven patients had a <2 mm margin at the time of irradiation. In addition, patients with 2–5 mm and <2 mm clear margins received total RT doses of 65 and 70 Gy respectively. Patients treated to doses of 70 Gy with electrons were found to have an adverse cosmetic outcome.

Solin et al. (1991) in a study of 697 women, also found no increased risk of recurrence in patients with involved margins. All patients with diffusely positive margins had a re-excision or mastectomy. Only patients with negative or focally positive margin were managed by breast conservation and RT and patients with a focally positive margin received a higher dose to the tumour bed of 65 Gy rather than 60 Gy. Median follow-up was only 4 years. This series has recently been updated with results on 1021 women at a median follow-up of 6 years. The same conclusions were reached.

In a published experience of 436 patients at Institute Gustave-Roussy an 'insufficient margin' was not found to increase risk of local recurrence (Clarke et al., 1985). This data set was immature with a mean follow-up of 5 years and only 50% of patients followed for 5 years. 'Insufficient margin' is not defined and may simply confirm the findings of others that tumour close to, but not involving the margin, or only focally involving the margin, does not increase risk of local recurrence.

The Joint Center for Radiation Therapy (JCRT) in Boston published experience of 343 women with a median follow-up of 9 years. They demonstrated a high risk of local recurrence in patients with more than focal margin involvement (>3 lowpower microscopy fields involved) despite RT to a median tumour bed dose of 63 Gy. Crude 5-year local recurrence was 28% versus 9% for focally positive margins and 2% for negative margins. They also demonstrated a further increase in risk for tumours with EIC in which they find local recurrence rates of 42% in the group with more than focal margin involvement and 6% for the negative margin group (Gage et al., 1996) (Table 8.2).

It would appear from these various retrospective series that a tumour close to but not involving the resection margin is not associated with an increased risk of local recurrence. Minor involvement of the margin, less than 3 low power fields, for example, does not indicate residual tumour bulk sufficient to increase risk of local recurrence following RT to total doses of around 65 Gy, if there is no extensive EIC. The presence of EIC predicts an increased risk of local recurrence (26%) if margins are positive. More extensive involvement of the margin with malignant cells is associated with 10-year local recurrence rates as high as 30% rising to over 40% in the presence of EIC.

The effect of radiotherapy dose escalation

With regard to the effect of increasing RT dose, the JCRT group found no evidence of a reduced risk of recurrence associated with increased doses of RT above 64 Gy (Gage et al., 1996). This concurs with the experience of others. Kurtz et al. (1990b) found a local recurrence rate of 21% in patients with tumour at the margin or an indeterminate margin despite a tumour bed dose of 70–85 Gy. Patients with clear margins had a local recurrence rate of 5%. The Netherlands NCI found an actuarial 5-year local recurrence rate of 16% when malignant cells were at the margin and 2% for complete excision, in their study of outcome in 1026 women. This was despite a tumour bed dose of 75 Gy. In contrast, Spivack et al. (1994), who did not include any patients with extensively involved margins, found that in those with focally positive margins doses of at least 66 Gy were associated with local recurrence rate of 8% compared with 22% for patients receiving less than 66 Gy. The Stanford group did include patients with diffusely involved margins in their series of 289 women and found that in those without negative margins, tumour bed doses of at least 66 Gy achieved a 5-year local control rate of 96% rather than 82% for lower doses. This had dropped to 85% at 10 years, suggesting that higher radiation dose may delay but not prevent local recurrence (Smitt et al., 1995).

In answer to our second question, RT dose escalation in the tumour bed to about 64–70 Gy results in acceptable levels of local recurrence in those with focally positive margins but dose escalation even as high as 85 Gy does not seem to compensate for the presence of a more extensively involved margin. As radiation

Table 8.2. Five-year crude rates of recurrence by presence of extensive intraduct component and margin status

Final margins	EIC Negative			EIC Positive		
	IBR	p-value	DM/RNF/DOC	IBR	p-value	DM/RNF/DOC
All negative	1% (2/75)		24% (42/175)	6% (2/34)		12% (4/34)
All positive	12% (12/97)	$p < 0.0001$	32% (31/97)	26% (9/34)	$p = 0.06$	15% (5/34)
Negative >1 mm	1% (1/93)		24% (22/93)	14% (2/14)		14% (2/14)
Negative <1 mm	25%(1/44)	$p = 0.78$	25% (11/44)	0% (0/10)	$p = 0.40$	0% (0/10)
Negative NOS	0% (0/38)		24% (9/38)	0% (0/10)		20% (2/10)
Focally positive	9% (6/65)		25% (16/65)	7% (1/14)		21% (3/14)
>Focally positive	19% (6/31)		45% (14/31)	42% (8/19)	$p = 0.08$	11% (2/19)
Positive NOS	0% (0/1)		100% (1/1)	0% (0/1)		0% (0/1)

EIC extensive intraduct component; IBR ipsilateral breast recurrence; DM/RNF/DOC distant failure, regional lymph node failure, or death from other causes; NOS 'not otherwise specified', or the exact distance is unknown.

The p values compare all negative to all positive, negative >1 mm to negative, 1 mm and focally positive to >focally positive.

Gage et al., 1996.

doses rise above 65 Gy probability of late radiation damage and poor cosmesis rise rapidly. A much better idea of the effects of radiation dose escalation on local recurrence and cosmesis will be obtained when the EORTC 22881 trial reports. This trial examines the role, and dose-effect of tumour bed boost irradiation in completely excised (15 Gy vs. none) and incompletely excised (10 Gy vs. 25 Gy) breast tumours.

The influence of systemic therapy on local recurrence following breast conservation

There is clear evidence that chemotherapy alone does not reduce local recurrence risk after BCS (Fisher et al., 1989, 1995). The data on the influence of systemic therapy in addition to adjuvant RT on local recurrence is scarce. Retrospective series are confounded by competing risks, with those selected for systemic therapy more likely to develop distant disease before local recurrence and thus do not have any local recurrence recorded. In addition, there is little data on those patients with positive margins. The JCRT have found treatment with adjuvant chemotherapy to be associated with reduced risk of local failure following BCS/RT and RT (Rose et al., 1989). However this paper does not include data on the status of the surgical margin. Randomized data from NSABP B-13 indicates that in patients with clear margins adjuvant chemotherapy does appear to reduce risk of ipsilateral breast recurrence from 13.4% to 2.6% at 8 years (Fisher et al., 1996). It should be noted, however, that a tumour bed boost was not used in this trial and the total tumour bed dose was only 50 Gy.

For patients with involved margins, a multivariate analysis of the Stanford series found the use of concurrent adjuvant chemotherapy to be independently associated with better local control in those with margins that were not >2 mm clear. In the group with margins positive, indeterminate or <2 mm clear local control was 98% compared with 86% for those who did not receive chemotherapy (Smitt et al., 1995). However, only 81 patients received chemotherapy and only 17 patients in the whole series of 289 women had more than focally positive margins. Other series including patients with involved margins have not found use of adjuvant chemotherapy to be associated with reduced local recurrence risk (Ryoo et al., 1989; Kurtz et al., 1990a; Anscher et al., 1993; Borger et al., 1994; Spivack et al., 1994; Touboul et al., 1999).

In answer to our third question there is, therefore, insufficient data available to conclude that adjuvant chemotherapy can normalize the high risk of local recurrence following BCS/RT and RT associated with a more than focally positive margin. Limited data suggests that use of adjuvant chemotherapy, at least if given either concurrently, following the radiotherapy or in a sandwich fashion, may further reduce risk of local recurrence in those with margins that are not more than focally positive (Rose et al., 1989; Smitt et al., 1995; Fisher et al., 1996).

The effect of re-excision

Finally, can re-excision normalize the risk of local recurrence in those with positive margins? Smitt has found that patients with focally positive margins were no more likely to have residual tumour found on re-excision (28%) than those with negative margins (25%). This was in marked contrast to those with more extensive or unknown margin involvement (46%). Patients with tumours with EIC had residual carcinoma in 82% of re-excisions. They also found re-excision to be associated with reduced risk of local recurrence, with those who achieved a negative final margin having 100% local control at 10 years compared with 78% for those that did not (Smitt et al., 1995). Anscher et al. (1993) found that of 63 patients who had re-excision for positive or indeterminate margins, 7 patients maintained a positive margin of whom 2 recurred (28%). Of those 56 patients who attained a negative margin only 1 recurred (2%) compared to 1 out of the 76 patients who had negative initial margins (1.5%). The fact that the high predictive value of EIC for recurrence is lost when margins are clear further suggests that complete re-excision reduces recurrence risk (Gage et al., 1996). It is possible that the act of re-excision may not itself alter prognosis but may identify a group who continue to have positive margins who have residual disease beyond the control of adjuvant RT. Women in this group may prefer a mastectomy and reconstruction as the large-volume re-excisions are associated with very poor cosmesis, particularly when the breast is small (Wazer et al., 1992).

Postmastectomy radiotherapy

Despite the widespread use of BCS in the management of early breast cancer a significant number of patients are unsuitable for this approach and are offered mastectomy. Many women who are now offered mastectomy rather than breast conservation tend to have larger tumours with adverse histopathological prognostic features. Despite the near complete removal of breast tissue that occurs at mastectomy, locoregional recurrence occurs in 30–40% of women with these adverse prognostic features. The chest wall is the commonest site of locoregional recurrence and this is thought to arise from tumour infiltration through dermal lymphatics. Unsurprisingly, the presence of tumour in axillary lymph nodes is the strongest indicator of risk of locoregional recurrence. High-grade, tumour diameter >4 cm and direct invasion of skin or pectoral fascia are also risk factors. Unlike breast recurrence following breast-conservation surgery, chest wall recurrence can only be controlled in about half of patients. Uncontrolled chest wall recurrence, which commonly progresses to encase the hemithorax, is one of the most distressing manifestations of advanced breast cancer and is difficult to adequately palliate.

Adjuvant RT may be used following surgery with two potential benefits: first, reduction in risk of locoregional recurrence; secondly, and more recently documented, is benefit in overall survival in both pre and postmenopausal women at high risk for recurrence treated with both adjuvant systemic therapy and modern adjuvant RT techniques.

A number of trials over the past 30 years have examined the effect of postoperative RT on these two endpoints. Unfortunately, trials have shown a great deal of heterogeneity with widely differing radiation volumes, techniques, volumes of normal tissue irradiation and RT dose/fractionation schedules. In order to achieve locoregional tumour eradication and prevent distant dissemination of disease RT must be delivered to the full extent of the predicted residual tumour burden without the inclusion of sufficient pulmonary or cardiac tissue sufficient to cause morbidity or mortality. It is also clear that locoregional RT cannot have any effect on survival in patients who already harbour micrometastatic disease and do not receive appropriate adjuvant systemic therapy. Many of the early trials were conducted before adjuvant systemic therapy had been shown to eradicate micrometastatic disease in some patients and before modern RT techniques which minimize normal tissue irradiation effects were widely used.

A meta-analysis of all randomized controlled trials (RCTs) started prior to 1975 and published in 1987, showed that postmastectomy RT was associated with a 66% reduction in risk of locoregional recurrence. RT was, however, associated with an excess mortality in those living more than 10 years after randomization. In this group the 25-year survival was 42% following RT and 51% following surgery alone. An update of the data was published in 1994, indicated that the excess mortality in the RT group was due to cardiac deaths and was balanced by a reduction in breast cancer mortality. In 1995 the EBCTCG initially published a meta-analysis of RCTs started prior to 1985; this has recently been updated (EBCTCG, 2000). This included 14 500 women randomized in 32 trials where primary surgery involved some form of mastectomy and 3000 women randomized in trials where surgery involved BCS. The use of RT was associated with a 66% reduction in risk of local recurrence. There was, however, no difference in 10-year overall survival, being 40.3% for RT and 41.4% for surgery alone. There was a statistically significant difference in OS associated with use of adjuvant RT, in those treated by mastectomy and axillary sampling (Odds Reduction (OR) $14\% \pm$ SD 7%, $P = 0.004$) in comparison with those treated by mastectomy alone (OR $3\% \pm$ SD 4%, $P =$ NS) or mastectomy and axillary clearance (OR $- 3\% \pm 4\%$

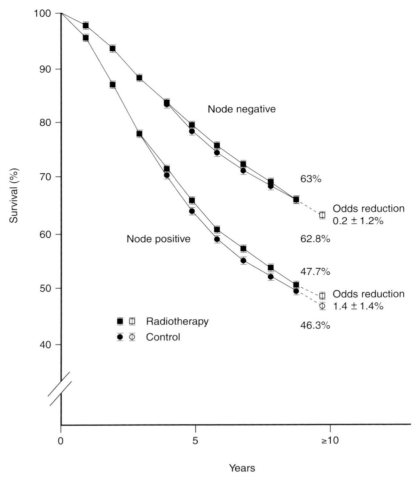

Figure 8.1　10-year survival among approximately 16 000 women in 35 randomized trials comparing surgery plus radiotherapy with surgery alone

SD, $P = $ NS). There was no significant heterogeneity among the four subgroups or between trials and thus no sound statistical evidence that, in relation to survival, RT benefited some surgical subgroups but not others. There was no evidence that RT affected overall survival in the presence or absence of involved axillary lymph nodes (EBCTCG, 1995) (Figure 8.1).

　RT was associated with a reduced risk of death due to breast cancer (OR 0.94; 95% CI: 0.88–1.00), i.e. 0–5 fewer deaths due to breast cancer per 100 women treated. However, there was an increased risk of death from other causes (OR 1.24; 95% CI: 1.09–1.42, $p = 0.002$). The relative increase in risk of death was the same in ages <50 yrs, 50–59 yrs and >60 years at the time of randomization. However, the absolute excess risk of death associated with RT was greater in those aged over 60 at randomization (4.2%) compared with those aged less than 50 (0.5%). Trials which included the irradiation of the internal mammary nodes, or use of older orthovoltage RT, were compared with those that did not. The former were thought to be associated with greater cardiac mortality. There was no evidence of this, with the proportionate increase in non-breast-cancer mortality being at least as great in the latter group. This does not indicate that cardiac irradiation did not affect non-breast-cancer mortality as inappropriately large chest wall radiation fields, and absence of cardiac shielding, may have increased cardiac damage in many of these trials, despite the lack of internal mammary or orthovoltage irradiation.

Use of RT was associated with a reduction in risk of breast cancer deaths (OR 0.94; 95% CI: 0.88–1.00). At the most optimistic extreme this would mean a 22% reduction in breast cancer deaths but is also statistically compatible with a negligibly small breast cancer survival benefit. It therefore seems that adjuvant RT after mastectomy may have a small beneficial effect on breast cancer mortality but this is negated by a small excess risk of cardiac mortality. This adverse effect is greatest in the older trials using large radiation fields, high biologically equivalent doses of radiation and radiation techniques with poor dose homogeneity (Cuzick et al., 1994) (Figures 8.2, 8.3).

It is important to note that modern RT techniques recognize the importance of minimizing the cardiac volume irradiated and use fractionated RT regimens that reduce normal tissue radiation late side-effects.

It is clear that adjuvant RT reduces the risk of locoregional recurrence following mastectomy. Any effect of RT on survival must be via the eradication of loco-regional disease and prevention of metastatic dissemination. As breast cancer metastasises at an early stage any survival benefit from RT will be seen in only a very small minority unless used in conjunction with adjuvant systemic therapy. The 1995 EBCTCG overview illustrates the heterogeneity of the examined trials with regard to systemic therapy (EBCTCG, 1995).

Three large randomized trials have recently reported long-term results of addition of postoperative RT to mastectomy in high-risk premenopausal women treated with CMF chemotherapy and high-risk postmenopausal women treated with tamoxifen.

In the Danish trial, 1789 premenopausal women were included who were defined as high risk by virtue of pathologically positive axillary lymph nodes, tumour >5 cm in diameter or invasion of the skin or the pectoral fascia (Overgaard et al., 1997). Following total mastectomy with stripping of the pectoral fascia and level I/II axillary dissection patients received 8–9 cycles of CMF chemotherapy. Women were randomized to RT and this was delivered to the chest

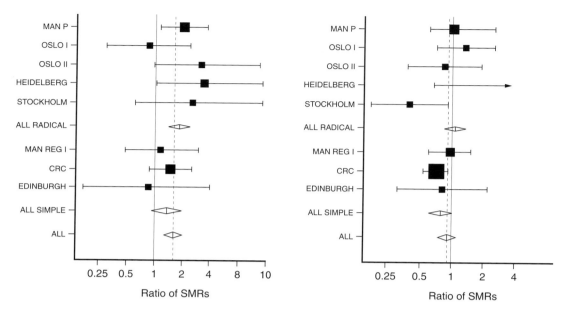

Figure 8.2   Cardiac and breast cancer mortality. Left panel: SMRs (radiotherapy/no radiotherapy) and 95% CIs by trial for cardiac mortality (after 10 years). Right panel: SMRs (radiotherapy/no radiotherapy) and 95% CIs by trial for breast cancer mortality (after 10 years)

wall, axilla, supra and infraclavicular nodes and the internal mammary nodes using a cardiac sparing technique. After a median follow-up of 114 months the use of RT was associated with a 21% absolute reduction in risk of local recurrence (9% vs. 32%, $p < 0.001$) and a 9% absolute increase in OS ($p < 0.001$) (Figure 8.3). The effect of RT on overall survival was irrespective of tumour size, node status, number of positive nodes or the histopathological grade (Table 8.3). A median of only seven nodes was removed by axillary dissection but this group has recently presented data showing the effect of RT to be the same in the subgroup of patients who had more than seven nodes resected (presented orally at BBG, Overgaard et al., Guildford, 1999).

The British Columbia trial also examined the effect of postoperative RT in premenopausal women with pathologically involved axillary lymph nodes treated with modified radical mastectomy, including level I/II axillary dissection and six cycles of CMF chemotherapy. This group also irradiated the axilla, supraclavicular fossa and IMC and used a relatively low biological equivalent radiation dose, which reduces late normal tissue damage. After a 15-year follow-up the use of RT was associated with a 20% absolute reduction in risk of locoregional recurrence (13% vs. 33%, $p = 0.003$), 17% absolute increase in disease-free survival (50% vs. 33%, $p = 0.007$) and in metastasis-free survival (51% vs. 34%, $p = 0.006$). Overall

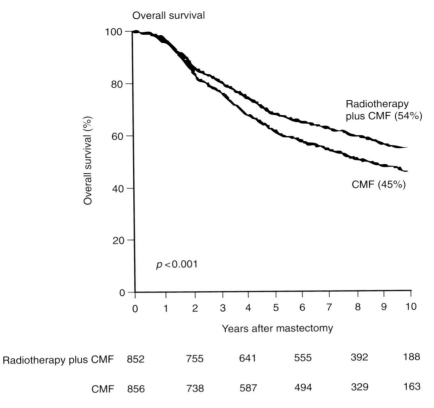

Figure 8.3   Kaplan–Meir estimates of overall survival among women treated with radiotherapy plus CMF and CMF alone

Note: Values in parentheses are overall survival at 10 years.

survival was improved by 8% at 15 years (54% vs. 46%, $p = 0.007$) (Ragaz et al., 1997). Overall survival data was recently updated at the San Antonio Breast Cancer meeting 1998, showing a statistically significant 30% reduction in risk of death (RR 0.7, $p = 0.002$) associated with use of RT. There was no difference in the relative benefit of RT in those women with 1–3 or >3 nodes involved. There was no excess cardiac morbidity or mortality in either of these trials.

These trials have received some criticism because the chemotherapy used, three-weekly intravenous CMF is considered suboptimal in comparison to more modern anthracycline-containing regimens. In the absence of data showing a reduction of risk of death of equivalent magnitude for anthracycline-containing adjuvant regimens over CMF, it seems unlikely that the use of these regimens would negate the 30% reduction of risk of death gained by use of RT seen in these trials. Both of these trials demonstrate that prevention of locoregional recurrence reduces metastatic disease and death.

Table 8.3. Cox multivariate proportional hazards analysis of the relative risk of any type of recurrence or death or of death from any cause

Variable	Any type of recurrence or death		Death	
	P Value	RR (95% CI)	P Value	RR (95% CI)
Tumour size (<21 mm, 21–50 mm, >50 mm)	<0.001	1.43 (1.30–1.58)	<0.001	1.49 (1.35–1.65)
No. of positive nodes (0, 1–3, >3)	<0.001	1.57 (1.36–1.81)	<0.001	1.75 (1.5–2.05)
Frequency of positive nodes (<34%, 34–67%, >67%)	<0.001	1.44 (1.30–1.58)	<0.001	1.38 (1.24–1.53)
Grade of anaplasia (I, II, III)	<0.001	1.44 (1.31–1.59)	<0.001	1.52 (1.37–1.70)
Age of 40–49 yr (vs. <40 yr and 50–59 yr)	<0.001	0.73 (0.64–0.83)	<0.001	0.76 (0.66–0.87)
Radiotherapy + CMF (vs. CMF alone)	<0.001	0.59 (0.51–0.67)	<0.001	0.71 (0.62–0.82)

The analysis included 1584 patients; RR relative risk; CI confidence interval.
Overgaard et al., 1997.

The effect of postmastectomy RT in postmenopausal women <70 years of age treated with adjuvant tamoxifen has recently been reported by the Danish Breast Cancer cooperative group (Overgaard et al., 1999): 1460 women were treated with total mastectomy and level I/II axillary dissection. All had either pathologically involved axillary lymph nodes, tumours >5 cm in diameter or involvement of skin or pectoral fascia. All received 30 mg tamoxifen daily for a year. Women were randomized to RT to the chest wall, axilla, supra/infraclavicular fossa and IMC or no RT. After a median follow-up of 119 months for survivors and 46 months for those who died, locoregional recurrence had occurred in 8% of the women who had RT arm and 35% of those who did not. RT was associated with a 9% absolute overall survival advantage at 10 years (45% vs. 36%, $p = 0.03$) (Figure 8.4). There was no difference in proportionate benefit of RT in those with large or small tumours or with few or many positive nodes. The median number of nodes removed was seven. The proportionate benefit of RT was identical in those who had more or less than eight nodes removed. The benefit of RT on overall survival only becomes apparent more than 4 years after randomization. There was no evidence of increased cardiac morbidity or mortality after 10 years of follow-up.

The duration of tamoxifen treatment and the absence of use of adjuvant chemotherapy would now be considered suboptimal. Whether the reduction in

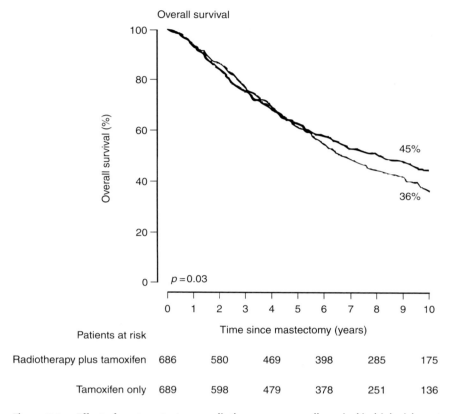

Figure 8.4   Effect of postmastectomy radiotherapy on overall survival in high-risk postmenopausal women

risk of local recurrence and subsequent improval in overall survival associated with RT would be nullified by the use of tamoxifen for 5 years is unknown. One would have to demonstrate a sustained 27% absolute improvement in loco-regional recurrence and 9% absolute improvement in survival compared with 1 year of tamoxifen alone to negate the observed advantage to RT.

These three randomized trials including 3500 women treated with more modern RT techniques and with adjuvant systemic therapy demonstrate very similar absolute improvements in locoregional recurrence and overall survival. Based on these data postmastectomy RT will prevent 1 death for every 11 women treated, and one locoregional recurrence for every 3–5 women treated.

It is possible that adequate systemic therapy for micrometastatic disease is required for the full impact of locoregional therapy to be manifest as improved overall survival. A recent meta-analysis has reported a systematic review of randomized trials that have examined the effectiveness of locoregional RT in patients treated by 'definitive' surgery and adjuvant systemic therapies (Whelan et al., 2000). It included 18 trials conducted between 1967 and 1999, involving a total of 6367 patients; most studies included both pre and postmenopausal women with node-positive breast cancer treated with modified radical mastectomy, and CMF or anthracycline-based chemotherapy. Radiation was shown to reduce the risk of locoregional recurrence (odds ratio, 0.25; 95% CI: 0.19–0.34) and mortality (odds ratio, 0.83; 95% CI: 0.74–0.94). Their study further supports the notion that, in the presence of effective systemic therapy, locoregional control may prevent secondary spread from regional sites and thus influence survival.

There are further questions raised by these trials. Most locoregional recurrences occur on the chest wall. We must determine whether the lymphatic components of the RT confer the survival advantage, as they are complex and involve greater normal tissue irradiation. The Canadian NCI are running a trial comparing chest wall irradiation alone with chest wall and supraclavicular fossa (SCF/axilla/IMC) irradiation. The EORTC will also be examining the effect of addition of IMC/ supraclavicular fields to chest wall irradiation.

There is no obvious reason why patients with positive lymph nodes treated by breast-conservation surgery should not gain a similar survival advantage from modern adjuvant RT in addition to systemic therapy. The Canadian NCI are also examining this by randomizing women to breast radiation with or without axilla/SCF/IMC irradiation.

Optimizing breast conservation with adjuvant radiotherapy

Current research is now focusing on optimizing the physical delivery of RT to maintain benefits of treatment, with reduced late toxicity. Active studies are addressing technical issues such as optimal dose fractionation, and improved homogeneity of dose delivery by intensity-modulation of beams (IMRT). Given the increasing proportion of women receiving both adjuvant chemotherapy and RT we need to define the most efficacious sequencing based on evidence. Finally, as the UK breast screening programme identifies a significant proportion of women with ductal carcinoma in situ or small (<2 cm) low-grade, node-negative cancers, we need to carefully examine the role of adjuvant RT in such good prognosis patients to be certain that treatment is efficacious.

Variation in UK radiotherapy practices for women with breast cancer: the START study

As a result of the empirical nature of development of RT practice, internationally it has become standard to treat women with early breast cancer with a schedule giving 46–50 Gray (Gy) total dose in 2.0 Gy fractions to the breast or chest wall. For reasons of resource, and patient convenience, in the UK there has been a practice of using fraction sizes of greater than 2.0 Gy, with a 'compensatory' reduction in total dose, and number of treatment visits. Over decades, experience has suggested that apparently similar levels of tumour control and late normal tissue effects can be achieved with empirically derived scheduling using several alternative fractionations. A national audit by the Royal College of Radiologists revealed three commonly used schedules: 50 Gy in 25 fractions over 5 weeks; 45 Gy in 20 fractions over 4 weeks and 40 Gy in 15 fractions over 3 weeks (Yarnold et al., 1995). Analysis suggests that these schedules are similar in their effects on breast normal tissues when adjustment is made for differences in fraction size and overall time using the linear-quadratic model of radiation effect. However, it is possible that this model does predict for important late effects in a range of critical adjacent normal tissues, for example, the brachial plexus, or coronary arteries. A major challenge in the RT of breast cancer is to deliver in a homogenious manner a dose likely to confer high tumour control rates, with low or ideally zero dose to nontarget structures. In practice, the anatomical contours of the breast or chest wall, and adjacent node groups create a complex challenge. Dose variations of greater than 10% across the breast results with 'standard' beam shaping. This is far in excess of that considered good clinical practice for curative RT in other tumour treatment scenarios. Similarly, junctions between adjacent treatment fields are difficult to maintain accurately due to patient movement, especially respiration.

The START study was designed to prospectively address the sensitivity of breast cancer and normal tissues to total dose and its fractionation. It represents one of the most important, comprehensively designed trials of adjuvant RT undertaken in breast cancer. Trial A tests the hypothesis that modest increases in fraction sizes of greater than 2.0 Gy (3.0 Gy, or 3.2 Gy) are as effective and safe with respect to tumour control and late toxicities in the use of RT to treat the chest wall or conserved breast. The pilot study was undertaken jointly between the Royal Marsden Hospital and the Gloucestershire Oncology Centre between 1986 and 1998; 1410 patients were randomized between three arms, testing 25 daily fractions of 2.0 Gy against 13 fractions of 3.0 Gy or 3.3 Gy on alternate days over 5 weeks. The same overall treatment time in all schedules controlled for differential effects of normal and tumour cell proliferation on outcome. An interim analysis conducted in 1998 on 1158 cases included detailed evaluation of late effects on the breast, skin, shoulder function and lymphoedema. It confirmed the expected dose–response relationship for late effects in the breast between 39–42.9 Gy. As only 318 of 1158 patients had received nodal irradiation it was considered inappropriate to reach conclusions as to the efficacy of larger than 2.0 Gy fractions to this critical region. There were also too few tumour events to give reliable information on the impact of such scheduling on breast cancer radiosensitivity.

The UK multicentre study was activated in April 1999. Endpoints of the study now prospectively record locoregional tumour control, physician-recorded normal tissue effects (and patient self-assessment/quality of life in a subset), second primary cancers, overall survival and disease-free survival. Patients showing unexpectedly severe acute or late normal tissue reactions will be recorded. All trial patients will be invited to participate in an associated study whereby blood is stored for future studies exploring biological determinants of radiosensitivity. A total of 2000 patients in addition to the 1410 entered in the pilot study will be needed to gain reliable comparisons of tumour control. Higher numbers may be required to generate acceptable estimates of radiosensitivity of differing normal tissues and their dependence on fraction size (so-called α/β values).

Trial B is a two-arm study comparing 40 Gy in 15 fractions of 2.67 Gy over 3 weeks with 50 Gy in 25 fractions of 2 Gy over 5 weeks. Retrospective studies suggest both schedules produce similar clinical effects, but much larger patient numbers are needed to detect small but clinically significant differences in tumour control or side-effects. This design will not contribute directly to our knowledge of the biomathematics of radiation effects as both fraction size and overall time are variables in both arms.

If the trial confirms that schedules using fraction sizes of >2.0 Gy are as efficacious as those using 2 Gy, the average number of visits for RT will be reduced, which will be welcomed by patients. If however, 2.0 Gy fraction sizes are optimal, the finding will have considerable financial implications for the NHS, requiring significant investment in both specialist staff and equipment!

Sequencing of chemotherapy and radiotherapy

The optimal timing and sequencing of adjuvant chemotherapy and RT following breast-conserving surgery or mastectomy has yet to be defined. Whilst early studies on perioperative chemotherapy suggested that early initiation of systemic therapy may improve survival (Nissen-Meyer et al., 1978), recent randomized data comparing neoadjuvant versus adjuvant chemotherapy have so far failed to demonstrate a survival advantage (Fisher et al., 1998). A small body of evidence would suggest that delaying chemotherapy might have a survival disadvantage, while delaying RT may increase local recurrence rate. Simultaneous treatment, especially with methotrexate or anthracycline-containing regimens enhances both acute and late RT toxicity. In the UK, current practice is evenly divided between 'sequential' (CT then RT) and 'synchronous' (CT, then RT, completion of CT). Several retrospective studies have reported a trend to higher local recurrence rates if RT is delayed to complete chemotherapy delivery (Recht et al., 1991; Hartsell et al., 1992; Buchholz et al., 1993; Slotman et al., 1994). Only one randomized study has specifically examined sequencing. Recht et al. reported a study in which 244 patients were randomized between CT followed by RT, versus the reverse sequence. It reported a higher local recurrence rate in the delayed RT arm (14% vs. 5%) $p = 0.07$) but the study was too small to give a definitive answer. Three studies have suggested that delaying CT by 4–6 weeks to complete RT may prejudice survival. Lara-Jimenez et al. (1991) reported actuarial survival rates at 10 years of 41%, 46% and 57% for a three-way randomization between RT–CT, compared with CT–RT, or CT–RT–CT respectively. In the study reported by Recht the 5-year actuarial rate of distant metastases was higher in those receiving RT prior to CT (36% vs. 25%, $p = 0.05$) with no significant differences in overall survival. The two recent studies suggesting an impact on survival of locoregional RT over and above CMF-based CT alone after mastectomy (Overgaard et al., 1997; Ragaz et al., 1997) both utilized 'sandwich' scheduling, with RT delivered between the first and second cycles of CT.

The SECRAB study is a UK-based, prospective, multicentre randomized study of 2000 women with early breast cancer who have a clear indication for both adjuvant CT and RT. Patients are randomized to either synchronous chemoRT, in which RT is given between the second and third cycles, or CT followed by RT. Permitted CT schedules include CMF (i.v. or oral) or hybrid anthracycline–CMF (Bonnadonna regimen) or epirubicin + CMF as in the National Breast Cancer study of epirubucin + CMF versus classical CMF adjuvant therapy (the NEAT study). Similarly, clinicians can elect to use their standard RT fractionation, including fraction sizes of 2–3 Gy. Irradiation of the IMC is not allowed and treatment of supraclavicular nodes discouraged due to uncertainty regarding potential for increased brachial plexus injury with synchronous therapy. The primary endpoint of the study is local tumour recurrence rate at 5 years. Important secondary endpoints include distant relapse and overall survival, acute toxicity causing delays or dose reduction, with substudy evaluation of cosmesis and quality of life.

Radiotherapy and postmastectomy breast reconstruction

Despite the success of conservative therapy for early breast cancer many patients still require or choose mastectomy. For these patients the option of immediate breast reconstruction offers an improved cosmesis, body image and quality of life (Noone et al., 1982; Dean et al., 1983; Stevens et al., 1984; Schain et al., 1985; Franchelli et al., 1995). There has in recent years been an increase in the number of reconstructions performed. As the indications for postmastectomy RT do not change with the presence of a breast reconstruction there are now more patients who require adjuvant postmastectomy RT who will have undergone reconstructive procedures.

How RT impacts on the success of a breast reconstruction has implications for the advice and information given to patients regarding optimal timing of the procedure, the techniques used and the likely outcome of the procedure in terms of cosmesis and complication rate. Were it demonstrated that RT had a significant negative effect on cosmesis or other quality of life areas then one would have to consider omitting or delaying the reconstruction in order to avoid this negative effect.

Radiotherapy and implant reconstruction

Implant reconstruction usually involves either subpectoral prosthesis implantation only or a latissimus dorsi (LD) myocutaneous flap with an underlying implant. Outcome measures in series reporting the results of implant reconstruction and RT vary and it is often difficult to compare figures. In addition, surgical techniques vary between institutions and individual surgeons, the type of implant may vary and there is likely to be significant publication bias. Surgical revision rates can include implant removal, capsulotomy, wound debridement and adjustment of implant position.

Papers that have directly compared irradiated and nonirradiated patients have reported conflicting results (Asplund, 1984; Lejour et al., 1988; Barreau-Pouhaer et al., 1992; Rosato & Dowden, 1994; Evans et al., 1995; Spear, 1995). A series from the Royal Marsden Hospital and St George's Hospital in London did not show an overall effect of RT on the need for revision. On further analysis it was found that this lack of effect was confined to the LD flap reconstructions, which made up the majority of those in the RT group. The requirement for surgical revision for the implant-only reconstructions, however, increased from 19% to 44% ($p = 0.029$) with the addition of RT ($p = 0.049$). This difference between the interaction of RT with LD flap and implant-only reconstructions has not been a consistent finding in the literature (Kuske et al., 1991; Evans et al., 1995). It can, however, be explained by the impact of stretching of the skin over the implant-only reconstructions impairing the blood flow in small vessels. This vascular effect may be exacerbated by RT resulting in increased fibrosis, a process common to all implants and which RT can also generate. Furthermore, there may in fact be little difference in the degree of fibrosis around the implants beneath LD flaps, but rather it might be masked by a padding effect due to the bulk of the myocutaneous flap.

The use of a boost dose and the regular use of skin bolus have been shown to impact on the outcome of reconstructions (Kuske et al., 1991; Victor et al., 1998). The native skin of the chest wall is, however, part of the target volume for postmastecomy RT and it is unclear what effect omitting the bolus might have. Fraction size has not been noted to impact on the outcome of irradiated reconstructions.

A number of authors have suggested delaying reconstruction in patients likely to require RT (Kuske et al., 1991; Barreau-Pouhaer et al., 1992; von Smitten & Sundell, 1992; Evans et al., 1995; Victor et al., 1998). This would certainly avoid direct irradiation of the prosthesis and also prevent irradiation during the period of capsule formation around the implant. There is no direct evidence in the literature to support the hypothesis that this would result in an improved complication rate, although the reported contracture rate tends to be lower in series with RT prior to reconstruction than in those with reconstruction prior to RT (Frazier & Noone, 1985; Rosato & Dowden, 1994; Evans et al., 1995; Spear, 1995; Ramon et al., 1997).

It should not be forgotten that there are a number of other factors that affect the outcome of reconstructions including surgical technique and expertise, choice of implant, appropriate antibacterial therapy and patient factors such as age and cigarette smoking. Furthermore, most implants that are removed because of capsule formation are successfully replaced with a good outcome.

Finally, cosmetic outcome has been directly compared for RT and non-RT patients in only one paper (von Smitten & Sundell, 1992). This reported significantly worse cosmesis with RT. In general, however, even with RT the proportion of patients with good or excellent cosmesis scores (albeit with various methods of assessment) is reasonably high (Stabile et al., 1980; Kuske et al., 1991; Chu et al., 1992; Jackson et al., 1994; Evans et al., 1995; Victor et al., 1998).

Dose distribution

The target volume for postmastectomy RT includes the skin of the chest wall and the superficial fascia of the underlying muscles. Does the presence of a breast prosthesis interfere with the dose distribution within this volume? A number of studies have investigated this question (McGinley et al., 1980; Shedbalkar et al., 1980; Krishnan et al., 1983; Kuske et al., 1991; Jackson et al., 1994) testing water and saline-filled expanders and silicone implants in a variety of experimental conditions. Whilst some minor variations from tissue equivalence have been detected, these papers concluded that there were no clinically relevant differences in dosimetry comparing silicone implants to tissue equivalent material. It is certainly not necessary to alter the field arrangements because of the presence of the implant.

Radiotherapy and TRAM flap reconstruction

Transverse rectus abdominis muscle (TRAM) myocutaneous flap reconstruction is usually performed without prosthesis implantation. A number of studies have reported significantly increased complication rates (mostly flap failure and fat necrosis) in patients with a history of prior RT (Hartrampf & Bennett, 1987; Banic et al., 1995; Watterson et al., 1995) and a worse cosmetic outcome (Kroll et al.,

Table 8.4. Current issues in the optimization of breast cancer radiotherapy

Tumour Group	Strategies
(1) 'Excellent prognosis', e.g. DCIS; small, low-grade, node-negative cancers	?Selective avoidance or decreased dose-intensity of post-operative radiotherapy ?Conformal or intensity modulated beams to minimize dose to normal tissue, e.g. heart
(2) 'Good prognosis', e.g. breast-conserving surgery, node-negative cancers	Greater attention to balance between radiotherapy intensity and surgical excision margins Improved cosmesis by evaluation of dose/fractionation issues; necessity for tumour bed boost; improved dose homogeneity
(3) 'Moderate prognosis', e.g. breast-conserving surgery, node-positive, locally advanced, operable by mastectomy ± reconstruction	Optimized dosimetry to chest wall/breast and regional nodes; analysis of contribution of components of regional treatment to control and survival; optimized sequencing with chemotherapy
(4) Locally advanced, inoperable or inflammatory	Optimized sequencing of treatment modalities; role of radiotherapy ± mastectomy after induction chemotherapy in inflammatory cancers

1995). Three studies have addressed the question of administering RT to such a reconstructed breast. Hunt et al. (1997) and Zimmerman et al. (1998) reported no complications in a total of 40 patients whilst Kuske et al. (1991) reported five complications in nine patients of whom eight had TRAM and one had gluteal flap transfers. In the Marsden/St George's series nine patients underwent 12 TRAM flap reconstructions. Eight women had received prior RT and two received postreconstruction RT. There have been no cases requiring surgical revision with a median follow-up of 16 months.

Conclusion

It is clear that RT and breast reconstruction can be safely combined. The difference between implant only and LD flap reconstruction when combined with RT is such that the former should only be offered to cancer patients with a very low likelihood of requiring RT. It must be remembered in evaluating the outcome that the alternative management in these patients is mastectomy without reconstruction and not reconstruction without RT.

Summary

Adjuvant RT has an established role in the reduction of risk of locoregional breast cancer recurrence, both postmastectomy and after breast conserving surgery. It may also impact on OS, adding to the benefits accruing to systemic adjuvant therapy. A summary of strategies aimed at optimizing the therapeutic ratio even further is contained in Table 8.4.

REFERENCES

Anscher, M.S., Jones, P., Prosnitz, L.R. et al. (1993). Local failure and margin status in early-stage breast carcinoma treated with conservation surgery and radiation therapy. *Annals of Surgery*, 218(1), 22–8.

Asplund, O. (1984). Capsular contracture in silicone gel and saline-filled breast implants after reconstruction. *Plastic and Reconstructive Surgery*, 73(2), 270–5.

Banic, A., Boeckx, W., Greulich, M. et al. (1995). Late results of breast reconstruction with free TRAM flaps: a prospective multicentric study. *Plastic and Reconstructive Surgery*, 95(7), 1195–204; discussion 1205–6.

Barreau-Pouhaer, L., Le, M.G., Rietjiens, M. et al. (1992). Risk factors for failure of immediate breast reconstruction with prosthesis after total mastectomy for breast cancer. *Cancer*, 70(5), 1145–51.

Blichert-Toft, M., Brincker, H., Andersen, J.A. et al. (1988). A Danish randomized trial comparing breast-preserving therapy with mastectomy in mammary carcinoma. Preliminary results. *Acta Oncologica*, 27(6A), 671–7.

Blichert-Toft, M., Rose, C., Andersen, J. et al. (1992). Danish randomised trial comparing breast conservation therapy with mastectomy: six years of life-table analysis. *Journal of the National Cancer Institute Monograms*, 11, 19–25.

Borger, J., Kemperman, H., Hart, A. et al. (1994). Risk factors in breast-conservation therapy. *Journal of Clinical Oncology*, 12(4), 653–60.

Boyages, J., Recht, A., Connolly, J.L. et al. (1990). Early breast cancer: predictors of breast recurrence for patients treated with conservative surgery and radiation therapy. *Radiotherapy Oncology*, 19(1), 29–41.

Buchholz, T.A., Austin-Seymour, M.M., Moe, R.E. et al. (1993). Effect of delay in radiation in the combined modality treatment of breast cancer. *International Journal of Radiation Oncology, Biology, Physics*, 26(1), 23–35.

Chu, F.C., Kaufmann, T.P., Dawson, G.A. et al. (1992). Radiation therapy of cancer in prosthetically augmented or reconstructed breasts. *Radiology*, 185(2), 429–33.

Clarke, D.H., Lê, M.G., Sarrazin, D. et al. (1985). Analysis of local-regional relapses in patients with early breast cancers treated by excision and radiotherapy: experience of the Institut Gustave-Roussy. *International Journal of Radiation Oncology, Biology, Physics*, 11(1), 137–45.

Cuzick, J., Stewart, H., Rutqvist, L. et al. (1994). Cause-specific mortality in long-term survivors of breast cancer who participated in trials of radiotherapy. *Journal of Clinical Oncology*, 12(3), 447–53.

Davis, B.W., Gelber, R.D., Goldhirsch, A. et al. (1986). Prognostic significance of tumor grade in clinical trials of adjuvant therapy for breast cancer with axillary lymph node metastasis. *Cancer*, 58(12), 2662–70.

Dean, C., Chetty, U. & Forrest, A.P. (1983). Effects of immediate breast reconstruction on psychosocial morbidity after mastectomy. *Lancet*, 1(8322), 459–62.

DiBiase, S J., Komarnicky, L.T., Schwartz, G.F. et al. (1998). The number of positive margins influences the outcome of women treated with breast preservation for early stage breast carcinoma. *Cancer*, 82(11), 2212–20.

Donegan, W.L., Perez-Mesa, C.M. & Watson, F.R. et al. (1966). A biostatistical study of locally recurrent breast carcinoma. *Surgery, Gynecology and Obstetrics*, 122(3): 529–40.

EBCTCG (1995). Effects of radiotherapy and surgery in early breast cancer: an overview of the randomized trials. Early Breast Cancer Trialists' Collaborative Group. *New England Journal of Medicine*, 333(22), 1444–55.

EBCTCG (2000). Favourable and unfavourable effects on long-term survival of radiotherapy for early breast cancer: an overview of the randomised trials. Early Breast Cancer Trialists' Collaborative Group. *Lancet*, 355 (9217), 1757–70.

Evans, G.R., Schusterman, M.A., Kroll, S.S. et al. (1995). Reconstruction and the radiated breast: is there a role for implants? *Plastic and Reconstructive Surgery*, 96(5): 1111–15; discussion, 1116–18.

Fisher, B., Redmond, C., Poisson, R. et al. (1989). Eight-year results of a randomized clinical trial comparing total mastectomy and lumpectomy with or without irradiation in the treatment of breast cancer. *New England Journal of Medicine*, 320(13), 822–8.

Fisher, B., Anderson, S., Redmond, C.K. et al. (1995). Reanalysis and results after 12 years of follow-up in a randomized clinical trial comparing total mastectomy with lumpectomy with or without irradiation in the treatment of breast cancer. *New England Journal of Medicine*, 333(22), 1456–61.

Fisher, B., Dignam, J., Mamounas, E.P. et al. (1996). Sequential methotrexate and fluorouracil for the treatment of node-negative breast cancer patients with estrogen receptor-negative tumors: eight-year results from National Surgical Adjuvant Breast and Bowel Project (NSABP) B-13 and first report of findings from NSABP B-19 comparing methotrexate and fluorouracil with conventional cyclophosphamide, methotrexate, and fluorouracil. *Journal of Clinical Oncology*, 14(7), 1982–92.

Fisher, B., Bryant J., Wolmark, N. et al. (1998). Effect of preoperative chemotherapy on the outcome of women with operable breast cancer. *Journal of Clinical Oncology*, 16(8), 2672–85.

Fourquet, A., Campana, F., Zafrani, B. et al. (1989). Prognostic factors of breast recurrence in the conservative management of early breast cancer: a 25-year follow-up. *International Journal of Radiation Oncology, Biology, Physics*, 17(4), 719–25.

Franchelli, S., Leone, M.S., Berrino, P. et al. (1995). Psychological evaluation of patients undergoing breast reconstruction using two different methods: autologous tissues versus prostheses. *Plastic and Reconstructive Surgery*, 95(7), 1213–18; discussion 1219–20.

Frazier, T.G. & Noone, R.B. (1985). An objective analysis of immediate simultaneous reconstruction in the treatment of primary carcinoma of the breast. *Cancer*, 55(6), 1202–5.

Gage, I., Schnitt, S.J., Nixon, A.J. et al. (1996). Pathologic margin involvement and the risk of recurrence in patients treated with breast-conserving therapy. *Cancer*, 78(9), 1921–8.

Halverson, K.J., Perez, C.A., Taylor, M.E. et al. (1993). Age as a prognostic factor for breast and regional nodal recurrence following breast conserving surgery and irradiation in stage I and II breast cancer. *International Journal of Radiation Oncology, Biology, Physics*, 27(5), 1045–50.

Hartrampf, C.R., Jr & Bennett, G.K. (1987). Autogenous tissue reconstruction in the mastectomy patient: a critical review of 300 patients. *Annals of Surgery*, 205(5), 508–19.

Hartsell, W., Recine, D. & Griem, K. (1992). Does delay in the initiation of radiation therapy adversely affect local control in treatment of the intact breast? (Abstract). *Radiotherapy Oncology*, 24, 37.

Hellman, S. (1997). Stopping metastases at their source. *New England Journal of Medicine*, 337(14), 996–7.

Holland, R., Veling, S.H., Mravunac, M. et al. (1985). Histologic multifocality of Tis, T1-2 breast carcinomas: implications for clinical trials of breast-conserving surgery. *Cancer*, 56(5), 979–90.

Hunt, K.K., Baldwin, B.J., Strom, E.A. et al. (1997). Feasibility of postmastectomy radiation therapy after TRAM flap breast reconstruction. *Annals of Surgical Oncology*, 4(5), 377–84.

Jackson, W.B., Goldson, A.L. & Staud, C. (1994). Postoperative irradiation following immediate breast reconstruction using a temporary tissue expander. *Journal of the National Medical Association*, 86(7), 538–42.

Krishnan, L., St George, F.J., Mansfield, C.M. et al. (1983). Effect of silicone gel breast prosthesis on electron and photon dose distributions. *Medical Physics*, 10(1), 96–9.

Kroll, S.S., Coffey, J.A. Jr, Winn, R.J. et al. (1995). A comparison of factors affecting aesthetic outcomes of TRAM flap breast reconstructions. *Plastic and Reconstructive Surgery*, 96(4), 860–4.

Kurtz, J.M., Spitalier, J.M., Amalric, R. et al. (1988). Mammary recurrences in women younger than forty. *International Journal of Radiation Oncology, Biology, Physics*, 15(2), 271–6.

Kurtz, J.M., Amalric, R., Brandone, H. et al. (1989). Local recurrence after breast-conserving surgery and radiotherapy: frequency, time course, and prognosis. *Cancer*, 63(10), 1912–17.

Kurtz, J.M., Jacquemier, J., Amalric, R. et al. (1990a). Risk factors for breast recurrence in premenopausal and postmenopausal patients with ductal cancers treated by conservation therapy. *Cancer*, 65(8), 1867–78.

Kurtz, J.M., Jacquemier, J., Amalric, R. et al. (1990b). Why are local recurrences after breast-conserving therapy more frequent in younger patients? *Journal of Clinical Oncology*, 8(4), 591–8.

Kuske, R.R., Schuster, R., Klein, E. et al. (1991). Radiotherapy and breast reconstruction: clinical results and dosimetry. *International Journal of Radiation Oncology, Biology, Physics*, 21(2), 339–46.

Lara-Jimenez, P., Puche, J.G. & Pedraza, V. (1991). Adjuvant combined modality treatment in high risk breast cancer patients: ten-year results. (Abstract). *Proceedings of the 5th EORTC Breast Cancer Working Conference*: A293.

Lejour, M., Jabri, M. & Deraemaecker, R. (1988). Analysis of long-term results of 326 breast reconstructions. *Clinics in Plastic Surgery*, 15(4), 689–701.

Lichter, A., Lippman, M., Danforth, D. et al. (1992). Mastectomy versus breast conserving therapy in the treatment of stage I and II carcinoma of the breast: a randomised trial of the National Cancer Institute. *Journal of Clinical Oncology*, 10, 976–83.

Matthews, R.H., McNeese, M.D., Montague, R.H. et al. (1988). Prognostic implications of age in breast cancer patients treated with tumorectomy and irradiation or with mastectomy. *International Journal of Radiation Oncology, Biology, Physics*, 14(4), 659–63.

McGinley, P.H., Powell, W.R. & Bostwick, J. (1980). Dosimetry of a silicone breast prosthesis. *Radiology*, 135(1), 223–4.

Nissen-Meyer R., Kjellgren, K., Malmio, K. et al. (1978). Surgical adjuvant chemotherapy: results with one short course with cyclophosphamide after mastectomy for breast cancer. *Cancer*, 41(6), 2088–98.

Noone, R.B., Frazier, T.G., Hayward, C.Z. et al. (1982). Patient acceptance of immediate reconstruction following mastectomy. *Plastic and Reconstructive Surgery*, 69(4), 632–40.

Ohtake, T., Abe, R., Kimijima, I. et al. (1995). Intraductal extension of primary invasive breast carcinoma treated by breast-conservative surgery: computer graphic three-dimensional reconstruction of the mammary duct–lobular systems. *Cancer*, 76(1), 32–45.

Osteen, R.T., Connolly, J.L., Recht, A. et al. (1987). Identification of patients at high risk for local recurrence after conservative surgery and radiation therapy for stage I or II breast cancer. *Archives of Surgery*, 122(11), 1248–52.

Overgaard, M., Hansen, P.S., Overgaard, J. et al. (1997). Postoperative radiotherapy in high-risk premenopausal women with breast cancer who receive adjuvant chemotherapy. Danish Breast Cancer Cooperative Group 82b Trial. *New England Journal of Medicine*, 337(14), 949–55.

Overgaard, M., Jensen, M.B., Overgaard, J. et al. (1999). Postoperative radiotherapy in high-risk postmenopausal breast-cancer patients given adjuvant tamoxifen: Danish Breast Cancer Cooperative Group DBCG 82c randomised trial. *Lancet*, 353, 1641–8.

Peterson, M.E., Schultz, D.J., Reynolds, C. et al. (1999). Outcomes in breast cancer patients relative to margin status after treatment with breast-conserving surgery and radiation therapy: the University of Pennsylvania experience. *International Journal of Radiation Oncology, Biology, Physics*, 43(5), 1029–35.

Ragaz, J., Jackson, S.M., Le, N. et al. (1997). Adjuvant radiotherapy and chemotherapy in node-positive premenopausal women with breast cancer. *New England Journal of Medicine*, 337(14), 956–62.

Ramon, Y., Ullmann, Y., Moscona, R. et al. (1997). Aesthetic results and patient satisfaction with immediate breast reconstruction using tissue expansion: a follow-up study. *Plastic and Reconstructive Surgery*, 99(3), 686–91.

Recht, A., Come, S.E., Gelman, R.S. et al. (1991). Integration of conservative surgery, radiotherapy, and chemotherapy for the treatment of early-stage, node-positive breast cancer: sequencing, timing, and outcome. *Journal of Clinical Oncology*, 9(9), 1662–7.

Rosato, R.M. & Dowden, R.V. (1994). Radiation therapy as a cause of capsular contracture. *Annals of Plastic Surgery*, 32(4), 342–5.

Rose, M.A., Henderson, I.C., Gelman, R. et al. (1989). Premenopausal breast cancer patients treated with conservative surgery, radiotherapy and adjuvant chemotherapy have a low risk of local failure. *International Journal of Radiation Oncology, Biology, Physics*, 17(4), 711–17.

Ryoo, M.C., Kagan, A.R., Wollin, M. et al. (1989). Prognostic factors for recurrence and cosmesis in 393 patients after radiation therapy for early mammary carcinoma. *Radiology*, 172(2), 555–9.

Sarrazin, D., Lê, M.G., Arriagada, R. et al. (1989). Ten-year results of a randomized trial comparing a conservative treatment to mastectomy in early breast cancer. *Radiotherapy and Oncology*, 14(3), 177–84.

Schain, W.S., Wellisch, D.K., Pasnau, R.O. et al. (1985). The sooner the better: a study of psychological factors in women undergoing immediate versus delayed breast reconstruction. *American Journal of Psychiatry*, 142(1), 40–6.

Schmidt-Ullrich, R., Wazer, D.E., Tercilla, O. et al. (1989). Tumor margin assessment as a guide to optimal conservation surgery and irradiation in early stage breast carcinoma. *International Journal of Radiation Oncology, Biology, Physics*, 17(4), 733–8.

Shedbalkar, A.R., Devata, A. & Padanilam, T. (1980). A study of effects of radiation on silicone prostheses. *Plastic and Reconstructive Surgery*, 65(6), 805–10.

Slotman, B.J., Meyer, O.W., Njo, K.H. et al. (1994). Importance of timing of radiotherapy in breast conserving treatment for early stage breast cancer. *Radiotherapy and Oncology*, 30(3), 206–12.

Smitt, M.C., Nowels, K.W., Zdeblick, M.J. et al. (1995). The importance of the lumpectomy surgical margin status in long-term results of breast conservation. *Cancer*, 76(2), 259–67.

Solin, L.J., Fowble, B.L., Schultz, D.J. et al. (1991). The significance of the pathology margins of the tumor excision on the outcome of patients treated with definitive irradiation for early stage breast cancer. *International Journal of Radiation Oncology, Biology, Physics*, 21(2), 279–87.

Spear, S. (1995). Reconstruction and the radiated breast: is there a role for implants? *Plastic and Reconstructive Surgery*, 96, 1116–18.

Spivack, B., Khanna, M.M., Tafra, L. et al. (1994). Margin status and local recurrence after breast-conserving surgery. *Archives of Surgery*, 129(9), 952–6; discussion 956–7.

Stabile, R.J., Santoro, E., Dispaltro, F. et al. (1980). Reconstructive breast surgery following mastectomy and adjunctive radiation therapy. *Cancer*, 45(11), 2738–43.

Stevens, L.A., McGrath, M.H., Druss, R.G. et al. (1984). The psychological impact of immediate breast reconstruction for women with early breast cancer. *Plastic and Reconstructive Surgery*, 73(4), 619–28.

Straus, K., Lichter, A., Lippman, M. et al. (1992). Results of the National Cancer Institute early breast cancer trial. *Journal of The National Cancer Institute. Monographs*, 11, 27–32.

Touboul, E., Buffat, L., Belkacemi, Y. et al. (1999). Local recurrences and distant metastases after breast-conserving surgery and radiation therapy for early breast cancer. *International Journal of Radiation Oncology, Biology, Physics*, 43(1), 25–38.

van Dongen, J.A., Bartelink, H., Fentiman, I.S. et al. (1992). Randomized clinical trial to assess the value of breast-conserving therapy in stage I and II breast cancer, EORTC 10801 trial. *Journal of the National Cancer Institute. Monographs*, 11, 15–18.

Van Limbergen, E., Rijnders, A., van der Schueren, E. et al. (1989). Cosmetic evaluation of breast conserving treatment for mammary cancer. 2. A quantitative analysis of the influence of radiation dose, fractionation schedules and surgical treatment techniques on cosmetic results. *Radiotherapy and Oncology*, 16(4), 253–67.

van Tienhoven, G., Voogd, A.C., Peterse, J.L. et al. (1999). Prognosis after treatment for loco-regional recurrence after mastectomy or breast conserving therapy in two randomised trials (EORTC 10801 and DBCG-82TM). EORTC Breast Cancer Cooperative Group and the Danish Breast Cancer Cooperative Group. *European Journal of Cancer*, 35(1), 32–8.

Veronesi, U., Banfi, A., Salvadori, B. et al. (1990a). Breast conservation is the treatment of choice in small breast cancer: long-term results of a randomized trial. *European Journal of Cancer*, 26(6), 668–70.

Veronesi, U., Volterrani, F., Luini, A. et al. (1990b). Quadrantectomy versus lumpectomy for small size breast cancer. *European Journal of Cancer*, 26(6), 671–3.

Victor, S.J., Brown, D.M., Horwitz, E.M. et al. (1998). Treatment outcome with radiation therapy after breast augmentation or reconstruction in patients with primary breast carcinoma. *Cancer*, 82(7), 1303–9.

von Smitten, K. & Sundell, B. (1992). The impact of adjuvant radiotherapy and cytotoxic chemotherapy on the outcome of immediate breast reconstruction by tissue expansion after mastectomy for breast cancer. *European Journal of Surgical Oncology*, 18(2), 119–23.

Watterson, P.A., Bostwick, J. 3rd, Hester, T.R. Jr et al. (1995). TRAM flap anatomy correlated with a 10-year clinical experience with 556 patients. *Plastic and Reconstructive Surgery*, 95(7), 1185–94.

Wazer, D.E., DiPetrillo, T., Schmidt-Ullrich, R. et al. (1992). Factors influencing cosmetic outcome and complication risk after conservative surgery and radiotherapy for early-stage breast carcinoma. *Journal of Clinical Oncology*, 10(3), 356–63.

Whelan, T.J., Julian J., Wright, J. et al. (2000). Does loco-regional radiation therapy improve survival in breast cancer? A meta-analysis. *Journal of Clinical Oncology*, 18(6), 1220–9.

Yarnold, J.R., Price, P. & Steel, G.G. (1995). Non-surgical management of early breast cancer in the United Kingdom: the role and practice of radiotherapy. Clinical Audit Sub-committee of the Faculty of Clinical Oncology, Royal College of Radiologists, and the Joint Council for Clinical Oncology. *Clinical Oncology*, 7(4), 219–22.

Zimmerman, R.P., Mark, R.J., Kim, A.I. et al. (1998). Radiation tolerance of transverse rectus abdominis myocutaneous-free flaps used in immediate breast reconstruction. *American Journal of Clinical Oncology*, 21(4), 381–5.

Predictors of response and resistance to medical therapy

Cell kinetic parameters and response to therapy

R.S. Camplejohn

Guy's, King's and St Thomas' School of Medicine, St Thomas' Hospital, London

Introduction

There has been a longstanding belief that measurements of cell proliferation should be useful in the management of cancer patients. Many cytotoxic drugs are more active against proliferating cells than nonproliferative ones and in the early 1970s Skipper and others suggested that response to chemotherapy of experimental tumours was related to their proliferative activity (Skipper, 1971). Further, clinical observations suggested that rapidly proliferating types of tumour (e.g. germ cell tumours and high-grade non-Hodgkin's lymphoma) are generally more responsive to chemotherapy and radiotherapy. These observations led to a plethora of studies investigating the relationship between cell kinetic parameters and response of tumours to chemotherapy and to schemes to try and take advantage of cell kinetics in the design of treatment schedules (Price et al., 1975). However, as early as 1977, Steel wrote 'although many clinical oncologists claim that their thinking has been influenced by research on tumour growth kinetics, it is hard to point to clear advances attributed to anything more than inspired clinical experimentation' (Steel, 1977). The lack of impact of cell kinetics on tumour treatment during this period was due to a variety of factors, including technical limitations in measuring cell proliferation in individual clinical tumours and to a failure to appreciate the degree of heterogeneity present in such tumours. Even up to the present day, it is difficult to point to real advances in patient management based on a knowledge of cell-proliferation-related parameters. This failure is still partly due to technical limitations in measuring cell proliferation in individual tumours and also to the failure to standardize the methods that are available. There is no shortage of methods which measure what can loosely be referred to as 'proliferation-related' parameters, on the contrary there are too many to review in the space available here. Most of these methods yield crude indices of proliferative activity such as the mitotic or labelling index, they do not give information concerning the *rate* of cell proliferation. An exception to this statement is a method involving simultaneous measurement by flow cytometry of DNA content and uptake of bromodeoxyuridine (BrdUrd), which will be discussed briefly later. Given the profusion of methods reported in the literature, pretty well all of which have been applied to breast cancer, we have decided to concentrate on one technique, namely DNA flow cytometry, which exemplifies both the problems and promise of such measurements. Reference will be made to other methods where appropriate and a brief discussion will be included of a number of recent immunohistochemical markers which show promise as predictors of response to treatment in breast cancer.

DNA flow cytometry

This technique has been chosen as an example for a number of reasons; it exemplifies the limitations and value of proliferative indices in patient management and there is a particularly large body of published work using this technique. Like most such methods there has, so far, been a failure to standardize both measurement techniques and data analysis despite efforts to achieve these objectives (Hiddemann et al., 1984). Despite these technical limitations, there is wide agreement that S-phase fraction (SPF) calculated from DNA histograms is a powerful prognostic marker in both node-positive and node-negative breast cancer (Macartney & Camplejohn, 1995). This finding was confirmed in a recent large single centre study carried out by one of us (Camplejohn et al., 1995). This study met a number, at least, of the necessary criteria for such clinical studies in that it was reasonably large (almost 900 patients) and DNA flow cytometric parameters were compared in a multivariate statistical analysis with a range of other important factors such as nodal status and tumour grade. Table 9a.1 gives abbreviated results of the multivariate analysis from this study; these results confirm that SPF is second only to nodal status as a significant prognostic marker and DNA ploidy is also shown to be an independent predictor of survival, although the magnitude of the effect is much less than for SPF. Interestingly, Zanon et al. (1998) suggested recently that a combination of SPF, DNA ploidy and tumour size may be predictive of axillary lymph node status in breast cancer.

SPF and other proliferative markers have withstood the test of time as prognostic markers when compared with more recent molecular and immunohistochemical markers (Ravaioli et al., 1998).

Similar claims concerning prognostic power in breast cancer have been made for a variety of proliferation-related parameters including mitotic index (Eskelinen et al., 1992), tritiated thymidine labelling index (Silvestrini, 1991) and a number of immunohistochemical markers.

Table 9a.1. Multivariate analysis of factors predictive for overall survival in a group of 802 cases of breast carcinoma

Variable name	X^2	p-value	Relative risk
Nodal status	141.0	<0.0001	3.6
SPF	26.7	<0.0001	2.8
Histological grade	21.9	<0.0001	2.2
Tumour size (<2 cm vs. >2 cm)	17.7	<0.0001	1.8
Diploid vs. aneuploid	11.2	0.0008	1.7
Menstrual status (peri vs. rest)	5.6	0.017	1.5

Data from Camplejohn et al., 1995.

Predictors of response to therapy

Adjuvant chemotherapy for node-negative breast cancer

A general marker of prognosis may not necessarily be of use in determining the most appropriate treatment for individual patients. However, the ability to define high-risk subgroups within a heterogeneous patient population may enable a better choice of treatment and such a situation appears to exist in node-negative breast cancer. The majority of node-negative patients have excellent survival prospects following surgical removal of their tumour, but there has been an increasing consensus in recent years that adjuvant therapy has a role for some node-negative women (O'Reilly & Richards, 1990; McGuire et al., 1990) (see also Chapter 7). There is good evidence that a proliferative marker such as SPF may have a role in defining those node-negative patients at high risk of relapse (O'Reilly et al., 1990a; Sigurdsson et al., 1990), who may benefit from adjuvant chemotherapy. It may well be that SPF needs to be combined with other parameters to get the best discrimination of high-risk patients. McGuire's group in the USA support the use of multiple parameters in decision-making relating to patient treatment (McGuire et al., 1990), whilst O'Reilly & Richards (1990) suggested that a combination of SPF and tumour size was adequate to define a high-risk group of patients.

Prediction of response to neoadjuvant chemotherapy

There is considerable interest in the use of preoperative (neoadjuvant) chemotherapy to downstage breast cancer and allow breast-conservation surgery in patients who would otherwise need mastectomy for local control of disease (Bonadonna et al., 1990) (see also Chapter 10). The data on the predictive power of proliferative markers and response to chemotherapy is more convincing for neoadjuvant

Table 9a.2. Summary of literature on the correlation between DNA ploidy/SPF and short-term response to primary chemotherapy

Study	Number of patients	Correlation with ploidy (p value)	Correlation with SPF (p value)
Bonadonna et al., 1990	92	NS	NS[a]
Briffod et al., 1989	35	0.008	—
Mathieu et al., 1995	66	<0.03	<0.02
O'Reilly et al., 1992	22	0.06	0.05
Remvikos et al., 1989	60	0.2	<0.002
Remvikos et al., 1993	92	—	<0.002
Spyratos et al., 1992	35	0.008	0.004

Note: It should be noted that data for SPF in particular is not available for all patients in the above studies and details of chemotherapy schedules and statistical analysis of data vary between the various studies; NS not significant.
[a]This finding was based on thymidine labelling index.

treatment than it is for adjuvant therapy. A series of reports published in the early 1990s suggest that pretreatment ploidy and SPF values predict clinical response to chemotherapy (see Table 9a.2).

Despite the small size of some of these studies, taken together they look fairly convincing. However, some authors have failed to find any predictive value of proliferative markers for patients receiving neoadjuvant therapy. For example, Makris et al. (1997) investigated a number of markers in 90 patients receiving chemoendocrine therapy. In this study only c-*erb*B-2 was predictive; SPF, Ki-67, DNA ploidy and p53 staining were not.

In addition to looking at the correlation between pretreatment DNA flow cytometric parameters and response to therapy, some studies have also attempted to monitor response to therapy by taking multiple sequential samples and examining changes in these measurements. A French group reported in a number of publications (Briffod et al., 1989; Briffod et al., 1992; Spyratos et al., 1992) that changes in DNA profiles predicted response to primary chemotherapy. In these studies, patients whose DNA profiles showed no change during treatment had a poor response to therapy, whilst two other groups of patients defined by the type of change seen, had better responses to therapy. In one of these studies a p value of 0.00005 is quoted for the correlation between objective regression and changes in DNA profiles seen during chemotherapy. O'Reilly et al. (1992) found no correlation between changes in DNA profiles and response to therapy but this observation was based on only 11 patients. Remvikos et al. (1993) did find a significant correlation between changes in DNA histograms and response to therapy in a study in which data was available sequentially for 71 patients ($p < 0.0001$). All the studies discussed above looked only at short-term response to therapy and there is no guarantee that SPF predicts long-term trends in survival and cure. Nevertheless, overall the data is suggestive that a simple proliferation-related measurement such as SPF may be a useful parameter to include in trials of neoadjuvant chemotherapy.

Adjuvant chemotherapy for node-positive breast cancer

There are studies in the literature which claim that proliferative indices may be correlated with the clinical outcome in patients receiving adjuvant chemotherapy. For example, Silvestrini et al. (1990) measured tritiated thymidine labelling index in quite a large cohort of patients (523) and found just such a correlation. However, overall, the case for proliferation-related parameters as predictors of response to adjuvant chemotherapy looks much weaker than for neoadjuvant therapy. Quite a number of DNA flow cytometric investigations have failed to find SPF useful as a predictor of response in such cases (see, e.g. O'Reilly et al., 1990b; Muss et al., 1994).

Hormonal therapy

The literature on proliferation-related markers and response to hormonal therapy is smaller than that on response to chemotherapy, but there are, nevertheless, some publications relating to this topic. Baildam and colleagues in two publications (Baildam et al., 1987a, 1987b) reported that tumours with tetraploid DNA content were most responsive to hormonal therapy with tamoxifen. Caution should be applied in relation to this finding, however, as we are unaware of any subsequent confirmation of this data and the studies of Baildam et al. appeared to have a number of technical problems. A more recent DNA flow cytometric study using sequential fine needle aspirates taken from 27 patients with primary breast cancer treated with tamoxifen, suggested that response could be predicted from changes in the DNA profiles during the early stages of therapy (Fernando et al., 1994). Two studies have also suggested that c-*erb*B-2 overexpression is a predictor of poor response to hormonal therapy in breast cancer (Wright et al., 1992; Borg et al., 1994).

Tumour p53 status as a possible predictor of response to therapy

The levels of expression of a large number of cellular proteins have been investigated as prognostic markers in breast cancer. Some of these proteins have also been studied as possible indicators of response to therapy, for example c-*erb*B-2, which as was discussed above, has been looked at in terms of chemo- as well as hormonal therapy (Muss et al., 1994). These authors suggested that c-*erb*B-2 overexpression was predictive for response to high-dose adjuvant treatment with cyclophosphamide, doxorubicin and fluorouracil. This finding has not been confirmed in some other studies but there is a suggestion that c-*erb*B-2 may predict response to tamoxifen (Ravaioli et al., 1998). Similar mixed evidence on the value of markers such as Bcl-2 and cyclins has also been published (Ravaioli et al., 1998). An interesting study on cyclin D1 has recently been published in which, surprisingly, overexpression is associated with a good prognosis and a good response to endocrine therapy (Barnes & Gillett, 1998).

In this brief section we are, however, going to use p53 as an example of ongoing research looking at response to chemotherapy; p53 is the gene mutated most frequently in clinical cancer with approximately a quarter of breast tumours having p53 mutations; p53 plays a central role in maintaining the genetic integrity of the cell by preventing cells with damaged DNA from proliferating further. A major way of achieving this is by causing damaged cells to be eliminated by induction of apoptosis (see Barnes & Camplejohn, 1996 for general review of p53). Many forms of chemotherapy exert their cytotoxic effects via the induction of apoptotic death and the tumour suppressor gene p53 appears to have major role in modulating this response (Lowe et al., 1993, 1994). Thus while apoptosis can be induced by cytotoxic treatments in cells lacking functional p53, the dose required to achieve this effect is much greater than that required for cells with functional p53. These experimental studies increasingly have been supported by clinical investigations which bolster the view that the p53 status of a tumour may be predictive of the response to chemotherapy. A number of studies, using im-munohistochemical or cytochemical methods, have suggested that p53 status and survival after therapy are linked in breast cancer (Allred et al., 1993; Koechli et al., 1994; Petty et al., 1994). There are, however, discrepant results in such im-munohistochemical studies (Makris et al., 1995; Mathieu et al., 1995), including a study carried out recently at Guy's Hospital, London, in which CMF treatment in a cohort of 277 patients was found to be of equal benefit in patients with p53-positive and p53-negative tumours (Dublin et al., 1997). Thus immunohis-tochemical studies have yielded inconsistent results and much of this is probably due to variations in tissue handling, staining and counting procedures (Barnes & Camplejohn, 1996). However, an additional complication stems from the fact that it is now known that immunohistochemical overexpression of p53 protein is not always a marker of mutation (Barnes & Camplejohn, 1996). Thus the application of different techniques to assess p53 status may also contribute to discrepant results concerning the role of p53 as a predictor of survival after chemotherapy. This possibility is supported by Aas et al. (1996) who, in a study of the relationship between p53 mutations and response of breast tumours to doxorubicin, found that specific mutations predicted response to chemotherapy but that immunohis-tochemical staining of p53 protein alone did not. Improved techniques for detecting p53 mutations have recently become available, for example one such improved technique involves the use of a yeast based assay of p53 function, which detected all p53 mutations present in a series of high-grade tumours (Duddy et al., 2000). A second new technique uses micro arrays to detect mutations (Ahrendt et al., 1999). Clearly, the value of p53 status and response to therapy is still uncertain but the biological importance of p53 to processes that influence response to therapeutic agents suggests that this is a topic worthy of more study and new detection methods for p53 mutations should enable the value of p53 status to be clarified in clinical cancer. Further, p53 may itself be a target for tumour therapy in the future (Bertelsen et al., 1995).

Potential predictors of response in clinical trials

Some of the studies discussed earlier in this chapter were performed on material from patients involved in clinical trials. However, in essentially all of them the proliferation-related measurements were not incorporated as an integral part of the trial. Further, in few if any of the studies were patients assigned randomly to treatment groups whose outcome was compared with a control arm. The lack of a control arm means that potential predictors of response are related to clinical outcome but it is difficult to separate their role as general prognostic markers (in the absence of treatment) from any value as predictors of response to the specific therapy given. Another problem in assessing parameters such as SPF or p53 status as predictors of response is the lack of standardization of measurement techniques. This problem is exacerbated by the plethora of potential predictors available. What is needed are large randomized trials, ideally with control arms, in which the putative response predictor is included in the initial design of the study. Furthermore, to gain maximum information a number of promising markers could be measured in the same study, for example flow cytometric assessment of SPF and ploidy could be combined with measurement of p53 and c-*erb*B-2 expression. In addition, as regards proliferation-related markers, it would be valuable to measure a parameter which actually gives information on the *rate* of cell proliferation. No data from any large trial on breast cancer which meets all of these criteria are available but a pilot study of BrdUrd labelling has been published (Stanton et al., 1996).

Work is under way on head and neck cancer which comes close to the ideal set out above. At present a phase III multicentre randomized trial of CHART (continuous, hyperfractionated, accelerated radiotherapy) is underway, incorporating multiparametric flow cytometry measuring DNA content and incorporation of BrdUrd. Although this method requires certain assumptions to be made, it does allow an estimate of potential doubling time (T_{POT}), a parameter related to the rate of proliferation, to be made from a single biopsy. The hypothesis being tested is that rapidly growing tumours should respond better to CHART, which involves three daily doses of radiation given over a short period with no breaks for weekends. CHART allows less time for tumour repopulation between doses of radiotherapy than conventional treatment schedules spread over many weeks with 72-hour gaps at weekends. The application of proliferative measurements to the CHART trial are described in detail by Wilson (1993).

Conclusion

In reference to the ability of proliferative markers to really influence the management of breast cancer patients the jury is still out. For patients with head and neck tumours, whilst it is not yet clear whether measurement of T_{POT}, as described above, will be useful for assigning patients to CHART or conventional radiotherapy schedules the carefully designed trial currently underway should, when finished, give a definitive answer to this question. Such definitive answers seem further off as regards the role of predictors of response to therapy of breast cancer, although the use of such predictors has some promise for neoadjuvant therapy and also for selection of high-risk groups of node-negative patients for adjuvant therapy.

REFERENCES

Ahrendt, S.A., Halachmi, S., Chow, J.T. et al. (1999). Rapid p53 sequence analysis in primary lung cancer using an oligonucleotide probe array. *Proceedings of the National Academy of Science USA*, 96, 7382–7.

Aas, T., Borresen, A.L., Geisler, S. et al. (1996). Specific P53 mutations are associated with de novo resistance to doxorubicin in breast cancer patients. *Nature Medicine*, 2, 811–14.

Allred, D.C., Clark, G.M., Elledge, R. et al. (1993). Association of p53 protein expression with tumor cell proliferation rate and clinical outcome in node-negative breast cancer. *Journal of the National Cancer Institute*, 85, 200–6.

Baildam, A.D., Zaloudik, J., Howell, A. et al. (1987a). DNA analysis by flow cytometry, response to endocrine treatment and prognosis in advanced carcinoma of the breast. *British Journal of Cancer*, 55, 553–9.

Baildam, A.D., Zaloudik, J., Howell, A. et al. (1987b). Effect of Tamoxifen upon cell DNA analysis by flow cytometry in primary carcinoma of the breast. *British Journal of Cancer*, 55, 561–6.

Barnes, D.M. & Camplejohn, R.S. (1996). p53, apoptosis and breast cancer. *Journal of Mammary Gland Biology and. Neoplasia*, 1, 163–75.

Barnes, D.M. & Gillett, C.E. (1998). Cyclin D1 in breast cancer. *Breast Cancer Research and Treatment*, 52, 1–15.

Bertelsen, A.H., Beaudry, G.A., Stoller, T.J. et al. (1995). Tumor suppressor genes: prospects for cancer therapies. *Biotechnology*, 13, 127–31.

Bonadonna, G., Veronesi, U., Brambilla, C. et al. (1990). Primary chemotherapy to avoid mastectomy in tumours with diameters of three centimeters or more. *Journal of the National Cancer Institute*, 82, 1539–45.

Borg, A., Baldetorp, B., Ferno, M. et al. (1994). ERBB2 amplification is associated with tamoxifen resistance in steroid-receptor positive breast cancer. *Cancer Letters*, 81, 137–44.

Briffod, M., Spyratos, F., Hacene, K. et al. (1992). Evaluation of breast carcinoma chemosensitivity by flow cytometric DNA analysis and computer assisted image analysis. *Cytometry*, 13, 250–8.

Briffod, M., Spyratos, F., Tubiana-Hulin, M. et al. (1989). Sequential cytopunctures during preoperative chemotherapy for primary breast carcinoma. *Cancer*, 63, 631–7.

Camplejohn, R.S., Ash, C.M., Gillett, C.E. et al. (1995). The prognostic significance of DNA flow cytometry in breast cancer: results from 881 patients treated in a single centre. *British Journal of Cancer*, 71, 140–5.

Dublin, E.A., Miles, D.W., Rubens, R.D. et al. (1997). p53 Immunohistochemical staining and survival after adjuvant chemotherapy for breast cancer. *International Journal of Cancer*, 74, 605–8.

Duddy, P.M., Hanby, A.M., Barnes, D.M. et al. (2000). Improving the Detection of *p53* Mutations in Breast Cancer by Use of the FASAY, a Functional Assay. *Journal of Molecular Diagnostics (American Journal of Pathology Part B)*, 2, 139–44.

Eskelinen, M., Lipponen, P., Papinaho, S. et al. (1992). DNA flow cytometry nuclear morphometry mitotic indices and steroid receptors as independent prognostic factors in female breast cancer. *International Journal of Cancer*, 51, 555–61.

Fernando, I.N., Titley, J.C., Powles, T.J. et al. (1994). Measurement of S-phase fraction and ploidy in sequential fine-needle aspirates from primary human breast tumours treated with tamoxifen. *British Journal of Cancer*, 70, 1211–16.

Hiddemann, W., Schumann, J., Andreeff, M. et al. (1984). Convention on nomenclature for DNA cytometry. *Cytometry*, 5, 445–6.

Koechli, O.R., Schaer, G.N., Seifert, B. et al. (1994). Mutant p53 protein associated with chemosensitivity in breast cancer specimens. *Lancet*, 344, 1647–8.

Lowe, S.W., Bodis, S., McClatchey, A. et al. (1994). p53 status and the efficacy of cancer therapy *in vivo*. *Science*, 266, 807–10.

Lowe, S.W., Ruley, H.E., Jacks, T. et al. (1993). p53-dependent apoptosis modulates the cytotoxicity of anti cancer agents. *Cell*, 74, 957–67.

Macartney, J.C. & Camplejohn, R.S. (1995). DNA ploidy analysis by flow cytometry. In *Quantitative Clinical Pathology*. Ed. P.W. Hamilton & D.C. Allen. Oxford: Blackwell Science, pp. 206–21.

Makris, A., Powles, T., Dowsett, M. et al. (1995). p53 protein overexpression and chemosensitivity in breast cancer. *International Journal of Molecular Medicine*, 345, 1181–2.

Makris, A., Powles, T.J., Dowsett, M. et al. (1997). Prediction of response to neoadjuvant chemoendocrine therapy in primary breast carcinomas. *Clinical Cancer Research*, 3, 593–600.

Mathieu, M.-C., Koscieiny, S., LeBihan, M.-L. et al. (1995). p53 protein overexpression and chemosensitivity in breast cancer. *International Journal of Molecular Medicine*, 345, 1182.

McGuire, W.L., Tandon, A.K., Allred, D.C. et al. (1990). How to use prognostic factors in axillary node-negative breast cancer patients. *Journal of the National Cancer Institute*, 82, 1006–15.

Muss, H.B., Thor, A.D., Berry, D.A. et al. (1994). c-*erb*B-2 expression and response to adjuvant therapy in women with node-positive early breast cancer. *New England Journal of Medicine*, 330, 1260–6.

O'Reilly, S.M., Camplejohn, R.S., Barnes, D.M. et al. (1990a). Node negative breast cancer: prognostic sub-groups defined by tumour size and flow cytometry. *Journal of Clinical Oncology*, 8, 2040–6.

O'Reilly, S.M., Camplejohn, R.S., Millis, R.R. et al. (1990b). Proliferative activity, histological grade and benefit from adjuvate chemotherapy in node positive breast cancer. *European Journal of Cancer*, 26, 1035–8.

O'Reilly, S.M., Camplejohn, R.S., Rubens, R.D. et al. (1992). DNA flow cytometry and response to preoperative chemotherapy for primary breast cancer. *European Journal of Cancer*, 28, 323–6.

O'Reilly, S.M. & Richards, M.A. (1990). Node negative breast cancer. Adjuvant chemotherapy should probably be reserved for patients at high risk of relapse. *British Medical Journal*, 300, 346–8.

Petty, R.D., Cree, I.A., Sutherland, L.A. et al. (1994). Expression of the p53 tumour suppressor gene product is a determinant of chemosensitivity. *Biochemical and Biophysical Research Communications*, 199, 264–70.

Price, L.A., Hill, B.T., Calvert, A.H. et al. (1975). Kinetically based multiple drug treatment for advanced head and neck cancer. *British Medical Journal*, 3, 10–11.

Ravaioli, A., Bagli, L., Zucchini, A. et al. (1998). Prognosis and prediction of response in breast cancer: the current role of the main biological markers. *Cell Proliferation*, 31, 113–26.

Remvikos, Y., Jouve, M., Beuzeboc, P. et al. (1993). Cell cycle modifications of breast cancers during neoadjuvant chemotherapy – a flow cytometry study on fine needle aspirates. *European Journal of Cancer*, 29A, 1843–8.

Sigurdsson, H., Baldetorp, B., Borg, A. et al. (1990). Indicators of prognosis in node-negative breast cancer. *New England Journal of Medicine*, 322, 1045–53.

Silvestrini, R. (1991). Feasibility and reproducibility of the [3H]-thymidine labelling index in breast cancer. *Cell Proliferation*, 24, 437–45.

Silvestrini, R., Daidone, M.G., Valagussa, P. et al. (1990). H-3-thymidine labeling index as a prognostic indicator in node-positive breast cancer. *Journal of Clinical Oncology*, 8, 1321–6.

Skipper, H.E. (1971). The cell cycle and chemotherapy of cancer. In *The Cell Cycle and Cancer*. Ed. R. Baserga. New York: Dekker.

Spyratos, F., Briffod, M., Tubiana-Hulin, M. et al. (1992). Sequential cytopunctures during preoperative chemotherapy for primary breast carcinoma; 2. DNA flow cytometry changes during chemotherapy, tumor regression and short-term follow-up. *Cancer*, 69, 470–5.

Stanton, P.D., Cooke, T.G., Forster, G. et al. (1996). Cell kinetics *in vivo* of human breast cancer. *British Journal of Surgery*, 83, 98–102.

Steel, G.G. (1977). *Growth Kinetics of Tumours*. Oxford: Clarendon Press.

Wilson, G.D. (1993). Limitations of the bromodeoxyuridine technique for measurement of tumour proliferation. In *Current Topics in Clinical Radiobiology of Tumors*. Ed. H. Beck-Bornholdt. Berlin: Springer-Verlag, pp. 27–43.

Wright, C., Nicholson, S., Angus, B. et al. (1992). Relationship between c-erbB-2 protein product expression and response to endocrine therapy in advanced breast cancer. *British Journal of Cancer*, 65, 118–21.

Zanon, C., Durando, A., Geuna, M. et al. (1998). Flow cytometry in breast cancer; prognostic and surgical indications of the sparing of axillary lymph node dissection. *American Journal of Clinical Oncology*, 21, 392–7.

Predictors of response and resistance to medical therapy: endocrine therapy

Zenon Rayter

Bristol Royal Infirmary, Bristol

Introduction

There is a substantial body of epidemiological evidence implicating oestrogens in the development of breast cancer (Henderson et al., 1988). In addition, there is a great deal of clinical and experimental evidence regarding the central role of oestrogens. It is now 100 years since the Glasgow surgeon, George Beatson, published his paper on the effect of oophorectomy on patients with metastatic breast cancer, observing regression of tumour in approximately 30% of cases (Beatson, 1896). Human breast cancer cell lines derived from patients' pleural or ascitic fluid have been used to demonstrate a proliferative response to physiological doses of oestrogens in vitro (Katzenellenbogen et al., 1987). The discovery of oestrogen receptors (ERs) in breast cancer (Jensen et al., 1968) gave fresh impetus to investigating the interrelationships between oestrogens and mammary cell growth. As a result, a variety of growth factors, oestrogen inducible proteins and oncogenes have been found to be influenced by oestrogen both in vitro and in vivo (Miller & Langdon, 1997).

The molecular mechanism by which oestadiol exerts its proliferative effects has also been extensively researched. It is suggested that oestradiol exerts its proliferative effects by regulating cyclins and cyclin-dependent kinases (Cdk). These enzymes regulate progression of the cell from G1 to S phase and therefore stimulation of these enzymes (Sherr, 1994), phosphorylation of the retinoblastoma protein and elimination of Cdk inhibitors (Foster & Wimalasena, 1996) allows cells to pass from G1 to S phase. Oestradiol also stimulates the oncogenes c-myc and p53, which are involved respectively in proliferation of cells (Dubik et al., 1987) and control of the cell cycle (Thompson et al., 1990). In MCF-7 cells oestradiol inhibits the expression of c-erbB-2 (Dati et al., 1990), an oncogene whose protein product is a putative growth factor receptor (Walker & Varley, 1993) and, when over-expressed, is associated with high proliferation (Tommasi et al., 1991). Oestradiol also increases the expression of the *bcl-2* gene which is involved in regulating apoptosis (Kandouz et al., 1996), an effect which may be involved in resistance to chemotherapy (Texeira et al., 1995).

Another important aspect of the discovery of ERs was that, for the first time, a biochemical marker existed which predicted, albeit imperfectly, response of breast tumours to endocrine therapy (Rayter, 1991; Stein et al., 1995). It is now apparent that the major pathway of the mechanism of response to almost all the major endocrine therapies is via the oestrogen receptor by the common mechanism of oestrogen deprivation (Stein et al., 1995). The structure and function of the ER is crucial to the understanding of the mechanism of action of oestrogens, the mechanism of action of endocrine therapies for breast cancer and the phenomenon of resistance to endocrine therapy. This phenomenon of endocrine resistance has necessitated the use of chemotherapy in the treatment of breast cancer both in the adjuvant setting and in the treatment of locally advanced or metastatic disease. Clearly breast cancers also become resistant to chemotherapy as metastatic disease is always incurable. Mechanisms of response and resistance to chemotherapy will also be discussed in Chapter 9c.

Recently, another form of oestrogen receptor has been discovered which has been designated ERβ (Kuiper et al., 1996). The classical ER has been designated ERα. A recent study has demonstrated that ERβ is expressed in approximately 50% of primary breast cancers and its expression is independent to that of ERα which is expressed in approximately 70% of breast cancers (Cullen et al., 1999). It is believed that all previous methods for detecting ER have identified only the ERα form and the following discussion on ER applies only to ERα. The clinical significance of ERβ is as yet unknown.

Oestrogen receptor (ER)

Structure and function of the oestrogen receptor

The ER is a 30 kDa molecule which is located in the nucleus of the cell (King & Greene, 1984) and is normally bound to a chaperone protein called heat shock protein (HSP), (Miller, 1996). ER consists of six regions, denoted A–F, each consisting of a different number of amino acids (Figure 9b.1). Sequence comparisons between oestrogen (Green et al., 1986), glucocorticoid (Hollenberg et al., 1985) and progesterone receptors (Conneely et al., 1986) and site directed mutation analysis (Kumar et al., 1986; Mader et al., 1989) have identified two functional domains important for ER function. Region E is the hormone-binding domain (Mader et al., 1989) whilst region C is a 66-amino acid region which binds to DNA and contains many cysteine, lysine and arginine residues (Green & Chambon, 1987). Cysteine residues in this C region tetrahedrally coordinate zinc

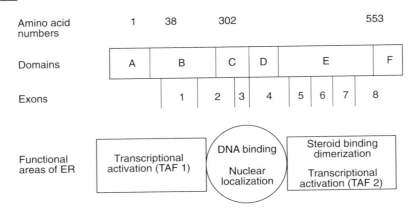

Figure 9b1   Schematic representation of ER

to form two 'zinc fingers' through which the interaction with DNA occurs (Ponglikitmongol et al., 1988). The C region of ER can be subdivided into two regions, C1 and C2. Oestrogen specificity of the DNA-binding domain lies in the N-terminal C1 finger and three amino acids located at the C-terminal side of the ER C1 finger play a key part in this specificity (Mader et al., 1989).

The region of DNA with which the zinc fingers interact is known as the oestrogen response element. When oestrogen binds to ER, the HSP is displaced leading to conformational changes and then dimerization of ER via the C-terminal domain which also contains the hormone-induced transcriptional factor, TAF 2. The N-terminal domain contains a second transcriptional activation function, TAF 1. The oestrogen–ER complex becomes much more tightly bound to the nucleus. The zinc fingers bind to the oestrogen response element of the DNA and this modulates transcription via TAF 1 and TAF 2. The receptor–DNA complex is then thought to interact with a series of other transcription factors to modulate gene function (Tora et al., 1989). The most obvious effect of the interaction of oestrogen with ER is on cell growth. Thus, oestrogen stimulates cell proliferation of ER-positive breast cancer cell lines (Darbre et al., 1989) and probably of ER-positive breast tumours (Markopoulos et al., 1988). There is a wide range of ER values found in breast cancer and this is partly due to differences in tumour cellularity and partly due to cell heterogeneity within the same tumour.

Measurement of ER

There are three major methods of measuring ER. The dextran-coated charcoal (DCC) adsorption steroid binding assay was the first method described. Quantitation of ER is described in detail elsewhere (McGuire & de la Garza, 1973) but will be described here briefly. Six paired tissue cytosol aliquots of the tumour are incubated with six known concentrations of tritium-labelled oestradiol in the presence or absence of diethylstilboestrol, an unlabelled competitor for ER. The differences in radiolabel concentrations between noncompeted and competed tubes following removal of unbound steroid with charcoal represents specifically bound radioligand. Scatchard analysis of this multipoint assay allows calculation of ER content in terms of fentomoles of receptor per milligram of cytosol protein (fmol/mg). A level < 10 fmol/mg cytosol protein is generally regarded as negative. The disadvantages of this method are that it requires a relatively large amount of tissue, is laborious and requires expensive equipment.

The ER immunocytochemical assay (ER-ICA) utilizes a monoclonal antibody which binds specifically to ER and utilizes a peroxidase-antiperoxidase detection system (Hawkins et al., 1988). Specific binding is detected by the addition of the chromogen diaminobenzidine tetrahydrochloride and hydrogen peroxide. After counterstaining with Harris haematoxylin, a staining intensity can be calculated by grading the intensity of staining and counting the percentage of cells stained. The advantage of this method is that no special equipment is required, it can be performed on very small samples of tumour and can even be performed on fine needle aspirates. The disadvantage of this method is that evaluation of staining intensity is subjective although this can be overcome by employing automated video analysis.

The ER enzyme immunoassay (ER-EIA) is based on an antibody sandwich technique. Breast tumour cytosols are incubated with an anti-ER monoclonal antibody. A second ER-specific antibody conjugated to peroxidase is added. Addition of an enzyme substrate produces a colour reaction the intensity of which is proportional to the amount of receptor. This method also requires only a small volume of tissue and requires little special equipment. Several studies have demonstrated very good correlations between the three methods of measurement of ER (Barnes et al., 1996; reviewed by Rayter, 1991). The other major advantage of immunocytochemistry over the previous methods of measurement (which required fresh or frozen tissue) is that it can be performed on paraffin sections, allowing retrospective analysis on archival material.

The commonest method of measurement of ER is by immunohistochemistry using a monoclonal antibody to ER. There is still some controversy as to how best to express ER in a semiquantitative way (Barnes et al., 1996) but it is likely that fine tuning the mode of assessment will eventually lead to a single definitive method which will become a universal standard.

ER as a predictor of hormone response

There is no doubt that ER status is useful in predicting response to antioestrogen therapy (McClelland et al., 1986; Williams et al., 1987; Hawkins et al., 1988;

Table 9b.1. Scoring system for steroid receptor expression in breast cancer

Score for proportion of cells staining	Score for staining intensity
0 = No nuclear staining	0 = No staining
1 = <1% nuclei staining	1 = Weak staining
2 = 1–10% nuclei staining	2 = Moderate staining
3 = 11–33% nuclei staining	3 = Strong staining
4 = 34–66% nuclei staining	
5 = 67–100% nuclei staining	

Adding the two scores gives a maximum of 8.

Gaskell et al., 1989; Oriani et al., 1989), whether ER status is assessed biochemically (Williams et al., 1987; Oriani et al., 1989) or immunohistochemically (McClelland et al., 1986; Hawkins et al., 1988; Gaskell et al., 1989; Barnes et al., 1996). Patients with ER-negative tumours have a response rate of the order of 10% (de Sombre et al., 1980; Williams et al., 1987). Higher response rates have been reported (Oriani et al., 1989) and a strong possibility existed that some figures for ER status included false-negative results. In patients with ER-positive tumours, reported rates of response have varied from 32% (Williams et al., 1987) to almost 80% (Gaskell et al., 1989; Oriani et al., 1989). There are several reasons for these large variations in response rates which include the cut-off value for positive ER status, method of measurement and interlaboratory variations. Several authors have reported that response is related to level of expression of ER. In patients whose tumours have high levels of ER (the definition of high varies from 25 to 200 fmol/mg), 60–80% of patients respond to endocrine manipulation (Williams et al., 1987; Oriani et al., 1989). These response rates are independent of menopausal status and in controlled clinical trials are similar to response rates for oophorectomy (Buchanan et al., 1986; Ingle et al., 1986).

Recently, a standardized working protocol has been published for the detection of ER and a scoring system for the intensity of staining which has been correlated to the likelihood of response to endocrine therapy (Leake et al., 2000). This describes the criteria which can be applied to the intensity of staining (Table 9b.1) which can also be used for other steroid receptors such as the progesterone receptor (PR). Experience of this scoring system in patients with advanced disease suggests the following:
- a score of 0 indicates that endocrine therapy will not work;
- a score of 2 or 3 indicates an approximately 20% chance of response to endocrine therapy;
- a score of 4–6 indicates an approximately 50% chance of response;

• a score of 7 or 8 indicates an approximately 75% chance of response.

The appropriate cut-off values for adjuvant therapy using immunohistochemistry have yet to be determined, although Harvey et al. (1999) have reported that with a similar scoring system, a value of >2 was the optimal cut-off point for predicting an improved outcome.

Oestrogen-regulated proteins predictive of hormone response

Progesterone receptor (PR)

Progesterone receptors are regulated by oestrogens (Horwitz & McGuire, 1978). The presence of PR is generally coupled to functional growth regulation by oestrogens in vivo and in vitro (Savouret et al., 1989). The structure of PR is unique amongst steroid receptors as it consists of a heterodimer of two separate steroid-binding proteins encoded by a single gene (Krett et al., 1988). As in the ER, it is bound to HSP and the steroid-binding subunits have a cysteine-rich region which coordinates zinc and binds to DNA. The carboxy-terminal region binds to progesterone. Tumours which possess both ER and PR are more likely to respond to endocrine treatment than tumours which are only ER positive (Rayter, 1991). However, some benefit from endocrine therapy has also been observed in PR-negative tumours (Clark & McGuire, 1983). It is of interest that the small group of patients with ER-negative but PR-positive tumours (approximately 2%) consistently show a response rate to hormonal therapy of approximately 54% (Clark & McGuire, 1983).

Oestrogen-inducible protein (pS2)

The oestrogen-inducible protein pS2 is also of interest. It is a small secretory protein with a molecular weight of 7 kDa (Nunez et al., 1987). It is induced by oestradiol in ER-positive breast cancer cells (Masiakowski et al., 1982). Located on chromosome 21q (Moison et al., 1988), the pS2 gene comprises three exons and two introns (Mori et al., 1990). It has structural similarities to insulin-like growth factors (IGF) I and II (Rio et al., 1987; Stack et al., 1988). Although its function is unknown, it is speculated that it may act in an autocrine or paracrine manner and that its expression may reflect tumour differentiation (Thompson et al., 1993). Many studies have confirmed a strong correlation with ER positivity (Rio et al., 1987; Stack et al., 1988; Thompson et al., 1993; Foekens et al., 1994).

One study has suggested that expression of pS2 mRNA by breast tumours is associated with improved survival and this is able to define a group of lymph-node positive patients who otherwise have a better prognosis than lymph-node-positive patients whose tumours do not express pS2 (Thompson et al., 1993). The cytosolic content of pS2 in primary breast tumour biopsies has also been shown to be a marker of favourable prognosis regarding response to adjuvant hormonal therapy (Predine et al., 1992; Spyratos et al., 1994) and time to relapse and death (Predine et al., 1992; Foekens et al., 1993). Similar results have been obtained when pS2 transcripts were analysed with respect to relapse-free survival (Thompson et al., 1993). However, when pS2 has been measured immunohistochemically, there was little or no prognostic value associated with its expression (Cappelletti et al., 1992; Henry et al., 1991; Thor et al., 1992). Most studies have, however, shown a correlation between immunohistochemical detection of expressed pS2 and response to endocrine therapy in patients with recurrent or advanced disease (Henry et al., 1991; Schwartz et al., 1991). In one of the largest studies to date, 230 patients who subsequently developed recurrent/advanced disease had cytosol pS2 (and ER and PR) measured in the primary tumour. None had received prior adjuvant endocrine treatment and first-line treatment for recurrent/advanced disease was with tamoxifen. Although pS2 expression was correlated with a longer progression-free survival, higher levels of pS2 were not associated with increased probability of response to tamoxifen as was the case with ER and PR (Foekens et al., 1994). However, in patients whose tumours had intermediate levels of expression of ER/PR (defined as >10 and <75 fmol/mg cytosol protein), pS2 was positively related to progression-free survival as well as postrelapse survival (Foekens et al., 1994). Expression of pS2 may have a role in selecting patients with intermediate levels of expression of steroid receptors for endocrine therapy, but this needs to be tested in a prospective manner. In conclusion, the current consensus seems to be that measurement of pS2 has little to add over and above that of ER although pS2 expression may have a role in defining a subset of patients with ER-positive tumours who on relapse are more likely to respond to antioestrogen therapy (Pichon & Milgrom, 1993).

Heat shock protein 27(HSP27)

HSP27 is a small molecular weight protein which is thought to have a role in thermotolerance and is found in both normal and malignant cells (Ciocca et al., 1993). It may also have a role in drug and endocrine resistance. Concentrations of HSP27 in breast tumours are quantitatively and qualitatively linked to ER expression (Dunn et al., 1993) but only weakly to PR expression (Ciocca et al., 1990). It has been reported that coexpression of ER and HSP27 in breast cancer increases the likelihood of response to hormone therapy as compared with patients expressing ER alone (Cano et al., 1986; King et al., 1986). However, HSP27 cannot be considered as a major determinant of endocrine response and its expression in breast cancer is not routinely undertaken.

Markers of lack of response to endocrine therapy

Epidermal growth factor receptor (EGFR) and c-erbB-2 (HER-2/neu)

Epidermal growth factor receptor (EGFR) and the proto-oncogene, c-erbB-2 show substantial homology and it is believed that EGFR is the protein product of c-erbB-2 (Downward et al., 1984). Both are transmembrane receptors whose function involves phosphorylation of tyrosine on their internal domains (Connelly & Stern, 1990). In addition, EGFR not only binds to EGF, but also transforming growth factor-alpha (TGF-α), both of which act as growth promoters of breast cancer cells (Dickson, 1990). A proportion of breast cancers overexpress EGFR and this expression is inversely proportional to expression of ER (Slamon et al., 1987; Nicholson et al., 1993). Tumour overexpression of both EGFR and c-erbB-2 appears to be related to aggressive behaviour of breast tumours and is predictive of poor disease-free and overall survival (Harris et al., 1992; Nicholson et al., 1991, 1993). Early studies had suggested that EGFR-positive tumours were associated with lack of response to hormone therapy (Nicholson et al., 1989, 1994a) and c-erbB-2-positive tumours have a poorer response to endocrine therapy than those which are c-erbB-2 negative (Nicholson et al., 1990). A study of 241 patients who had relapsed and were treated with first-line endocrine therapy supported these observations (Houston et al., 1999). A recent meta-analysis of published data from seven studies comparing more than 1100 patients showed a 2.46 odds ratio of disease progression on hormonal therapy for HER-2-positive patients compared with HER-2 negative patients (De Laurentiis et al., 2000). Of even greater concern has been the suggestion that in patients whose tumours coexpress both ER and HER-2, adjuvant tamoxifen therapy leads to a worse outcome compared with patients not receiving tamoxifen (Bianco et al., 2000). This needs to be confirmed in a prospective randomized trial.

Urokinase

Urokinase-type plasminogen activator (uPA) is a proteolytic enzyme thought to be involved in the process of tumour cell invasion. Its activity during the metastatic process may be regulated by an inhibitor, plasminogen activator inhibitor-1 (PAI-1). In one study, 235 tamoxifen-naive patients who relapsed were treated with tamoxifen; those patients with high levels of uPA in the primary tumour were associated with a shorter duration of response to tamoxifen and a shorter survival compared with patients with uPA negative tumours (Foekens et al., 1995). However, this only achieved a statistical significance in those patients whose tumours expressed intermediate levels of expression of ER/PR.

Transforming growth factor α

TGFα has been shown to stimulate breast cancer cell growth in vitro, although oestradiol is still required for cell growth to occur (Clarke et al., 1989). In a small study of human tumours whose endocrine sensitivity was known, high levels of TGFα expression were associated with lack of response to hormone therapy and this was independent of ER or EGFR expression (Nicholson et al., 1994b).

Prolactin

Prolactin levels in one study have been correlated with resistance to antioestrogens given in an adjuvant setting (Bhatavdekar et al., 1994). Tamoxifen normally lowers serum prolactin, but prolactin levels remained high in patients who relapsed compared with patients who did not relapse, when the serum prolactin levels remained low. Although there is some experimental work which may support this association (Manni et al., 1985), there is, at present, no other corroborative evidence.

Prostate-specific antigen (PSA)

PSA is a serine protease which may play a role in several cancers, notably prostate cancer and breast cancer. In breast cancer, low level of expression in the tumour is related to larger tumours, postmenopausal status and ER-negative tumours. In patients with recurrent breast cancer, it has been shown that high levels of PSA were significantly associated with a poor response to tamoxifen (Foekens et al., 1999). However, measurement of PSA in breast cancer is not routinely performed and further confirmation of these results is warranted.

Mechanisms of endocrine resistance

Since the observation by Beatson that some patients with advanced breast cancer respond to bilateral oophorectomy (Beatson, 1896), it has been appreciated that the majority of patients are resistant to hormonal manipulation. Even those patients with metastatic breast cancer initially sensitive to oestrogen withdrawal or antagonism, will ultimately become resistant to endocrine therapy and will eventually die of their disease. There has been growing interest in the mechanisms of resistance to endocrine therapy for two major reasons. First, greater knowledge of hormone resistance may lead to new strategies to overcome endocrine resistance to the patient's advantage. Secondly, greater understanding of the mechanisms of endocrine resistance may lead to a better understanding of steroid receptor-mediated control mechanisms of cell function and the interplay between steroid and peptide growth factors in the control of cell proliferation. It is likely that the mechanisms of endocrine resistance for any individual patient will vary with the clinical situation.

Breast cancers which lack ER are very unlikely to respond to oestrogen withdrawal or antioestrogens (Rayter, 1991). However, many breast cancers may express ER and/or PR, yet still be unresponsive to endocrine therapy. The development of breast cancer cell lines for study in vitro which show similar patterns of hormone sensitivity, dependency and independency to those observed clinically, has allowed the elucidation of a wide variety of mechanisms by which breast cancer cells can become independent of hormones despite, apparently, still possessing the cellular machinery which allowed them to respond to endocrine therapy initially. The types of cell lines which have been developed include the following:

(1) wild type cells with different inherent hormone sensitivities;
(2) sublines derived from the continuous growth or passage of wild type cells under differing selective conditions;
(3) genetically engineered phenotypes of dependency/sensitivity, independency/ sensitivity and total autonomy (Miller & Langdon, 1997). These in vitro systems suggest that progression to hormone independence may occur by a variety of mechanisms and that ER function may be normal, abnormal or lost. Not all of these in vitro mechanisms have been confirmed in vivo in humans. However, altered regulation of specific subsets of ER-regulated genes are strongly implicated. Some of these genes such as those encoding for EGFR, laminin receptor and cathepsin D, appear to be central to the mechanisms of other processes such as angiogenesis, cell mobility, invasion and metastasis. Therefore, it is not surprising that the breast cancer cell line MCF-7, normally highly oestradiol dependent, exhibits increased invasiveness and metastatic potential in vivo with the development of hormone independence and insensitivity (Clarke et al., 1994). The following mechanisms may be theoretically involved in the phenomenon of hormone resistance.

Oestrogen receptor mechanisms
Absence of oestrogen receptor

Approximately 10–30% of human breast cancers have either undetectable or very low levels of expression of ER. It is not clear whether these tumours arise from ER-negative cells or whether they arise from ER-positive cells which have lost their receptor. However, the fact that a similar proportion of in situ breast cancers express ER as invasive cancers suggests that if ER-negative tumours arise from ER-positive cells, then loss of ER is a very early event. Tumours which are ER negative are usually associated with high levels of expression of EGFR and the c-erbB-2 oncogene protein. Histologically, these tumours are more likely to be of high histological grade and exhibit a high proliferation rate. It is not surprising that such tumours rarely respond to endocrine therapy.

Exon variants and deletions

The ER consists of 8 exons (Figure 9b.1) and recently, several groups have reported variant forms of ER mRNA in primary human breast cancers and in breast cancer cell lines (Barrett-Lee et al., 1987; Fuqua et al., 1991; Fuqua, 1993; Miksicek et al., 1993). To date, the variant ER mRNAs have only been found in the presence of the normal ER mRNA and it appears that the variant mRNA is produced by alternative splicing of the normal ER mRNA. When tumours with the receptor phenotype ER+/ER− were examined by isolating RNA from these tumours, transcripts with exon 7 deletions were identified in most of them (Fuqua et al., 1991, 1992). When this variant was transcribed in yeast containing an ER hormone response element, it was able to inhibit the activity of wild type ER. Exon 7 forms part of the hormone binding domain and does not bind oestrogen but is able to inhibit the activity of wild type ER in a dominant-negative fashion. Subsequent work has shown that the exon 7 variant is present in most ER-positive tumours, but is present in higher concentrations in ER+/PR− tumours compared with ER+/PR− tumours. This may indicate a dose effect of the exon 7 variant not only on PR expression but also on antioestrogen sensitivity.

In ER−/PR+ tumours, Fuqua et al. (1991) demonstrated ER with a deletion of exon 5. This is also part of the hormone binding domain and is capable of binding the oestrogen response element of ER, causing activation of transcription in a dominant-positive manner. Transfection studies into MCF-7 cells have shown the exon 5-deleted ER variant to cause increased production of PR positive cells, enhanced colony formation in semisolid media and enhanced growth in nude mice in the absence of the normally required oestrogen supplementation. MCF-7 cells transfected with the exon 5-deleted ER variant are resistant to tamoxifen but are inhibited by pure antioestrogens. This ER variant has also been shown to be present in some ER+/PR+ tumours and increased amounts of this variant have now been detected in the tumours of some patients resistant to tamoxifen. However, not all studies have been able to demonstrate the presence of an exon 5 deletion with resistance to oestrogen deprivation (Zhang et al., 1993).

Most breast tumours have been found to contain variant ERs with deletions of exons 3 and 4 which occur in the C and D domains of the ER. They do not inhibit the binding activity of wild type ER. However, it has been shown in the human breast cancer cell line T47-D that the exon 3 variant inhibited transcriptional activation in a dominant-negative manner when cotransfected with wild type ER (Miksicek et al., 1993). This effect probably occurs through protein–protein interactions rather than directly interacting with ER as the exon 3 variant cannot bind its response element.

Mutations of the hormone binding domain

The hormone binding domain of the ER also contains functions for transactivation, nuclear binding and dimerization. It contains the amino acids 302–553 and at least six mutations have been described. Thus, alteration of amino acid 380 leads to increased sensitivity to oestradiol despite an unaltered receptor affinity (Katzenellenbogen et al., 1993). When ERs containing a mutation at amino acid 400 were tranfected into the ER-negative human breast cancer cell line MDA-MB-231, addition of oestradiol inhibited growth of the cells, whereas 4-hydroxy tamoxifen (4-OH TAM) stimulated growth and the steroidal antioestrogen ICI 164,384 inhibited growth (Jiang et al., 1992). Other single amino acid mutations in the hormone binding domain of ER occur which may have differing results. These observations suggest that oestradiol may not bind as well to the mutated ER as some antioestrogens, or where binding does occur, the mutated ER may not allow transactivation to occur or may form inactive heterodimers with wild type ER. Although these studies of ER in vitro are interesting, there is yet no evidence for specific mutations in the ER of human tumours to explain resistance to endocrine therapy in the clinical setting.

Tumour cell elimination of antioestrogens

Breast cancer cells may acquire resistance to antioestrogens by elimination of tamoxifen in much the same way as cytotoxic agents are removed from the cell by the action of p-glycoprotein. The evidence in support of this theory of resistance is the observation in nude mice that tumours which have become resistant to tamoxifen have lower intratumoral levels of tamoxifen than responsive tumours (Osborne et al., 1991). In addition, two groups have found that levels of tamoxifen and its antioestrogenic metabolites are low in resistant tumours (Osborne et al., 1992; Johnston et al., 1993). Whether this difference in intratumour tamoxifen levels is important is still open to question, especially as it has been shown in a similar mouse model that even low levels of tamoxifen in apparently tamoxifen-resistant tumours may stimulate growth of the tumour (Gottardis et al., 1989).

Clonal selection

There is evidence to suggest that tamoxifen can act as an agonist in human breast cancer by causing the proliferation of a subpopulation of breast cancer cells which 'see' tamoxifen as an oestrogen (Baildam et al., 1987; Graham et al., 1992). In support of this mechanism as a cause of resistance are the observations of a 'withdrawal' response of the tumour on cessation of tamoxifen therapy. Such withdrawal responses have been recorded in a human breast cancer cell line (MCF-7) grown in nude mice (Gottardis & Jordan, 1988; Gottardis et al., 1989), and in 10–30% of patients with advanced breast cancer (Canney et al., 1987; Howell et al., 1992). One explanation of this effect is that within an endocrine-responsive tumour there may be clones of cells with different sensitivities to tamoxifen. Cellular heterogeneity of breast cancers has been well documented both in regard to hormone sensitivity and hormone receptors (Greene et al., 1984; Hamm & Allegra, 1988). Selective cell kill has also been demonstrated after successful endocrine therapy and responses to second-line endocrine manipulation are more likely in tumours which have responded to first-line endocrine therapy (Stoll, 1988). These data would be compatible with a successive destruction of cellular populations with differing hormone sensitivity. However, clinical observations are not entirely compatible with the clonal selection theory as the major and only mechanism by which endocrine resistance occurs. For example, if ER status is a marker of hormone dependence and relapse following initial successful endocrine therapy is due to proliferation of ER-negative clones, the resulting hormone independent tumour should be ER poor or negative. Although this occasionally occurs (Taylor et al., 1982) most relapsed tumours remain ER positive (Hawkins et al., 1990; Johnston et al., 1995). They may also continue to express oestrogen-regulated proteins such as PR and pS2 (Johnston et al., 1995). It is therefore likely that other mechanisms come into play which lead to endocrine resistance.

Acquisition of steroidogenic metabolic pathways

Some breast cancers may acquire the ability to synthesize oestrogens (Miller & Forrest, 1974; Miller et al., 1990). This may allow tumours to become independent of external sources of oestrogen. However, in the clinical setting, there is little evidence that endocrine resistance is associated with enhanced capacity for oestrogen biosynthesis or that hormone-independent cancers are more likely to synthesize oestrogen than hormone-dependent cancers (Miller et al., 1990). An alternative may be the ability of breast cancers to convert tamoxifen to oestrogenic metabolites. Pathways of tamoxifen metabolism within breast tumour cells have been described (Murphy et al., 1990) and tamoxifen can be converted to metabolite E which is a weak oestrogen. This may undergo isomerization to a more powerful oestrogen capable of stimulating breast cancer cell growth (Osborne et al., 1992). However, this mechanism of tamoxifen agonism has been questioned as tumour progression still continued in nude mice even if the mice were treated with a nonisomerizable analogue, suggesting that tamoxifen itself was the agonist (Wolf et al., 1993).

Constitutive production of mitogens

The transition from an oestrogen-dependent to an oestrogen-independent growth state has been postulated to occur through the mechanism of oestrogen-induced growth factors which have become constitutive. The known mitogenic properties of transforming growth factors suggests them for this role. Studies using exogenous TGF-α or antibodies/antisense oligonucleotides against TGF-α have suggested that TGF-α acted as an autocrine stimulus to breast cancer cells. Furthermore, levels of TGF-α mRNA were elevated in oestrogen-independent cell lines compared with those that are oestrogen-dependent (Murphy & Dotzlaw, 1989). However, the observation that transfection of the TGF-α gene into an oestrogen-dependent cell line did not alter the oestrogenic requirement for cell growth suggests that other growth factors are involved (Clarke et al., 1989), such as the insulin-like growth factors (IGFs). IGF-II expression is closely linked to hormone sensitivity (Nicholson et al., 1992) and in certain cell lines and xenografts, it is constitutively expressed (Nicholson et al., 1993).

One transforming growth factor, TGF-β, is growth inhibitory to breast cancer cells and high constitutive levels of TGF-β activity have been reported in media conditioned by hormone-independent breast cancer cells (Dickson et al., 1986). Loss of oestrogen sensitivity may be associated with increased responsiveness to TGF-β1 and with a marked increase in TGF-β1 mRNA (King et al., 1989). The introduction of TGF-β1 cDNA into a hormone-sensitive cell line has been reported to produce oestrogen-independent tumours in nude mice (Arteaga et al., 1993).

Messenger system interactions

Interactions between ER-mediated pathways and polypeptide growth factor pathways could theoretically also result in tamoxifen resistance. Thus, increasing the levels of cyclic AMP in tumour cells may alter the cellular response to tamoxifen, converting it from an antioestrogen to a weak oestrogen agonist (Katzenellenbogen, 1996). The mechanism by which this occurs is not fully defined, but a possible mechanism may be by increasing phosphorylation of ER or proteins involved in the ER response pathway. Changes in phosphorylation status of cells may determine the biological activity of ER as well as the effectiveness of antioestrogens as oestrogen antagonists (Fujimoto & Katzenellenbogen, 1994). Another mechanism by which resistance may occur is by the interaction of specific proteins which interact with the ER/oestrogen response element complex which may influence transcriptional activation (Tonetti & Jordan, 1995).

Effects of oncogenes on cell cycle control

Aberrant expression of oncogenes (for example, c-*myc* and cyclin D1) and tumour suppressor genes (for example, p53) are relatively common in breast cancer (Callahan et al., 1992; Shiu et al., 1993; Deng et al., 1994). These have key roles in cell cycle progression. In particular, cyclin D1 has a central role in the progression of breast cancer cells (Musgrove et al., 1994) and the fact that cyclin D1 mRNA levels decline rapidly after antioestrogen treatment of breast cancer (Musgrove et al., 1993; Watts et al., 1994) suggests that cyclin D1 may be important in mediating antioestrogen growth inhibition and the development of endocrine resistance. Failure of antioestrogens to inhibit cyclin D1 because of constitutive upregulation or overexpression may result in continuous cyclin D1/CDK activation and cell cycle progression even in the presence of a growth inhibitor (Daly et al., 1994; Janes et al., 1994). Overexpression of cyclin D1 is well described in breast cancer cell lines (Gillett et al., 1994). Its relevance in the development of endocrine resistance of human breast cancer in vivo requires further study.

Alteration of secreted proteins

Differences in the pattern of secreted proteins have been observed between tamoxifen-responsive and tamoxifen-resistant cell lines. In particular, tamoxifen resistance may be associated with the lack of upregulation of the synthesis of a 42 kDa protein with presumed growth inhibitory functions (Lykkesfeldt et al., 1994). Pure antioestrogens which exert normal upregulation of the protein also inhibit growth of tamoxifen-resistant cells. Another protein which is selectively alerted in tamoxifen-resistant cells is the type I IGF receptor (Wiseman et al., 1993).

The use of steroid receptors in clinical trials

It can be seen from the above discussion that steroid receptors have been extremely valuable predictive markers for response to endocrine agents. A predictive factor is any measurement associated with response or lack of response to a particular therapy. Most of the indications regarding adjuvant endocrine therapy have been deduced retrospectively from controlled clinical trials in which the effect of ER status has been calculated. Thus, from the data published by the Early Breast Cancer Trials Collaborative Group (EBCTCG, 1998), adjuvant tamoxifen has been shown to be beneficial in all patients whose tumours are ER positive irrespective of age. Indeed, the proportional risk reductions for recurrence and mortality for women younger than 50 who received tamoxifen for 5 years were 45% and 32% respectively. This compares favourably with the results for women older than 59 who obtained a 54% and 33% reduction in recurrence and mortality respectively. In women with node-negative breast cancer treated with adjuvant chemotherapy followed by adjuvant tamoxifen irrespective of ER status, patients receiving tamoxifen did not gain any benefit if their tumours did not express ER and, if anything, did slightly worse (Hutchins et al., 1998). Similar findings regarding the predictive value of steroid receptors in advanced disease can be found.

How should steroid receptors be used in clinical trials? First, the receptor status of the tumour should be determined, probably by immunocytochemical methods. ER-positive patients could then be selected for trials involving new endocrine agents. A variety of new endocrine agents have recently been discovered, the most important of which are the new aromatase inhibitors such as anastrazole, letrozole and exemestane and the new pure antioestrogen Faslodex (Astrazeneca, UK). Each of these agents needs to be tested in the areas of neoadjuvant, adjuvant and advanced treatment settings and it is clear from the data presented that tumour expression of ER is the most logical method of patient selection. Not only do each of these agents require testing against tamoxifen in each of these settings, but it is conceivable that combinations of endocrine therapies may work better than single-agent therapies as has recently been demonstrated in ER-positive premenopausal women taking a combination of LHRH inhibitors plus tamoxifen in the adjuvant setting (Rutqvist, 1999). The ATAC study, which has recently closed to accrual, is an example of combination endocrine therapy in which postmenopausal women with ER-positive (or ER unknown) tumours were randomized to tamoxifen, tamoxifen plus anastrazole or anastrazole for 5 years adjuvant therapy.

Another area of interest where ER expression is important is in the potential to inhibit contralateral breast cancers in women who have already had one breast cancer successfully treated. Thus, the above study by Hutchins et al. (1998) suggested that women who have had ER-negative breast cancer may not exhibit the expected reduction in contralateral breast cancer previously reported by the EBCBCG (1998). This requires confirmation in a prospective randomized controlled trial. This naturally leads on to whether ER expression by normal human breast predicts for prevention or delay in the appearance of breast cancers in a preventative setting. The recently reported NSABP P1 study of primary prevention of breast cancer in normal women at increased risk showed a 45% reduction in the incidence of breast cancer in women taking tamoxifen for 5 years (Fisher et al., 1998). Careful study of the data suggests that only ER-positive tumours were prevented. The role of ER expression in the normal breast and its role in chemoprevention is as yet entirely unknown.

A further role in ER receptor measurement in clinical trials is the duration of adjuvant endocrine therapy. The EBCTCG meta-analysis also provides strong evidence for the use of tamoxifen therapy for at least 5 years (EBCTCG, 1998). The proportional risk reduction in recurrence was 21%, 28% and 50% for 1, 2 and 5 years respectively. Subset analysis, although not as statistically robust, suggests that the risk reduction is greater in patients whose tumours were ER positive compared with patients in whom the ER was unknown and it seems reasonable to measure ER expression if patients are to be asked to take an adjuvant agent which is known to increase the risk of endometrial cancer (Chapter 2). The data regarding longer duration of adjuvant endocrine therapy is contradictory but the aTTom (adjuvant tamoxifen treatment offer more?) study in which patients are randomized to receive tamoxifen for a further 5 years after uncertainty arises in the duration of tamoxifen therapy should provide a definitive answer. It again seems reasonable that if women are to be asked to take an adjuvant therapy for this length of time, ER expression of the tumour should be measured. Similar studies examining duration of adjuvant endocrine therapies using the newer endocrine agents will also need to be performed.

There is a suggestion that women whose tumours do not express ER and receive adjuvant tamoxifen may do worse than if they received no adjuvant endocrine therapy (Hutchins et al., 1998). It has been speculated that this may be due to the expression of the HER-2/*neu* oncogene in ER-negative tumours and a recent retrospective study seems to support this hypothesis (Bianco et al., 2000). However, retrospective studies have been conflicting on whether HER-2/*neu* expression confers resistance to endocrine therapy (Carlomagno et al., 1996; Elledge et al., 1996). Clinical trials need to be constructed to examine the interaction of ER and HER-2/*neu* in patients treated in the neoadjuvant, adjuvant and advanced settings with currently available endocrine agents. A recent study of patients with metastatic breast cancer whose tumours overexpressed HER-2/*neu* has confirmed an increase in response to chemotherapy with the addition of Herceptin® (a humanized monoclonal antibody to the HER-2 receptor protein) to 50% compared with a response of 35% to chemotherapy alone (Slamon et al., 2001). It therefore seems logical to test this monoclonal antibody in patients with recurrent disease with HER-2-positive tumours with and without an endocrine agent in both ER-positive and ER-negative patients. It also seems logical to extend this to the adjuvant setting. Finally, the role of the newly discovered form of ER, ERβ will also need to be investigated.

Conclusion

A great deal of progress has been made over the last 25 years regarding the molecular mechanisms of breast cancer progression and inhibition with endocrine agents. Steroid receptor analysis should now be routine and its expression can now be used as a good guide to therapy in the advanced and adjuvant settings. The role of HER-2/*neu* in relation to steroid receptors requires further evaluation. Although the mechanisms of resistance to endocrine therapy are scientifically interesting and important, they do not yet play an important role in the management of the individual patient.

REFERENCES

Arteaga, C.L., Carty-Dugger, T., Moses, H.L. et al. (1993). Transforming growth factor beta 1 can induce estrogen-independent tumorigenicity of human breast cancer cells in athymic mice. *Cell Growth and Differentiation*, 4, 193–201.

Baildam, A.D., Zaloudik, J., Howell, A. et al. (1987). DNA analysis by flow cytometry, response to endocrine treatment and prognosis in advanced carcinoma of the breast. *British Journal of Cancer*, 55, 553–9.

Barnes, D.M., Harris, W.H., Smith, P. et al. (1996). Immunohistochemical determination of oestrogen receptor: a comparison of different methods of assessment of staining and correlation with clinical outcomes of breast cancer patients. *British Journal of Cancer*, 74, 1445–51.

Barrett-Lee, P.J., Travers, M.T., McClelland, R.A. et al. (1987). Characterization of estrogen receptor messenger RNA in human breast cancer. *Cancer Research*, 47, 6653–9.

Beatson, G.T. (1896). On the treatment of inoperable cases of carcinoma of the mamma: suggestions for a new method of treatment with illustrative cases. *Lancet*, ii, 104–7.

Bhatavdekar, J.M., Patel, D.D., Karelia, N.H. et al. (1994). Can plasma prolactin predict tamoxifen resistance in patients with advanced breast cancer? *European Journal of Surgical Oncology*, 20, 118–21.

Bianco, A.R., De Laurentiis, M., Carlomagno, C. et al. (2000). HER-2 overexpression predicts adjuvant tamoxifen failure for early breast cancer (EBC): complete data at 20 years of the Naples GUN randomised trial. *Proceedings of the American Society of Clinical Oncology*, 19, 75a, Abstract 289.

Buchanan, R.B., Blamey, R.W., Durrant, K.R. et al. (1986). A randomized comparison of tamoxifen with surgical oophorectomy in premenopausal patients with advanced breast cancer. *Journal of Clinical Oncology*, 4, 1326–30.

Callahan, R., Cropp, C.S., Merlo, G.R. et al. (1992). Somatic mutations in human breast cancer – a status report. *Cancer*, 69, 1582–8.

Canney, P.A. Griffiths, T., Latief, T.N. et al. (1987). Clinical significance of tamoxifen withdrawal response. (Letter.) *Lancet*, i, 36.

Cano, A., Coffer, A. I., Adatia, R. et al. (1986). Histochemical studies with an estrogen receptor-related protein in human breast tumors. *Cancer Research*, 46, 6475–80.

Capalletti, V., Coradini, D., Scanziani, E. et al. (1992). Prognostic relevance of pS2 status in association with steroid receptor status and proliferative activity in node-negative breast cancer. *European Journal of Cancer*, 28A, 1315–18.

Carlomagno, C., Perrone, F., Gallo, C. et al. (1996). c-*erb*B-2 overexpression decreases the benefit of adjuvant tamoxifen in early stage breast cancer without axillary node metastases. *Journal of Clinical Oncology*, 14, 2702–8.

Ciocca, D.R., Stato, A.O. & Amprino de Castro, M.M. (1990). Colocalization of estrogen and progesterone receptors with an estrogen-regulated heat shock protein in paraffin sections of human breast and endometrial cancer tissue. *Breast Cancer Research and Treatment*, 16, 243–51.

Ciocca, D.R., Osterreich, S., Chamness, G.C. et al. (1993). Biological and clinical implications of heat shock protein 27000 (Hsp27): a review. *Journal of the National Cancer Institute*, 85, 1558–70.

Clark, G.M. & McGuire, W.L. (1983). Progesterone receptors and human breast cancer. *Breast Cancer Research and Treatment*, 3, 157–63.

Clarke, R., Brunner, N., Katz, D. et al. (1989). The effects of a constitutive expression of transforming growth factor-α on the growth of MCF-7 human breast cancer cells *in vitro* and *in vivo*. *Molecular Endocrinology*, 3, 372–80.

Clarke, R., Skaar, T., Baumann, K. et al. (1994). Hormonal carcinogenesis in breast cancer: cellular and molecular studies of malignant progression. *Breast Cancer Research and Treatment*, 31, 237–48.

Conneely, O.M., Sullivan, W.P., Toft, D.O. et al. (1986). Molecular cloning of the chicken progesterone receptor. *Science*, 46, 389–99.

Connelly, P.A. & Stern, D.F. (1990). The epidermal growth factor receptor and the product of the *neu* protooncogene are members of a receptor tyrosine phosphorylation cascade. *Proceedings of the National Academy of Science USA*, 87, 6047–57.

Cullen, R., Maguire, T.M., McDermott, E. et al. (1999). Estrogen receptor-beta: a new form of estrogen receptor in breast cancer. *European Journal of Cancer*, 35, Suppl. 4, 84.

Daly, R.J., Binder, M.D. & Sutherland, R.L. (1994). Overexpression of the Grb2 gene in human breast cancer cell lines. *Oncogene*, 9, 2723–7.

Darbre, P.D., Glover, J.F. & King, R.J.B. (1989). Effects of steroids and their antagonists on breast cancer cells: therapeutic implications. *Recent Results in Cancer Research*, 113, 16–28.

Dati, C., Antoniotti, S., Taverna, D. et al. (1990). Inhibition of c-erbB2m oncogene expression by estrogens in human breast cancer cells. *Oncogene*, 5, 1001–6.

De Laurentiis, M., Arpino, G., Massarelli, E. et al. (2000). A meta analysis of the interaction between HER 2 and the response to endocrine therapy (ET) in metastatic breast cancer (MBC). *Proceedings of the American Society of Clinical Oncology*, 19, 78a, Abstract 300.

Deng, G., Chen, L.C., Schott, D.R. et al. (1994). Loss of heterozygocity and p53 gene mutations in breast cancer. *Cancer Research*, 54, 499–505.

deSombre, E.R., Greene, G.L. & Jensen, E.V. (1980). Estrogen receptors and hormone dependence of breast cancer. In: *Breast Cancer: New Concepts in Etiology and Control*, 1st edn, ed. M.J. Brennan, C.M. McGrath & M.A. Rich, p. 69. New York: Academic Press.

Dickson, R.B. (1990). Stimulating and inhibitory growth factors and breast cancer. *Journal of Steroid Biochemistry and Molecular Biology*, 37, 795–811.

Dickson, R.B., Bates, S.E., McManaway, M.E. et al. (1986). Characterisation of estrogen responsive transforming activity in human breast cancer cell lines. *Cancer Research*, 46, 1707–13.

Downward, J., Yarden, Y., Scrace, G. et al. (1984). Close similarity of epidermal growth factor receptor and c-erbB oncogene protein sequence. *Nature*, 307, 521–7.

Dubik, D., Dembinski, T.C. & Shiu, R.P.O. (1987). Stimulation of c-myc oncogene expression associated with estrogen-induced proliferation of human breast cancer cells. *Cancer Research*, 47, 6517–21.

Dunn, D.K., Whelan, R.D.H., Hill, B. et al. (1993). Relationship of HSP27 and oestrogen receptor in hormone sensitive and insensitive cell lines. *Journal of Steroid Biochemistry and Molecular Biology*, 46, 469–79.

EBCTCG (1998). Tamoxifen for early breast cancer: an overview of the randomised trials. *Lancet*, 351, 1451–67.

Elledge, R., Green, S., Ciocca, D. et al. (1996). HER-2 neu expression does not predict response to tamoxifen in ER-positive metastatic breast cancer. *Breast Cancer Research and Treatment*, 41, 289, Abstract 518.

Fisher, B., Constantino, J.P., Wickerham, D.L. et al. (1998). Tamoxifen for prevention of breast cancer: report of the National Surgical Adjuvant Breast and Bowel Project P-1 study. *Journal of the National Cancer Institute*, 90, 1371–81.

Foekens, J.A., van Putten, W.L.J., Portengen, H. et al. (1993). Prognostic value of pS2 and cathepsin D in 710 human primary breast tumours: multivariate analysis. *Journal of Clinical Oncology*, 11, 899–908.

Foekens, J.A., Portengen, H., Look, M.P. et al. (1994). Relationship of pS2 with response to tamoxifen therapy in patients with recurrent breast cancer. *British Journal of Cancer*, 70, 1217–23.

Foekens, J.A., Look, M.P., Peters, H.A. et al. (1995). Urokinase-type plasminogen activator and its inhibitor PAI-1: predictors of poor response to tamoxifen therapy in recurrent breast cancer. *Journal of the National Cancer Institute*, 87(10), 751–6.

Foekens, J.A., Diamandis, E.P., Yu, H. et al. (1999). Expression of prostate-specific antigen (PSA) correlates with poor response to tamoxifen therapy in recurrent breast cancer. *British Journal of Cancer*, 79, 888–94.

Foster, K.S. & Wimalasena, J. (1996). Estrogen regulates activity of cyclin-dependant kinases and retinoblastoma protein phosphorylation in breast cancer cells. *Molecular Endocrinology*, 10, 488–98.

Fujimoto, N. & Katzenellenbogen, B.S. (1994). Alteration in the agonist/antagonist balance of antiestrogens by activation of protein kinase A signalling pathways in breast cancer cells: antiestrogen-selectivity and promoter-dependence. *Molecular Endocrinology*, 8, 296–304.

Fuqua, S.A.W. (1993). Abnormalities of the estrogen receptor in breast cancer – introduction. *Breast Cancer Research and Treatment*, 26, 117–18.

Fuqua, S.A.W., Fitzgerald, S.D., Chamness, G.C. et al. (1991). Variant human breast tumor estrogen receptor with constitutive transcriptional activity. *Cancer Research*, 51, 105–9.

Fuqua, S.A.W., Fitzgerald, S.D., Allred, D.C. et al. (1992). Inhibition of estrogen receptor action by a naturally occurring variant in human breast tumours. *Cancer Research*, 52, 483–6.

Gaskell, D.J., Hawkins, R.A., Dangster, K. et al. (1989). Relation between immunocytochemical estimation of oestrogen receptor in elderly patients with primary breast cancer and response to tamoxifen. *Lancet*, i, 1044–6.

Gillett, C., Fantl, V. & Smith, R. (1994). Amplification and overexpression of cyclin D1 in breast cancer detected by immunohistochemical staining. *Cancer Research*, 54, 1812–17.

Gottardis, M.M. & Jordan, V.C. (1988). Development of tamoxifen-stimulated growth of MCF-7 tumours in athymic mice after long-term antiestrogen administration. *Cancer Research*, 48, 5183–7.

Gottardis, M.M., Jiang, S.Y., Jeng, M.H. et al. (1989). Inhibition of tamoxifen-stimulated growth of an MCF-7 tumour variant in athymic mice by novel steroidal anti-oestrogens. *Cancer Research*, 49, 4090–3.

Graham, M.L. II, Smith, J.A., Jewett, P.B. et al. (1992). Heterogeneity of progesterone receptor content and remodelling by tamoxifen characterize subpopulations of cultured human breast cancer cells: analysis by quantitative dual parameter flow cytometry. *Cancer Research*, 52, 593–602.

Green, S. & Chambon, P. (1987). Oestradiol induction of a glucocorticoid-responsive gene by a chimaeric receptor. *Nature*, 325, 75–8.

Green, S., Walter, P., Kumar, V. et al. (1986). Human oestrogen receptor with DNA: sequence, expression and homology to v-erb A. *Nature*, 320, 134–9.

Greene, G.L., Sobel, N.B., King, W.J. et al. (1984). Immunochemical studies of estrogen receptors. *Journal of Steroid Biochemistry*, 20, 51–6.

Hamm, J.T. & Allegra, J.C. (1988). Loss of hormonal responsiveness in cancer. In: *Endocrine Management of Cancer-Biological Cases*, ed. B.A. Stoll, pp. 61–71. Basle: Karger Press.

Harris, A.L., Nicholson, S., Sainsbury, J.R.C. et al. (1992). Epidermal growth factor receptor and other oncogenes as prognostic markers. *National Cancer Institute Monographs*, 11, 181–7.

Harvey, J.M., Clark, G.M., Osborne, C.K. et al. (1999). Estrogen receptor status by immunohistochemistry is superior to the ligand-binding assays for predicting response to adjuvant therapy in breast cancer. *Journal of Clinical Oncology*, 17, 1475–85.

Hawkins, R.A., Sangster, K., Tesdale, A. et al. (1988). The cytochemical detection of oestrogen receptors in fine needle aspirates of breast cancer; correlation with biochemical assay and prediction of response to endocrine therapy. *British Journal of Cancer*, 58, 77–80.

Hawkins, R.A., Tesdale, A.L., Anderson, E.D.C. et al. (1990). Does the oestrogen receptor concentration of a breast cancer change during systemic therapy? *British Journal of Cancer*, 6, 877–80.

Henderson, B. E., Ross, R. & Bernstein, L. (1988). Estrogens as a cause of human cancer: the Richard and Hinda Rosenthal Foundation award lecture. *Cancer Research*, 48, 246–53.

Henry, J.A., Piggott, N.H., Mallick, U.K. et al. (1991). pNR–2/PS2 immunohistochemical staining in breast cancer: correlation with prognostic factors and endocrine response. *British Journal of Cancer*, 63, 615–22.

Hollenberg, S.M., Weinberger, C., Ong, E.S. et al. (1985). Primary structure and expression of a functional human glucocorticoid receptor with DNA. *Nature*, 318, 635–41.

Horwitz, K.B. & McGuire, W.L. (1978). Estrogen control of progesterone receptor in human breast cancer. *Journal of Biological Chemistry*, 253, 223–8.

Houston, S.J., Plunkett, T.A., Barnes, D.M. et al. (1999). Overexpression of c-erbB2 is an independent marker of resistance to endocrine therapy in advanced breast cancer. *British Journal of Cancer*, 79, 1220–6.

Howell, A., Dodwell, D.J., Anderson, H. et al. (1992). Response after withdrawal of tamoxifen and progestogens in advanced breast cancer. *Annals of Oncology*, 3, 611–17.

Hutchins, L., Green, S., Ravdin, P. et al. (1998). CMF versus CAF with and without tamoxifen in high-risk node-negative breast cancer patients and a natural history follow up study in low-risk node-negative patients: first results of intergroup trial INT 0102. *Proceedings of the American Society of Clinical Oncology*, 17.1a, Abstract 2.

Ingle, J.N., Krook, J.E., Green, S.J. et al. (1986). Randomized trial of bilateral oophorectomy versus tamoxifen in premenopausal women with metastatic breast cancer. *Journal of Clinical Oncology*, 4, 178–85.

Janes, P.W., Daly, R.J., de Fazio, A. et al. (1994). Activation of the Ras signalling pathway in human breast cancer cells overexpressing erbB–2. *Oncogene*, 19, 3601–8.

Jensen, E.V., Suzuki, T., Kawashima, T. et al. (1968). A two-step mechanism for the interaction of oestradiol with rat uterus. *Proceedings of the National Academy of Science*, 59, 632–8.

Jiang, S.-Y., Langan-Fahey, S.M., Stella, A. et al. (1992). Point mutation of estrogen receptor (ER) at the ligand binding domain changes the pharmacology of antiestrogens in ER-negative breast cancer cells stably expressing cDNAs for ER. *Molecular Endocrinology*, 6, 2167–74.

Johnston, S.R.D., Haynes, B.P., Smith, I.E. et al. (1993). Acquired tamoxifen resistance in human breast cancer and reduced intra-tumoral drug concentration. *Lancet*, 342, 1521–2.

Johnston, S.R.D., Saccani-Jotti, G., Smith, I.E. et al. (1995). Change in oestrogen receptor expression and function in tamoxifen-resistant breast cancer. *Endocrine Related Cancer*, 2, 105–10.

Kandouz, M., Siromachkova, M., Jacob, D. et al. (1996). Antagonism between estradiol and progestin on bcl-2 expression in breast cancer cells. *International Journal of Cancer*, 68, 120–5.

Katzenellenbogen, B.S. (1996). Estrogen receptors: bioactivities and interactions with cell signalling pathways. *Biology of Reproduction*, 54, 287–93.

Katzenellenbogen, B.S., Kendra, K.L., Norman, K.N. et al. (1987). Proliferation, hormone responsiveness and estrogen-receptor content of MCF-7 human breast cancer cells grown in the short-term and long-term absence of estrogen. *Cancer Research*, 47, 4355–60.

Katzenellenbogen, B.S., Fang, H.B., Ince, A. et al. (1993). Estrogen receptors: ligand discrimination and antiestrogen action. *Breast Cancer Research and Treatment*, 27, 17–26.

King, W.J. & Greene, G.L. (1984). Monoclonal antibodies localise oestrogen receptor in the nucleus of target cells. *Nature*, 307, 745–7.

King, R.J., Cano, A., Finley, J. et al. (1986). Immunological probes for oestradiol receptors in human breast tumours. *Journal of Steroid Biochemistry*, 24, 369–72.

King, R.J.B., Wang, D.Y., Daly, R.J. et al. (1989). Approaches to studying the role of growth factors in the progression of breast tumours from the steroid sensitive to insensitive state. *Journal of Steroid Biochemistry*, 34, 133–8.

Krett, N.L., Wei, L.L., Francis, M.D. et al. (1988). Human progesterone A-receptors can be synthesised intracellularly and are biologically functional. *Biochemical and Biophysical Research Communications*, 157, 278–85.

Kuiper, G.G., Enmark, E., Pelto-Huikko, M. et al. (1996). Cloning of a novel estrogen receptor expressed in rat prostate and ovary. *Proceedings of the National Academy of Science, USA*, 93, 5925–30.

Kumar, V., Green, S., Staub, A. et al. (1986). Localisation of the oestradiol-binding and putative DNA-binding domains of the human oestrogen receptor. *EMBO Journal*, 5, 2231–6.

Leake, R., Barnes, D., Pinder, S. et al. (2000). Immunohistochemical detection of steroid receptors in breast cancer: a working protocol. *Journal of Clinical Pathology*, 53, 634–5.

Lykkesfeldt, A.E., Madsen, M.W. & Briand, P. (1994). Altered expression of estrogen-regulated genes in a tamoxifen-resistant and ICI 164,383 and ICI 182,780 sensitive human breast cancer cell line MCF-7TAM^{R}1[1]. *Cancer Research*, 54, 1587–95.

Mader, S., Kumar, V., de Verneuil, H. et al. (1989). Three amino acids of the oestrogen receptor are essential to its ability to distinguish an oestrogen from a glucocorticoid responsive element. *Nature*, 338, 271–4.

Manni, A., Pontari, M. & Wright, C. (1985). Autocrine stimulation by prolactin of hormone-responsive breast cancer growth in cultures. *Endocrinology*, 117, 2040–3.

Markopoulos, C., Berger, U., Wilson, P. et al. (1988). Oestrogen receptor content of normal breast cells and breast carcinoma throughout the menstrual cycle. *British Medical Journal*, 296, 1349–51.

Masiakowski, P., Breathnach, R., Bloch, J. et al. (1982). Cloning of cDNA sequences of hormone-regulated genes from the MCF-7 human breast cancer cell line. *Nucleic Acids Research*, 10, 7895–903.

McClelland, R.A., Berger, U., Miller, L.S. et al. (1986). Immunocytochemical assay for estrogen receptor: relationship to outcome of therapy in patients with advanced breast cancer. *Cancer Research*, 46 (Suppl.), 4241s–3s.

McGuire, W.L. & de la Garza, M. (1973). Similarity of the estrogen receptor in human and rat mammary carcinoma. *Journal of Clinical Endocrinology and Metabolism*, 36, 548–52.

Miksicek, R.J., Lei, Y. & Wang, Y. (1993). Exon skipping gives rise to alternatively spliced forms of the estrogen receptor in breast tumor cells. *Breast Cancer Research and Treatment*, 26, 163–74.

Miller, W.R. (1996). Steroid hormones and cancer: (I) Basic biology and endocrinology. *European Journal of Surgical Oncology*, 22, 627–37.

Miller, W.R. & Forrest, A.P.M. (1974). Oestradiol synthesis from C19 steroids by human breast cancer. *British Journal of Cancer*, 33, 16–18.

Miller, W.R., Anderson, T.J. & Jack, W.J. (1990). Relationship between tumour aromatase activity, tumour characteristics and response to therapy. *Journal of Steroid Biochemistry and Molecular Biology*, 37, 1055–9.

Miller, W.R. & Langdon, S.P. (1997). Steroid hormones and cancer: lessons from experimental systems. *European Journal of Surgical Oncology*, 23, 72–83.

Moison, J.P., Mattei, M.G. & Mandel, J. (1988). Chromosome localisation and polymorphism of an oestrogen-inducible gene specifically expressed in some breast cancers. *Human Genetics*, 79, 168–71.

Mori, K., Fujii, R., Kida, N. et al. (1990). Complete primary structure of the human estrogen-responsive gene (pS2) product. *Journal of Biochemistry*, 107, 73–6.

Murphy, L.C. & Dotzlaw, H. (1989). Endogenous growth factor expression in T-47D human breast cancer cells associated with reduced sensitivity to antiproliferative effects of progestins and antiestrogens. *Cancer Research*, 49, 599–604.

Murphy, C.S., Langan-Fahey, S.M., McCague, R. et al. (1990). Structure–function relationships of hydroxylated metabolites of tamoxifen that control the proliferation of estrogen responsive T47D breast cancer cells *in vitro*. *Molecular Pharmacology*, 38, 737–43.

Musgrove, E.A., Hamilton, J.A., Lee, C.S.L. et al. (1993) Growth factor steroid and steroid antagonist regulation of cyclin gene expression associated with changes in T-47D human breast cancer cell cycle progression. *Molecular Cell Biology*, 13, 3577–87.

Musgrove, E.A., Lee, C.S.L., Buckley, M.F et al. (1994). Cyclin D1 induction in breast cancer cells shortens G1 and is sufficient for cells arrested in G1 to complete the cell cycle. *Proceedings of the National Academy of Science USA*, 91, 8022–6.

Nicholson, S., Sainsbury, J.R., Halcrow, P. et al. (1989). Expression of epidermal growth factor receptors associated with lack of response to endocrine therapy in recurrent breast cancer. *Lancet*, 1(8631), 182–5.

Nicholson, S., Wright, C., Sainsbury, J.R.C. et al. (1990). Epidermal growth factor receptor (EGFr) as a marker for poor prognosis in node-negative breast cancer patients: NEU and tamoxifen failure. *Journal of Steroid Biochemistry and Molecular Biology*, 6, 811–14.

Nicholson, S., Richard, J., Sainsbury, J.R.C. et al. (1991). Epidermal growth factor receptor (EGFR): results of a 6-year follow-up study in operable breast cancer with emphasis on the node-negative group. *British Journal of Cancer*, 63, 146–50.

Nicholson, R.I., McClelland, R.A., Finlay, P. et al. (1992). IGF-I and IGF-II expression in human breast cancer xenografts: relationship to hormone independence. *Breast Cancer Research and Treatment*, 22, 39–45.

Nicholson, R.I., McClelland, R.A., Finlay, P. et al. (1993). Relationship between EGF-R, c-erbB2 protein expression and Ki67 immunostaining in breast cancer and hormone sensitivity. *European Journal of Cancer*, 29A, 1018–23.

Nicholson, R.I., McClelland, R.A., Gee, J.M.W. et al. (1994a). Epidermal growth factor expression in breast cancer: association with response to endocrine therapy. *Breast Cancer Research and Treatment*, 29, 117–25.

Nicholson, R.I., McClelland, R.A., Gee, J.M.W. et al. (1994b). Transforming growth factor α and endocrine sensitivity in breast cancer. *Cancer Research*, 54, 1684–9.

Nunez, A.M., Jacolew, S., Briand, J.P. et al. (1987). Characterization of the estrogen-induced pS2 protein secreted by the human breast cancer cell line MCF-7. *Endocrinology*, 121, 1759–65.

Oriani, S., Bohm, S., Baeli, A. et al. (1989). Clinical response and survival according to oestrogen receptor levels after bilateral ovariectomy in advanced breast cancer. *European Journal of Surgical Oncology*, 15, 39–42.

Osborne, C.K., Coronardo, E., Allred, D.C. et al. (1991). Acquired tamoxifen resistance: correlation with reduced breast tumour levels of tamoxifen and isomerisation of trans-4-hydroxytamoxifen. *Journal of the National Cancer Institute*, 83, 1477–82.

Osborne, C.K., Wiebe, V.J., McGuire, W.L. et al. (1992). Tamoxifen and the isomers of 4-hydroxytamoxifen in tamoxifen-resistant tumours from breast cancer patients. *Journal of Clinical Oncology*, 10, 304–10.

Pichon, M.F. & Milgrom, E. (1993). Clinical significance of the estrogen regulated pS2 protein in mammary tumors. *Critical Reviews in Oncology and Haematology*, 15, 13–21.

Poglikitmongol, M., Green, S. & Chambon, P. (1988). Genomic organisation of the human oestrogen receptor gene. *EMBO Journal*, 7, 3385–8.

Predine, J., Spyratos, F., Prud'homme, J.F. et al. (1992). Enzyme-linked immunosorbent assay of pS2 in breast cancers, benign tumours and normal tissues. *Cancer*, 69, 2116–23.

Rayter, Z. (1991). Steroid receptors in breast cancer. *British Journal of Surgery*, 78, 528–35.

Rio, M.C., Bellocq, J.P., Gairard, B. et al. (1987). Specific expression of the pS2 gene in subclasses of breast cancers in comparison with expression of the estrogen and progesterone receptors and the oncogene ERB B2. *Proceedings of the National Academy of Science USA*, 84, 9243–7.

Rutqvist, L. (1999). Zoladex and tamoxifen as adjuvant therapy in premenopausal breast cancer: a randomised trial by the Cancer Research Campaign (CRC) Breast Cancer Trials Group, the Stockholm Breast Cancer Study Group, the South East Sweden Breast Cancer Group and the Gruppo Interdisciplinare Valutazione Interventi in Oncologia. *Proceedings of ASCO*, 18, 67a, Abstract 251.

Savouret, J.F., Misrahi, M., Loosfelt, H. et al. (1989). Molecular and cellular biology of mammalian progesterone receptors. *Recent Progress in Hormone Research*, 45, 65–111.

Schwartz, L.H., Koerner, F.C., Edgerton, S.M. et al. (1991). pS2 expression and response to hormonal therapy in patients with advanced breast cancer. *Cancer Research*, 51, 624–8.

Sherr, C.J. (1994). G1 phase progression: cycling on cue. *Cell*, 79, 551–5.

Shiu, R.P.C., Watson, P.H. & Dubik, D. (1993). c-myc oncogene expression in estrogen-dependent and independent breast cancer. *Clinical Chemistry*, 39, 353–5.

Slamon, D.J., Clark, G.M., Wong, S.G. et al. (1987). Human breast cancer: correlation of relapse and survival with amplification of the HER-2/neu oncogene. *Science*, 235, 177–82.

Slamon, D.J., Leyland-Jones, B., Shak, S. et al. (2001). Use of chemotherapy plus a monoclonal antibody against HER 2 for metastatic breast cancer that overexpresses HER 2. *New England Journal of Medicine*, 344, 783–92.

Spyratos, F., Andrieu, C., Hacene, K. et al. (1994). pS2 and response to adjuvant hormone therapy in primary breast cancer. *British Journal of Cancer*, 69, 394–7.

Stack, G., Kumar, V., Green, S. et al. (1988). Structure and function of the pS2 gene and estrogen receptor in human breast cancer cells. In: *Breast Cancer: Cellular and Molecular Biology*. 1st edn, ed. M.E. Lippmann & R.B. Dickson, pp. 185–206. Boston: Kluwer.

Stein, R.C., Coombes, R.C. & Howell, A. (1995). The basis of hormonal therapy for breast cancer. In *Oxford Textbook of Oncology*, vol. I, ed. M. Peckham, H.M. Pinedo & U. Veronesi, pp. 629–48. Oxford: Oxford Medical Publications.

Stoll, B.A. (1988). Second endocrine response in breast, prostatic and endometrial cancers. *Reviews of Endocrine Related Cancers*, 30, 19–25.

Taylor, R.E., Powles, T.J., Humphreys, J. et al. (1982). Effects of endocrine therapy on steroid receptor content of breast cancer. *British Journal of Cancer*, 45, 80–5.

Texeira, C., Reed, J.C. & Pratt, M.A.C. (1995). Estrogen promotes chemotherapeutic drug resistance by a mechanism involving bcl-2 proto-oncogene expression in human breast cancer cells. *Cancer Research*, 55, 3902–7.

Thompson, A.M., Steel, C.M., Foster, M.E. et al. (1990). Gene expression in oestrogen-dependant human breast cancer xenograft tumours. *British Journal of Cancer*, 62, 78–84.

Thompson, A.M., Hawkins, R.A., Elton, R.A. et al. (1993). pS2 is an independant factor of good prognosis in primary breast cancer. *British Journal of Cancer*, 68, 93–6.

Thor, A.D., Koerner, F.C., Edgerton, S.M. et al. (1992). pS2 expression in primary breast carcinomas: relationship to clinical and histological features and survival. *Breast Cancer Research and Treatment*, 21, 111–19.

Tommasi, S., Paradiaso, A., Mangia, A. et al. (1991). Biological correlation between HER2/neu and proliferative activity in human breast cancer. *Anticancer Research*, 11, 1395–400.

Tonetti, D.A. & Jordan, V.C. (1995). Possible mechanisms in the emergence of tamoxifen-resistant breast cancer. *Anti-Cancer Drugs*, 6, 498–507.

Tora, L., White, J., Brou, C. et al. (1989). The human estrogen receptor has two independent nonacid transcriptional activation functions. *Cell*, 59, 477–87.

Walker, R.A. & Varley, J.M. (1993). The molecular pathology of human breast cancer. *Cancer Surveys*, 16, 31–57.

Watts, C.K.W., Sweeney, K.J.E., Walters, A. et al. (1994). Antiestrogen regulation of cell cycle progression and cyclin D1 gene expression in MCF-7 human breast cancer cells. *Breast Cancer Research and Treatment*, 31, 95–105.

Williams, M.R., Todd, J.H., Ellis, I.O. et al. (1987). Oestrogen receptors in primary and advanced breast cancer: an eight year review of 704 cases. *British Journal of Cancer*, 55, 67–73.

Wiseman, L.R., Johnson, M.D., Wakeling, A.E. et al. (1993). Type I IGF receptor and acquired tamoxifen resistance in oestrogen-responsive human breast cancer cells. *European Journal of Cancer*, 29A, 2256–64.

Wolf, D.M., Langan-Fahey, S.M., Parker, C.J. et al. (1993). Investigation of the mechanism of tamoxifen-stimulated breast tumour growth with non-isomerisable analogues of tamoxifen and metabolites. *Journal of the National Cancer Institute*, 85, 806–12.

Zhang, Q.X., Borg, A. & Fuqua, S.A.W. (1993). An exon 5 deletion variant of the estrogen receptor frequently coexpressed with wild-type estrogen receptor in human breast cancer. *Cancer Research*, 53, 5882–4.

Predictors of response and resistance to medical therapy: chemotherapy

Stephen R.D. Johnston

The Royal Marsden Hospital, Fulham Road, London

Introduction

Resistance to chemotherapy invariably occurs in breast cancer patients being treated for metastatic disease. As with hormonal therapy, resistance may be either 'intrinsic', manifest as a failure to respond to initial therapy, or 'acquired', seen as progression after a variable length of time in patients who initially respond to cytotoxic therapy. In the adjuvant setting resistance to chemotherapy is inferred by rapid relapse following completion of therapy. In vitro models have established that cancer cells exhibit varying degrees of intrinsic drug-specific resistance, but may also acquire the same phenotype following long-term exposure to a given agent. Many of the established mechanisms of resistance are associated with genetic abnormalities such as activation of dominantly active oncogenes, or loss of tumour suppressor genes. Both patterns of intrinsic and acquired resistance are consistent with a model of cumulative genetic change during the development and progression of breast cancer.

Although many of the mechanisms involved in chemoresistance have been investigated extensively in vitro, other factors such as systemic drug metabolism and bioavailability may influence the likelihood of tumour response/resistance in vivo. Clinical studies have been used to verify whether a given genetic or biochemical change observed in experimental studies of drug resistance is relevant to clinical practice. There are several limitations in this approach when studying biological markers of resistance, not least the methodologic problems in analysing clinical specimens (for example, protein vs. RNA analysis, type of antibody used, tissue fixation) and sampling errors due to heterogeneous expression within human tumours. Markers of resistance have been correlated retrospectively with clinical outcome in large randomized trials of adjuvant therapy, and many such studies have defined novel biological 'prognostic' markers. Unlike oestrogen receptor expression and endocrine therapy, none of the potential determinants of chemoresistance have influenced clinical management to date. A more promising approach has emerged from the recent use of chemotherapy drugs as primary medical (neoadjuvant) therapy. Clinical studies are now underway to directly determine whether biological markers are 'predictive' of drug response/resistance, raising the possibility that in future individual treatment could be tailored, depending on the molecular profile of the tumour.

Laboratory studies – potential mechanisms for drug resistance

The most frequently used chemotherapy drugs in breast cancer are cyclophosphamide (C), methotrexate (M), 5-fluorouracil (5-FU), doxorubicin (A) and epirubicin (E). These represent various classes of cytotoxic agent (i.e. alkylating agents, antimetabolites, anthracycline antibiotics) which have different mechanisms of action including a direct effect on DNA by intercalation (A, E) or cross-linking (C), inhibition of DNA synthesis by purine depletion (M) or inhibition of thymidylate synthetase (M, F), and inhibition of RNA synthesis (A, E, F). By combining these drugs in established regimens (i.e. CMF, CAF, FEC or AC) maximal cytotoxic effect is achieved by utilizing each drug's different mechanism of action. In addition this approach can maximize clinical response by overcoming any intrinsic resistance within a tumour to a given specific drug. More recently, two new classes of drug have been introduced into clinical practice which target microtubular function, namely the taxanes (T) and the third-generation vinca alkaloids (V). Non-cross resistance with the previously mentioned drugs is becoming apparent from recently reported clinical studies.

Mechanisms for chemoresistance in breast cancer may be considered either as 'proximal' in association with impaired delivery of the drug to its target, 'drug specific' due to alteration of the target enzyme/protein, or 'distal' manifest as changes in the final common response pathway following cytotoxic exposure which includes cell-cycle arrest and/or programmed cell death (apoptosis). In general, acquired resistance is often associated with the development of proximal or drug-specific mechanisms of resistance, while intrinsic resistance may be associated with established mutations or amplification of distal apoptosis-regulating oncogenes.

Proximal mechanisms

The multidrug resistance phenotype (MDR) is associated with several intracellular mechanisms by which cancer cells reduce their vulnerability to various different cytotoxic agents, and thus survive. The most consistent finding is overexpression of a 170 kD transmembrane protein (P-glycoprotein) due to amplification of the *MDR1* gene, which results in energy-dependent drug efflux and thus decreased intracellular drug accumulation (Endicott & Ling, 1989). As a consequence, cross resistance of such cells in vitro can be demonstrated to several structurally unrelated drugs, including anthracyclines, taxanes and vinca alkaloids. There is much discrepancy amongst the studies of either *MDR1* gene expression or P-170 protein expression in human breast cancer samples (Goldstein, 1995). In general, untreated breast carcinomas have a low level of *MDR1* gene expression, although this may increase significantly in acquired resistance following treatment. Prospective studies are necessary to establish the role of *MDR1* gene expression in clinical drug resistance. Alternative drug transporters are now known to exist including the family of ATP dependent multidrug resistance-associated proteins (MRP) initially identified in a multidrug-resistant lung cancer cell line which did not express P-glycoprotein (Cole et al., 1992).

The MDR phenotype may also be associated with other phenotypic changes, including upregulation of intracellular glutathione-associated detoxification processes. Enzymes exist within cells to protect them from environmental toxins and carcinogens, including glutathione S-transferase (GST) which mediates the conjugation of glutathione to toxic drug intermediates resulting in increased water solubility and drug elimination, and glutathione peroxidase (GSHPx) which exists to detoxify organic and inorganic peroxides and limit the damaging effect of oxygen free radicals. The GSTs are involved in metabolism of several antineoplastic drugs, including alkylating agents and anthracyclines. Four different isoforms of GST exist (α, πp, μ, θ), each containing multiple subunits (Mannervik et al., 1992). In terms of extra-hepatic GST isoforms the most extensively studied enzyme is GST P1.1 which is expressed in normal and malignant breast tissue (Di Illo et al., 1985), and may be regulated either by the growth state of cells or steroid hormones (Hatayama et al., 1986). Immunohistochemical studies have shown GST P1.1 to be expressed in normal breast epithelium, while in human breast carcinomas its expression is inversely associated with oestrogen receptor (ER) expression (Gilbert et al., 1993). Initial studies suggested increased expression of GST P1.1 in hormone-dependent MCF-7 human breast cancer cells selected in vitro for resistance to doxorubicin (Batist et al., 1986). However, several subsequent studies failed to see altered drug sensitivity or metabolism following transfection of GST P1.1 into breast cancer cells (Moscow et al., 1989; Fairchild et al., 1990). From these and other studies it appears that increased expression of GST P1.1 alone is not sufficient to cause resistance in vitro.

The selenium-dependent GSHPx enzymes utilise glutathione to reduce both hydrogen peroxide and complex organic hydroperoxides which may be toxic to the cell. Oxidative metabolism of drugs such as doxorubicin and mitomycin-C produces fatty acids and lipid hydroperoxides, byproducts which may contribute to the cytotoxic action of these drugs. Consequently up-regulation of GSHPx, noted in multidrug-resistant MCF-7 cells, may in part, induce drug resistance to doxorubicin through intracellular elimination and detoxification of its metabolites (Kramer et al., 1990; Sinha et al., 1989).

Drug-specific targets

Altered expression of an enzyme which is the principal target for the mechanism of action of a given cytotoxic drug can modulate chemosensitivity. For example, topoisomerase II is a critical enzyme involved in DNA conformation which catalyses the concerted breaking and rejoining of double-stranded DNA during transcription, replication and recombination (Wang, 1985). The anthracyclines (i.e. doxorubicin) and epipodophyllotoxins inhibit topoisomerase II function, interrupting the process of breakage and reunion of DNA and generating cytotoxic double-strand breaks. Two isoforms (α and β) of the enzyme exist, and drug resistance has been associated in vitro with reduced enzyme activity secondary to either mutation (Deffie et al., 1989) or reduced topoisomerase II expression (Lefevre et al., 1991).

The fluoropyrimidine 5-fluorouracil (5-FU) is a commonly used active drug in breast cancer; 5-FU is metabolized within the cell to its active metabolite fluorodeoxy uridine monophosphate (FdUMP) which inhibits the target enzyme thymidylate synthase (TS). As a consequence thymidylate formation and both RNA and DNA synthesis is impaired. Resistance to 5-FU may develop through several mechanisms, including increased levels of the target enzyme TS, alteration in the binding affinity of TS for FdUMP, or decreased intracellular pools of the reduced folate substrate. Amplification of the *TS* gene and increased enzyme activity has been associated with resistance to 5-FU in human breast cancer cell lines *in vitro* (Chu et al., 1990). Treatment with 5-FU may induce increased *TS* gene expression as an adaptive response mechanism. In a study of serial cutaneous tumour biopsies from metastatic breast cancer patients, TS enzyme levels were elevated threefold following treatment with 5-FU (Swain et al., 1989), although correlation with clinical resistance to the drug was not demonstrated.

The taxanes (paclitaxel and docetaxel) are cytotoxic as a consequence of their stabilization of polymerized microtubules which thus prevents cell cycle progression through the G2/M phase. Altered expression of the various isotypes of β-tubulin has been postulated as a mechanism of resistance to paclitaxel. In particular, increased expression of the Hβ4 and Hβ5 isotypes has been associated with resistance to paclitaxel in both human sarcoma and prostate cancer cell lines (Dumontete et al., 1996; Ranganathan et al., 1998), and in a series of 11 paclitaxel-sensitive and resistant human ovarian carcinoma samples (Kavallaris et al., 1997). Point mutations in β-isotubulin have also been identified which may alter the paclitaxel-binding-site, interfering with the degree of microtubular stabilization (Giannakakou et al., 1997). At present, evidence for these mechanisms of resistance to taxanes in human breast cancer is limited.

Distal response: apoptosis regulatory oncogenes

There is increasing evidence that several chemotherapy agents ultimately act through induction of programmed cell death (apoptosis). Genes which regulate this process such as *Bcl-2* and *p53* may therefore play a critical role in determining cell sensitivity and resistance to cytotoxic agents (Lowe et al., 1993a; Chiou et al., 1994).

Bcl-2

The Bcl-2 (B cell lymphoma/leukaemia-2) gene was initially cloned from a 14:18 translocation break point associated with 85% of follicular lymphoma and 20% of diffuse B cell lymphoma. As a consequence the *Bcl-2* gene is moved from its normal chromosomal location on chromosome 18 into juxtaposition with heavy chain immunoglobulin promoter on chromosome 14, resulting in overproduction of Bcl-2 m-RNA and its encoded 26 kD protein (Tsujimoto & Croce, 1986). Subsequently, *Bcl-2* was found to protect cells from a variety of apoptotic signals including glucocorticoids, γ-irradiation, phorbol esters and chemotherapy-induced cell death (Miyashita & Reed, 1993; Strasser et al., 1994). Antisense mediated reduction in Bcl-2 gene expression was shown to accelerate the rate of cell death in the setting of growth factor withdrawal (Reed et al., 1990). All of these observations suggested a critical role for Bcl-2 in blocking a final common pathway leading to cell death. It is now recognized that Bcl-2 belongs to a growing family of apoptosis-regulating gene products. Broadly, these fall into two categories: antiapoptotic proteins including Bcl-2, Bcl-xl, Mcl-1, Bcl-w, Brag-1, and proapoptotic cell-death-promoting proteins such as Bax, Bcl-xs, Bak, Bad, Bik, Bid, Hrk (Reed, 1994).

Recent discoveries have suggested that Bcl-2 family proteins modulate the process of apoptosis by alteration of the mitochondrial permeability through interaction with related and nonrelated proteins (Figure 9c.1). For example, formation of Bax homodimers facilitates ion channels in the mitochondrial membrane to release cytochrome c which activates the caspase cascade (Kelekar & Thompson, 1998), ultimately resulting in proteolytic activation of the downstream effector caspases (caspase 3, 6 and 7) which cleave key proteins and trigger cell disintegration (Nunez et al., 1998). In contrast, Bcl-2 will bind to bax and prevent release of cytochrome c, thus preventing the triggering of apoptosis. Cytotoxic agents, through their action on targets within DNA, may alter this balance in favour of promoting apoptosis either by inducing p53 which directly transactivates and upregulates Bax expression (Yin et al., 1997), or by inactivating

Bcl-2 through phosphorylation as has been observed with paclitaxel (Haldar et al., 1996). In addition, recent interest has focused on the survival factors (i.e. peptide growth factors) which may impact on the interaction of Bcl-2 family proteins within the mitochondrial membrane. These may lead to suppression of apoptosis via the PI3-kinase/AKT pathway which inactivates and sequesters Bad, thus promoting Bcl-xl homodimer formation which is antiapoptotic (Datta et al., 1997).

Several experimental models have shown that modulation of the Bcl-2 family of proteins can alter sensitivity to cytotoxic agents in breast cancer. MCF-7 breast cancer cells transfected with Bcl-2 demonstrated a marked increase in resistance to doxorubicin, whereas modulation of Bcl-2 expression by antisense transcripts restored chemosensitivity (Teixeira et al., 1995). In contrast, expression of proapoptotic proteins appeared to enhance cytotoxicity. MCF-7 breast cancer cells, known to express high endogenous levels of the antiapoptotic protein Bcl-xl, transfected with the proapoptotic protein Bcl-x_s induced a marked increase in chemosensitivity to paclitaxel (Sumantran et al., 1995). Our increased understanding of the molecular biology of these proteins may impact on our understanding of certain aspects of cytotoxic drug resistance, which ultimately may allow therapeutic strategies to emerge to overcome such resistance.

Gene p53

The p53 gene codes for a sequence-specific DNA transcription factor that activates the expression of a number of well-defined target genes. Wild type p53 can transcriptionally transactivate genes involved in cell cycle arrest (e.g. *p21*), those involved in DNA repair machinery (e.g. *GADD45*), or apoptosis-regulating genes (e.g. *Bax and Fas*) (Harris, 1996). Thus, following DNA damage, p53 may induce cell cycle arrest allowing DNA repair before proceeding through the cell cycle or inducing apoptosis if the damage is severe. These two functions appear to be separable; in tumour cell lines lacking p53 in which inducible restoration of p53 results in cell cycle arrest and apoptosis, *Bcl-2* gene transfer blocks apoptosis but not cell cycle arrest (Ryan et al., 1994; Wang et al., 1993). Although the exact role of p53 in induction of apoptosis has not been defined, its central role has been implied by a series of observations. Expression of wild type p53 has been shown to initiate apoptosis in a variety of cell lines in which p53 is either absent or mutated, although the existence of p53-independent mechanisms is supported by normal development of p53 knock-out mice (Lowe et al., 1993b). There is some evidence to suggest that p53 directly modulates apoptosis-regulating proteins, as restoration of p53 in a murine leukemia cell line was associated with increased Bax m-RNA and protein, accompanied by decreased Bcl-2 levels (Miyashita et al., 1994; Miyashita & Reed, 1996).

In breast cancer the *p53* gene is mutated predominantly within exons 4–8 and 9–10 which code for the DNA-binding and tetramerization domains of the protein, respectively (Levine, 1997). Point mutations or deletions result in a truncated or abnormal nuclear p53 protein which can be detected immunohistochemically in approximately 20–40% of primary breast carcinomas (Cattoretti et al., 1988; Allred et al., 1993). In vitro studies have shown that resistance to a variety of chemotherapy drugs results from p53 inactivation, although the relationship is not always that clear (Brown & Wouters, 1998). The presence of wild type p53 enhances the sensitivity of the cell to DNA damaging agents, and in situations where p53 has been lost (mutated or null), restoration of p53 enhances drug responses (Weller, 1998). However, the relationship is complex as there is evidence in vitro that different p53 mutations may induce differential effects on the sensitivity of cells to chemotherapy agents (Blandino et al., 1999).

There is emerging evidence that mutant p53 may determine the rate of onset of apoptosis, but not whether apoptosis is induced in response to a cytotoxic insult. It is known that apoptosis may still occur in the absence of a functional *p53* gene (Stahler & Rommer, 1998). Likewise, the response to the antimicrotubule agent paclitaxel may be somewhat varied in different cells containing mutated p53. In human fibroblasts inactivation of p53 conferred a six- to ninefold increase in sensitivity to paclitaxel (Wahl, 1996; Hawkins et al., 1996), whereas others have shown that ovarian carcinoma cells with nonfunctional p53 became resistant to paclitaxel (Wu & El-Diery, 1996). Therefore some cells may remain sensitive to the cytotoxic or proapoptotic action of paclitaxel independent of p53 status, which may in part be due to direct inactivation by phosphorylation of the antiapoptotic protein Bcla-2 (Haldar et al., 1996) (Figure 9c.1).

Extrachromosomal DNA and drug resistance

There is emerging evidence that human tumours, including many human breast cancer cell lines and tumour samples, contain extrachromosomal DNA referred to microscopically as double minutes (Von Hoff & McGill, 1995). These double minutes can carry amplified copies of genes, including oncogenes (e.g. c-*erb*B-2, c-*myc*) and drug resistance genes (e.g. *mdr*-1, DHFR, thymidylate synthase). In addition to identifiable double minutes, submicroscopic circular supercoiled pieces of extrachromosomal DNA (episomes) which range in size from 120 to 750 kilobase pairs are also known to contain amplified genes (Ruiz et al., 1989). Both forms are thought to develop during DNA replication following a damaging insult such as UV irradiation which induces a deletion. The deleted DNA circularizes to form an episome, may multimerize to form a double minute, and ultimately may be reincorporated into chromosomal DNA. It is probable that during malignant transformation this extrachromosomal source of DNA accumulates several critical

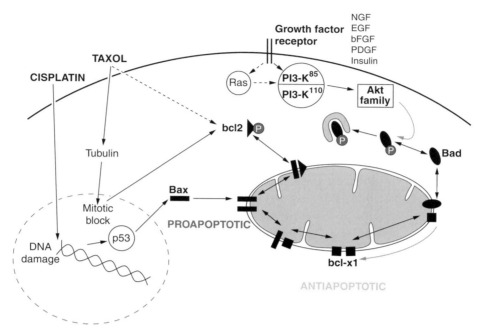

Figure 9c1   Effects of chemotherapy and growth factor-survival factors on the balance of pro-apoptotic (i.e. Bax) and anti-apoptotic (i.e. *Bcl*-xl) regulatory homodimers in the mitochondrial membrane, mediated via the phosphorylation status of *Bcl*-2 and Bad, respectively.

genes involved in tumour progression. For example, mdm-2, a protein which binds to and inactivates the tumour suppressor p53, was first identified in double-minute DNA isolated from transformed mouse cells (Cahilly-Snyder et al., 1987). Likewise, malignant cells within a tumour which contain amplified extrachromosomal drug resistance genes may be selected for during cytotoxic chemotherapy treatment, accounting for the emergence of acquired resistance.

Clinical studies – predictive markers of chemotherapy response/resistance

HER-2/*neu*

Overexpression of c-*erb*B-2 (also known as HER2/*neu*), a type 1 tyrosine kinase growth factor receptor, occurs in up to 30% of human breast cancers. Gene amplification which results in c-*erb*B-2 overexpression was initially associated with a poor clinical outcome (Slamon et al., 1987). Recently, several retrospective studies have addressed whether c-*erb*B-2 is a predictor of either resistance or sensitivity to specific chemotherapeutic agents in the adjuvant setting. Initial reports had suggested that while patients with c-*erb*B-2 negative tumours derived significant benefit from adjuvant CMF chemotherapy, those with either gene amplification or overexpressed levels of c-*erb*B-2 protein showed no benefit from such therapy (Gusterson et al., 1992; Allred et al., 1992). Although these initial reports were interpreted as c-*erb*B-2 expression being associated with chemoresistance, such studies require prospective validation in order to detect any treatment interaction with c-*erb*B-2 status.

In contrast to these previous results with CMF, tumours with high expression of c-*erb*B-2 seemed to benefit from dose-intensive anthracycline-based chemotherapy such as CAF (cyclophosphamide, adriamycin, 5-fluorouracil) (Muss et al., 1994). In that study, 1550 lymph-node-positive patients were randomly assigned to CAF in three different dose schedules. It has since been debated that the top dose, namely 600:60:600 mg/m^2 of CAF, respectively, represents standard doses such that in effect the trial compared conventional versus suboptimal dose CAF chemotherapy. Regardless of this, the results showed a significant benefit of anthracycline-based chemotherapy in terms of disease-free and overall survival for those with c-*erb*B-2 positive tumours. In a recent update of their initial report with longer follow-up (median 10.4 years) and an additional 595 patients, the interaction between dose of CAF and c-*erb*B-2 was still present, although not statistically significant (Thor et al., 1998). However, at the same time the NSABP reported a retrospective series of 638 patients given adjuvant chemotherapy with or without doxorubicin (NSABP B-11) in which a preferential benefit from doxorubicin was seen in patients with c-*erb*B-2 positive breast cancer (Paik et al., 1998). In this trial formal tests of interaction beween doxorubicin and c-*erb*B-2 expression were statistically significant for disease-free survival ($p = 0.02$), although not for overall survival.

The biological basis for c-*erb*B-2 predicting resistance or sensitivity to individual chemotherapy drugs remains unclear. An association of c-*erb*B-2 overexpression with topoisomerase II expression has been suggested, an enzyme which alters the topological state of DNA and is thus a target for doxorubicin which inhibits DNA replication following double-strand DNA cleavage (Jarvinen et al., 1996). Increased levels of topoisomerase II alpha expression in vitro are associated with enhanced sensitivity to doxorubicin, and it has been suggested that as the chromosome location (17q21–22) is similar to that for c-*erb*B-2, coamplification of both genes may explain any modulation of chemosensitivity seen in some c-*erb*B-2 positive tumours (Harris & Carmichael, 1995).

Changes in cell proliferation and apoptosis

Cytotoxic chemotherapy is being used increasingly as primary medical therapy for patients with large (>3 cm) operable breast cancer (see Chapter 10). The measurement of biological markers in this setting provides an opportunity to learn more about response and guide the appropriate use of systemic treatment. In particular, early changes in these markers during therapy might predict for long-term outcome and prove more effective than current clinical or pathological factors. Chemotherapy-induced changes in cell proliferation (i.e. expression of Ki-67, a proliferation-related antigen expressed in late G1, S, G2 and M phases of the cell cycle, detected by MIB-1 labelling) and apoptosis (detected by TUNEL, an in situ end-labelling assay) have been examined following neoadjuvant chemo-therapy in operable breast cancer. Rapid induction of apoptosis has been observed after only 24 hours of preoperative chemotherapy (Ellis et al., 1997), which may occur through pathways dependent on or independent of the p53 status (Wosikowski et al., 1995). Likewise, Ki-67 scores were reduced, although at the early timepoint of 24 hours only 9/35 patients demonstrated a > 50% fall (Archer et al., 1998). Measurements of reduction in cell proliferation after 21 days chemo-therapy have shown a greater association with clinical response, with all nonres-ponders (chemoresistance) showing an actual increase in Ki-67 (Assersohn et al., 1998). It is possible that expression of cyclin dependent kinases and their inhibi-tors may prove more sensitive early indicators of growth inhibition following chemotherapy than Ki-67. At present these preliminary observations require confirmation from larger randomized clinical trials of neoadjuvant chemother-apy, in particular to see whether any early changes in cell growth detected by Ki-67 and TUNEL can predict for the final clinical response and improved overall survival. If so, this would allow use of these surrogate biomarkers of clinical response to help in the selection of patients for whom this approach would be advantageous, and identify patients with more chemoresistant disease who may benefit from novel therapeutic approaches (see below) (see Chapter 9a).

Bcl-2

Initial clinical studies of Bcl-2 expression in breast cancer reported expression in 40–70% of primary tumours which was associated with a more favourable clinical prognosis (Nathan et al., 1993; Silvestrini et al., 1994). This appeared to be inconsistent with its biological behaviour as an antiapoptotic protein associated with resistance to therapy. Subsequent studies have shown a clear association with ER expression (Leek et al., 1994; Gee et al., 1994), and it is widely believed that its expression is either associated with or regulated by steroid hormones in ER-positive tumours. In terms of adjuvant chemotherapy and outcome as measured by relapse-free and overall survival, no data exist which address whether Bcl-2 is associated with a worse prognosis in relation to whether or not patients received chemotherapy.

There are very few clinical data which have looked at Bcl-2 expression in the pretreatment samples as a predictor of response or resistance to chemotherapy. However, residual cells in primary human breast carcinomas which remain following completion of neoadjuvant chemotherapy may represent chemoresistant clones which have survived cytotoxic drug exposure. It has been shown in such samples that rates of cell proliferation and apoptosis (surrogate markers of tumour growth) are much lower, suggestive of quiescent or dormant cells, while levels of Bcl-2 (both number of positive samples and level of expression) were increased compared with pretreatment values (Ellis et al., 1998). This would be consistent with the hypothesis stated above that Bcl-2 may be associated with resistance to chemotherapy. It is unclear from such studies whether these changes in Bcl-2 protein expression in surviving cells are selected for during therapy, and thus represent clonal selection of resistant cells (acquired resistance).

p53

Clinical evidence emerged recently which suggested that p53 status may determine chemosensitivity to doxorubicin in primary breast cancer (Aas et al., 1996). In this Norwegian study, 63 patients with locally advanced breast cancer received doxorubicin monotherapy, with p53 status determined in a pretreatment open biopsy specimen both by constant denaturant gel electrophoresis with direct sequencing and protein immunohistochemical staining. A total of 18 patients (29%) had p53 mutations, and tumours with mutations within the critical DNA-binding domain were strongly associated with *de novo* resistance to doxorubicin; 4/11 with L2/L3 domain mutations progressed on doxorubicin compared with only 2/52 (4%) without ($p < 0.01$). Patients with such mutations within their tumours were more likely to have a poor survival.

Other studies have proved less convincing in relation to p53 status and chemoresponsiveness in human breast cancer. While mutations in p53 have been associated with poor prognosis in patients with breast cancer treated by primary surgery (Elledge et al., 1993; Andersen et al., 1993), a correlation with outcome in those receiving adjuvant chemotherapy or radiotherapy has not always been apparent (Bergh et al., 1995). In one other study of patients with primary breast cancer treated with neoadjuvant chemotherapy, p53 mutations (determined by denaturing gradient gel electrophoresis and direct sequencing) were found in 31% of primary tumours (Chevillard et al., 1997). While most patients with wild-type p53 responded to chemotherapy, mutant p53 status was not associated with a worse clinical outcome in terms of distant disease-free or overall survival. Unlike the Norwegian study (Aas et al., 1996) which assessed response to a single drug (doxorubicin), most other studies have used two or three drug combinations making any interaction between p53 status and specific chemoresponsiveness more difficult to assess.

Opportunities for therapy

Modulation of chemoresistance

Identification of drug-specific mechanisms of resistance has resulted in the development of strategies aimed at modulating chemosensitivity. Agents such as verapamil, quinidine and tamoxifen have been identified which can reverse the MDR phenotype in vitro through competition for binding to p-glycoprotein. Despite numerous preclinical data, clinical trials to overcome chemoresistance in vivo have been disappointing (Goldstein, 1995). Alternative approaches have been directed both at the target site for drug action and preventing drug metabolism. For example, the reduced folate 5-formyltetrahydrofolate (leucovorin) is thought to enhance 5-FU activity by stabilizing the ternary complex formed between TS, FdUMP and the reduced folate substrate. A clinical trial of 5-FU with or without leucovorin in chemorefractory breast cancer showed that leucovorin significantly increased the percentage of tumour TS inactivation, which correlated with likelihood of response to 5-FU (Swain et al., 1989).

Targeted therapy

The finding of specific abnormalities in some of the above genes in association with resistance to conventional therapy may offer new opportunities for targeted therapies in this subgroup of patients. In particular, trastuzumab (Herceptin) is a humanized monoclonal antibody which has been developed against the external domain of c-erbB-2 (also known as HER-2/neu). Following evidence of preclinical efficacy in HER-2 overexpressing tumours, phase II studies in advanced metastatic breast cancer showed evidence of clinical activity and good tolerability (Cobleigh et al., 1999). More recent studies have demonstrated objective tumour response rates of 26% as first-line therapy in HER-2 positive metastatic breast cancer, with an additional 10% demonstrating stable disease for at least 6 months (Vogel et al., 2000). Furthermore, randomized clinical trials have shown a significantly improved response rate for the addition of Herceptin to chemotherapy, either anthracycline-based chemotherapy or paclitaxel, in women with advanced HER-2 positive breast cancer (Slamon et al., 2001). Whether this is an additive effect, or represents modulation of response to cytotoxic therapy in the setting of confirmed drug resistance remains unclear. The benefit for addition of Herceptin was associated with a significant improvement in overall survival from a median of 20.9 months to 25.4 months ($p = 0.045$) (Norton et al., 1999). Further development of this antibody in combination with cytotoxic chemotherapy, especially paclitaxel, is now proposed in the adjuvant setting.

Direct gene therapy strategies have been conceived which are aimed at restoring wild-type p53 to tumours in which the gene is mutated. At present, clinical trials have been undertaken in squamous cell cancers of the lung or head and neck (Roth & Cristiano, 1997), and strategies for metastatic breast cancer are limited (Ruppert et al., 1997). Antisense oligonucleotides against chemoresistant cells which overexpress Bcl-2 represents an alternative method of overcoming chemoresistance, and phase I trials in follicular lymphoma have shown good tolerability and selective modulation of protein expression (Webb et al., 1997). Our greater understanding of the molecular biological changes in breast cancer may yield further opportunities for novel therapies, some of which may allow treatment to bypass existing mechanisms of resistance to conventional cytotoxic drugs.

Conclusion

The problem of resistance to drug therapy in breast cancer is encountered in the clinic on a regular basis, and to a large extent this may be responsible for the limitations of current therapies, especially in the setting of metastatic disease. The ability to overcome drug resistance and prolong the time to progression following a successful response to therapy would be of enormous benefit to both the clinician and the patient. Progress in this field can only be made by enhancing our basic understanding of the biology of response and resistance to current chemotherapy drugs, and, as a consequence, developing novel modulators of resistance mechanisms. The promise that we can achieve this is now finally reaching the clinic, and expectations remain high that further biological agents will be developed for use in conjunction with current standard cytotoxic drugs.

REFERENCES

Aas, T., Borresen, A.-L., Geisler, S. et al. (1996). Specific p53 mutations are associated with de-novo resistance to doxorubicin in breast cancer patients. *Nature Medicine*, 2, 811–14.

Allred, D.C., Clark, G.M., Elledge, R. et al. (1993). Association of p53 protein expression with tumour cell proliferation rate and clinical outcome in node-negative breast cancer. *Journal of the National Cancer Institute*, 85, 200–6.

Allred, D.C., Clark, G.M., Tandon, A.K. et al. (1992). HER2/neu in node-negative breast cancer: prognostic significance of overexpression influenced by the presence of in situ carcinoma. *Journal of Clinical Oncology*, 10, 599–605.

Andersen, T.I., Holm, R., Nesland, J.M. et al. (1993). Prognostic significance of TP53 alterations in breast carcinoma. *British Journal of Cancer*, 68, 540–8.

Archer, C.D., Ellis, P.A., Dowsett, M. et al. (1998). C-erbB2 positivity correlates with poor apoptotic response to chemotherapy in primary breast cancer. *Breast Cancer Research and Treatment*, 50, Abstract 237.

Assersohn, L., Powles, T.J., Dowsett, M. et al. (1998). Changes in MIB-1 expression relate to response in patients receiving primary medical therapy for carcinoma of the breast. *Breast Cancer Research and Treatment*, 50, Abstract 239.

Batist, G., Tulpule, A., Sinha, B.K. et al. (1986). Over-expression of a novel anionic glutathione transferase in multi-drug resistant human breast cancer cells. *Journal of Biological Chemistry*, 261, 15 544–9.

Bergh, J., Norberg, T., Sjogren, S. et al. (1995). Complete sequencing of the p53 gene provides prognostic information in breast cancer patients, particularly in relation to adjuvant systemic therapy and radiotherapy. *Nature Medicine*, 1, 1029–34.

Blandino, G., Levine, A.J. & Oren, M. (1999). Mutant p53 gain of function: differential effects of different p53 mutations on resistance of cultured cells to chemotherapy. *Oncogene*, 18, 477–85.

Brown, J.M. & Wouters, B.G. (1998). Apoptosis, p53 and tumour cell sensitivity to anticancer agents. *Cancer Research*, 59, 1391–9.

Cahilly-Snyder, L., Yang-Feng, T., Franke, U. et al. (1987). Molecular analysis and chromosomal mapping of amplified genes isolated from a transformed mouse 383 cell line. *Somatic Cell and Molecular Genetics*, 13, 235–44.

Cattoreti, G., Rilke, F., Andreola, S. et al. (1998). p53 expression in breast cancer. *International Journal of Cancer*, 41, 178–83.

Chevillard, S., Lebeau, J., Pouillart, P. et al. (1997). Biological and clinical significance of concurrent p53 gene alterations, MDR1 gene expression, and S-phase fraction analyses in breast cancer patients treated with primary chemotherapy or radiotherapy. *Clinical Cancer Research*, 3, 2471–8.

Chiou, S.K., Rao, L. & White, E. (1994). Bcl-2 blocks p53 dependent apoptosis. *Molecular Cell Biology*, 14, 2556–63.

Chu, E., Drake, J.C., Koeller, D.M. et al. (1990). Induction of thymidylate synthase associated with multidrug resistance in human breast and colon cancer cell lines. *Molecular Pharmacology*, 39, 136–43.

Cobleigh, M.A., Vogel, C.L., Tripathy, D. et al. (1999). Multinational study of the efficacy and safety of humanised anti-HER2 monoclonal antibody in women who have HER-2-overexpressing metastatic breast cancer that has progressed after chemotherapy for metastatic disease. *Journal of Clinical Oncology*, 17, 2639–48.

Cole, S.P.C., Bhardwaj, G., Gerlach, J.H. et al. (1992). Overexpression of a transporter gene in multidrug-resistant human lung cancer cell line. *Science*, 258, 1650–4.

Datta, S.R., Dudeck, K., Tao, X. et al. (1997). Akt phosphorylation of Bad couples survival signals to the cell intrinsic death machinery. *Cell*, 91, 231–41.

Deffie, A.M., Bosman, D.J. & Goldenberg, G.J. (1989). Evidence for a mutant allele of the gene for DNA topoisomerase II in adriamycin-resistant P388 murine leukaemia cells. *Cancer Research*, 49, 6879–82.

Di Illo, C., Sacchetta, P., Del Boccio, G. et al. (1985). Glutathione peroxidase, glutathione S-transferase and glutathione reductase activities in normal and neoplastic human breast tissue. *Cancer Letters*, 29, 37–42.

Dumontete, C., Steger, K.A., Beketic-Oreskovic, L. et al. (1996). Resistance mechanism in human sarcoma mutants derived by single-step exposure to paclitaxel (Taxol). *Cancer Research*, 56, 1091–7.

Elledge, R.M., Fuqua, S.A., Clark, G.M. et al. (1993). Prognostic significance of p53 gene alterations in node-negative breast cancer. *Breast Cancer Research and Treatment*, 26, 225–35.

Ellis, P.A., Smith, I.E., Detre, S. et al. (1998). Reduced apoptosis and proliferation and increased Bcl-2 in residual breast cancer following pre-operative breast cancer. *Breast Cancer Research and Treatment*, 48, 107–16.

Ellis, P.A., Smith, I.E., McCarthy, K. et al. (1997). Pre-operative chemotherapy induces apoptosis in early breast cancer. *Lancet*, 349, 849.

Endicott, J. & Ling, V. (1989). The biochemistry of P-glycoprotein-mediated multidrug resistance. *Annual Reviews in Biochemistry*, 58, 137–71.

Fairchild, C.R., Moscow, J.A., O'Brien, E.E. et al. (1990). Multidrug resistance in cells transfected with human genes encoding a variant P-glycoprotein and glutathione S-transferase-pi. *Molecular Pharmacology*, 37, 801–9.

Gee, J., Robertson, J.F.R., Ellis, I.O. et al. (1994). Immunocytochemical localisation of Bcl-2 protein in human breast cancers and its relationship to a series of prognostic markers and response to endocrine therapy. *International Journal of Cancer*, 59, 619–28.

Giannakakou, P., Sackett, D.L. & Kong, Y.K. (1997). Paclitaxel-resistant human ovarian cancer cells have mutant beta tubulin that exhibit impaired paclitaxel-driven polymerization. *Journal of Biological Chemistry*, 272, 17 118–25.

Gilbert, L., Elwood, L.J., Merino, M. et al. (1993). A pilot study of pi-class glutathione S-transferase expression in breast cancer: correlation with estrogen receptor expression and prognosis in node-negative breast cancer. *Journal of Clinical Oncology*, 11, 49–58.

Goldstein, L.J. (1995). Multidrug resistance in breast cancer. In: *Drug and hormonal resistance in breast cancer*. Eds. R.B. Dickson & M.E. Lippmann. New York: Ellis Horwood, 219–48.

Gusterson, B.A., Gelber, R.D., Goldhirsch, A. et al. (1992). Prognostic importance of c-erbB2 expression in breast cancer. International (Ludwig) Breast Cancer Study Group. *Journal of Clinical Oncology*, 10, 1049–56.

Haldar, S., Chintapalli, & Croce, C.M. (1996). Taxol induces Bcl-2 phosphorylation and death of prostate cancer cells. *Cancer Research*, 56, 1253–5.

Harris, A.L. & Carmichael, J. (1995). Topoisomerase inhibitors and muliple drug resistance mechanisms in human breast cancer. In *Drug and hormonal resistance in breast cancer*. Eds R.B. Dickson & M.E. Lippmann. New York: Ellis Horwood, 303–22.

Harris, C.C. (1996). Structure and function of the p53 tumour suppressor gene: clues for rational cancer therapeutic strategies. *Journal of the National Cancer Institute*, 88, 1442–55.

Hatayama, I., Satoh, K., Sato, K. et al. (1986). Developmental and hormonal regulation of the major form of hepatic glutathione S-transferase in male mice. *Biochemical and Biophysical Research Communications*, 140, 581–8.

Hawkins, D.S., Demers, G.W. & Galloway, D.A. (1996). Inactivation of p53 enhances sensitivity to multiple chemotherapeutic agents. *Cancer Research*, 56, 892–8.

Jarvinen, T.A., Kononene, J., Pelto-Huikko, M. et al. (1996). Expression of topoisomerase II alpha is associated with rapid cell proliferation, aneuploidy, and c-erbB2 overexpression in breast cancer. *American Journal of Pathology*, 148, 2073–82.

Kavallaris, M., Bukhart, C.A., Regl, D.L. et al. (1997). Taxol-resistant epithelial ovarian tumors are associated with altered expression of specific beta-tubulin isotypes. *Journal of Clinical Investigation*, 100, 1282–93.

Kelekar, A. & Thompson, C.B. (1998). Bcl-2 family proteins: the role of the BH3 domain in apoptosis. *Trends in Cell Biology*, 8, 324–30.

Kramer, R.A., Zakher, J. & Kim, G. (1990). Role of glutathione redox cycle in acquired and de-novo multidrug resistance. *Science*, 241, 694–7.

Leek, R.D., Kaklamanis, L., Pezzella, F. et al. (1994). Bcl-2 in normal human breast carcinoma, association with oestrogen receptor-positive, epidermal growth factor-negative tumours and in-situ cancer. *British Journal of Cancer*, 69, 135–9.

Lefevre, D., Riou, J.-F., Ahomadegbe, J.C. et al. (1991). Study of molecular markers of resistance to mAMSA in a human breast cancer cell line. Decrease of topisomerase II and increase of both topoisomerase I and acidic glutathione S transferase. *Biochemical Pharmacology*, 41, 1967–79.

Levine, A.J. (1997). p53, the cellular gatekeeper for growth and division. *Cell*, 88, 323–31.

Lowe, S.W., Ruley, H.E., Jacks, T. et al. (1993a). p53-dependent apoptosis modulates the cytotoxicity of anticancer agents. *Cell*, 74, 957–67.

Lowe, S.W., Smith, S.W., Osborne, B.A. et al. (1993b). P53 is required for radiation-induced apoptosis in mouse thymocytes. *Nature*, 362, 847–9.

Mannervik, B., Awasthi, Y.C., Board, P.G. et al. (1992). Nomenclature for human glutathione transferases. *Biochemistry*, 282, 305–8.

Miyashita, T., Krajewska, M., Wang, H.G. et al. (1994). Tumour suppressor p53 is a regulator of Bcl–2 and bax gene expression *in vitro* and *in vivo*. *Oncogene*, 9, 1799–805.

Miyashita, T. & Reed, J.C. (1993). Bcl-2 oncoprotein blocks chemotherapy-induced apoptosis in a human leukemia cell line. *Blood*, 81, 151–7.

Miyashita, T. & Reed, J.C. (1996). Tumour suppressor p53 is a direct transcriptional activator of the human bax gene. *Cell*, 80, 293–9.

Moscow, J.A., Fairchild, C.R., Madden, M.J. et al. (1989). Expression of anionic glutathione-S-transferase and P-glycoprotein genes in human tissues and tumors. *Cancer Research*, 49, 1422–8.

Muss, H.B., Thor, A.D., Berry, D.A. et al. (1994). c-erbB2 expression and response to adjuvant therapy in women with node-positive early breast cancer. *New England Journal of Medicine*, 330, 1260–6.

Nathan, B., Anbazhagan, R., Dyer, M. et al. (1993). Expression of Bcl-2 like immunoreactivity in the normal breast and in breast cancer. *The Breast*, 2, 134–7.

Norton, L., Slamon, D., Leyland-Jones, B. et al. (1999). Overall survival advantage to simulta-neous chemotherapy plus the humanised anti-HER2 monoclonal antibody Herceptin in HER2 overexpressing metastatic breast cancer. *Proceedings of the American Society of Clinical Oncology*, 18, Abstract 483.

Nunez, G., Benedict, M.A., Hu, Y. et al. (1998). Caspases; the proteases of the apoptotic pathway. *Oncogene*, 17, 3237–45.

Paik, S., Bryant, J., Park, C. et al. (1998). erbB2 and response to doxorubicin in patients with axillary lymph node-positive, hormone receptor-negative breast cancer. *Journal of the National Cancer Institute*, 90, 1361–70.

Ranganathan, S., Colarusso, P.J., Dexter, D.W. et al. (1998). Altered beta-tubulin isotype expression in paclitaxel-resistant human prostate carcinoma cells. *British Journal of Cancer*, 77, 562–6.

Reed, J.C. (1994). Bcl-2 and the regulation of programmed cell death. *Journal of Cell Biology*, 124, 1–6.

Reed, J.C., Subasinghe, C., Haldar, S. et al. (1990). *Antisense*-mediated inhibition of Bcl-2 protooncogene expression and leukemic cell growth and survival: comparisons of phosphodiester and phosphorothioate oligodeoxynucleotides. *Cancer Research*, 50, 6565–70.

Roth, J.A. & Cristiano, R.J. (1997). Gene therapy for cancer; what have we done and where are we going? *Journal of the National Cancer Institute*, 88, 21–39.

Ruiz, J.C., Choi, K., Von Hoff, D.D. et al. (1989). Autonomously replicating episomes contain mdr-1 genes in a multidrug-resistant human cell line. *Molecular Cell Biology*, 9, 109–15.

Ruppert, J.M., Wright, M. & Rosenfeld, M. (1997). Gene therapy strategies for carcinoma of the breast. *Breast Cancer Research and Treatment*, 44, 93–114.

Ryan, J.J., Gottlieb, C.A. & Clarke, M.F. (1994). C-myc and Bcl-2 modulate p53 function by altering p53 subcellular trafficking during the cell cycle. *Proceedings of the National Academy of Sciences of the United States of America*, 91, 5878–82.

Silvestrini, R., Verenoni, S., Daidone, M.G. et al. (1994). The Bcl-2 protein: a prognostic indicator strongly related to p53 protein in lymph node-negative breast cancer patients. *Journal of the National Cancer Institute*, 86, 499–504.

Sinha, B.K., Mimnaugh, E.G., Rajagopalan, S. et al. (1989). Adriamycin activation and oxygen free radical formation in human breast tumour cells; protective role of glutathione peroxidase in adriamycin resistance. *Cancer Research*, 49, 3844–8.

Slamon, D.J., Clark, G.M., Wong, S.G. et al. (1987). Human breast cancer: correlation of relapse and survival with amplification of HER2/neu oncogene. *Science*, 235, 177–82.

Slamon, D., Leyland-Jones, B., Shak, S. et al. (2001). Use of chemotherapy plus a monoclonal antibody against HER2 for metastatic breast cancer that overexpresses HER2 *New England Journal of Medicine*, 344, 783–92.

Stahler, F. & Rommer, K. (1998). Mutant p53 can provoke apoptosis in p53 deficient cells with delayed kinetics relative to wt p53. *Oncogene*, 17, 3507–12.

Strasser, A., Harris, A.W., Jacks, T. et al. (1994). DNA damage can induce apoptosis in proliferating lymphoid cells via p53-independent mechanisms inhibitable by Bcl-2. *Cell*, 79, 329–39.

Sumantran, V.N., Ealovega, M.W., Nunez, G. et al. (1995). Overexpression of Bcl-xs sensitizes MCF-7 cells to chemotherapy induced apoptosis. *Cancer Research*, 55, 2507–10.

Swain, S.M., Lippman, M.E., Egan, E.F. et al. (1989). Fluorouracil and high-dose leucovorin in previously treated patients with metastatic breast cancer. *Journal of Clinical Oncology*, 7, 890–9.

Teixeira, C., Reed, J.C. & Pratt, M.A.C. (1995). Estrogen promotes chemotherapeutic drug resistance by a mechanism involving Bcl-2 proto-oncogene expression in human breast cancer cells. *Cancer Research*, 55, 3902–7.

Thor, A.D., Berry, D.A., Budman, D.R. et al. (1998). erbB2, p53, and the efficacy of adjuvant therapy in lymph-node positive breast cancer. *Journal of the National Cancer Institute*, 90, 1346–60.

Tsujimoto, Y. & Croce, C.M. (1986). Analysis of the structure, transcripts, and protein products of Bcl-2, the gene involved in human follicular lymphoma. *Proceedings of the National Academy of Sciences of the United States of America*, 83, 5214–18.

Vogel, C.L., Cobleigh, M., Tripathy, D. et al. (2000). First-line, non-hormonal, treatment of women with HER-2 overexpressing metastatic breast cancer with Herceptin (trastuzumab, humanised anti-HER2 antibody). *Proceedings of the American Society of Clinical Oncology*, 19, 71a, Abstract 275.

Von Hoff, D.D. & McGill, J. (1995). Drug resistance and tumor progression can be mediated by extrachromosomal DNA. In *Drug and hormonal resistance in breast cancer*. Ed. R.B. Dickson & H.E. Lippmann. New York: Ellis Horwood, 267–81.

Wahl, A.F. (1996). Loss of normal p53 function confers sensitisation to Taxol by increasing G2/M arrest and apoptosis. *Nature Medicine*, 2, 72–9.

Wang, J.C. (1985). DNA topoisomerases. *Annual Review of Biochemistry*, 54, 665–97.

Wang, Y., Szekely, L., Okan, I. et al. (1993). Wild type p53-triggered apoptosis is inhibited by Bcl-2 in a v-myc-induced T-cell lymphomal line. *Oncogene*, 8, 3427–31.

Webb, A., Cunningham, D., Cotter, F. et al. (1997). Bcl-2 antisense therapy in patients with Non-Hodgkins Lymphoma. *Lancet*, 349, 1137–41.

Weller, M. (1998). Predicting response to chemotherapy; the role of p53. *Cell and Tissue Research*, 292, 435–45.

Wosikowski, K., Regis, J.T., Robey, R.W. et al. (1995). Normal p53 status and function despite the development of drug resistance in human breast cancer cells. *Cell Growth Differentiation*, 6, 1395–403.

Wu, S.G. & El-Diery, W.S. (1996). p53 and chemosensitivity. *Nature Medicine*, 2, 255–6.

Yin, C., Knudson, C.M., Korsmeyer, S.J. et al. (1997). Bax suppresses tumorigenesis and stimulates apoptosis *in vivo*. *Nature*, 385, 637.

10

Primary medical therapy in breast cancer

Janine L. Mansi

Department of Medical Oncology, St George's Hospital, Blackshaw Road, London

Introduction

The definition of locally advanced breast cancer includes patients with large tumours, extensive regional lymph node involvement, or direct involvement of the skin or underlying chest wall. These tumours thus include stage IIIA and IIIB breast cancer as well as inflammatory breast cancer and involvement of the supraclavicular nodes (stage IV). Haagensen & Stout (1943) were the first to describe the clinical signs and then confirmed that these patients had a uniformly poor prognosis with no cures at 5 years in 120 patients treated with radical mastectomy (and 49% developing a local recurrence by 5 years) (Haagensen, 1971). Radiotherapy alone then became the standard treatment (Baclesse, 1949), with a local tumour control rate of 28% to 74% at 5 years and a 5-year survival of between 12% to 38% (Bouchard, 1965; Fletcher, 1972; Zucali et al., 1976; Langlands et al., 1976; Bruckman et al., 1979; Treurniet-Donker et al., 1980; Bedwinek et al., 1982; Balawajder et al., 1983). Some of these more recent studies compared radiation alone with a combination of surgery and radiotherapy and confirmed that the 5-year survival could be improved to between 35% and 55% (Fletcher, 1972; Zucali et al., 1976; Bruckman et al., 1979; Bedwinek et al., 1982; Balawajder et al., 1983).

Since the early 1980s there has been an increasing trend to offer systemic chemotherapy (so-called primary medical therapy or neoadjuvant therapy) as part of the multimodality approach. As a result of this it was found that a proportion of women could be offered conservative surgery and thus avoid a mastectomy. Over the last decade this approach has been extended to women with earlier stage tumours, i.e. stage II who would otherwise require a mastectomy as their definitive surgical management. Thus women are increasingly being offered the choice of primary chemotherapy as initial treatment to decrease the size of the tumour and increase the potential for conservative surgery. This can avoid mastectomy in some 90% of women. In addition, this sequence of treatment offers the opportunity of determining whether the patient has a chemosensitive tumour, with the option of stopping chemotherapy early or changing to a different regimen of non-cross-resistant drugs if there is no response. Local control does not appear to be compromised, provided surgery and radiotherapy are given after chemotherapy. Moreover, as the number of women being offered adjuvant chemotherapy increases, this approach simply represents an alternative in the order of therapeutic options with the added advantage of the potential for breast conservation.

The unique opportunity to study the biology of early breast cancer using the in situ cancer as a human tumour model is also facilitated, which may provide information by which future therapies can be tailored.

Primary medical therapy in locally advanced breast cancer

The rationale for giving chemotherapy as initial treatment came from its use in locally advanced inoperable tumours (De Lena et al., 1978). In this study adriamycin and vincristine were given initially followed by radiotherapy to the primary tumour. Their results demonstrated an improvement in relapse-free and overall survival compared with an historical control group who received radiotherapy alone (Zucali et al., 1976).

De Lena et al. (1981) subsequently set out to evaluate the relative contributions of radiotherapy or surgery to primary chemotherapy in a randomized trial. The study was limited to women with T3b or T4 tumours with or without axillary lymphadenopathy (N0-2), but did not include inflammatory breast cancer or those women with supraclavicular lymphadenopathy; 132 women were randomized to receive three cycles of adriamycin and vincristine followed by either a radical mastectomy or radiotherapy, and then a further seven cycles of adriamycin and vincristine. The relapse-free survival was 22 months for the radiotherapy group and 15 months for the surgical group, but this was not statistically significant ($p = 0.58$). Moreover, the overall survival was identical between the two groups (50% at 4 years). This finding was supported by Perloff et al. (1988). In this study the median disease-free interval was 29.2 months in the group of 43 women who were randomized to surgery and 24.4 months in the 44 randomized to radiotherapy ($p = 0.5$), with no difference in overall survival (median 39.3 months for surgery and 39.0 months for radiotherapy).

Since then there have been a large number of relatively small studies evaluating the multimodality concept. There has been a diversity of different chemotherapy regimens and schedules (many adjuvantly as well as prior to local treatment), i.e. after definitive surgery/radiotherapy, followed by radiotherapy with or without surgery (Lippman et al., 1986; Morrow et al., 1986; Schwartz et al., 1987; Swain et al., 1987; Hobar et al., 1988; Rubens et al., 1989; Gardin et al., 1995; Kuerer et al., 1999; Zambetti et al., 1999). Most, but not all, of these studies include inflammatory breast cancer (Lippman et al., 1986; Morrow et al., 1986; Schwartz et al., 1987; Swain et al., 1987; Hobar et al., 1988; Rubens et al., 1989; Gardin et al., 1995) and supraclavicular lymphadenopathy (Morrow et al., 1986; Swain et al., 1987; Hobar et al., 1988; Kuerer et al., 1999), and some have added hormone therapy to the regimen (Lippman et al., 1986; Morrow et al., 1986; Swain et al., 1987; Rubens et al., 1989).

What is clear from these studies is that chemotherapy can downstage tumours from being inoperable to operable, that primary breast cancer is an extremely chemosensitive tumour, and that local recurrence rates can be decreased by this combined modality approach. Because of the broad range of characteristics for most of the studies it is difficult to determine the effect on overall survival. Schwartz et al. (1987) projected a 5-year disease-free and overall survival of 65% and 85% respectively in patients who responded to primary chemotherapy. Zambetti et al. (1999) reported on a series of 88 women who after a median follow-up of 52 months had a relapse-free and overall survival of 52% and 62%. Kuerer et al. (1999) also recently reported on their group of 372 patients with locally advanced breast cancer (this included stages IIA to IV [supraclavicular lymphadenopathy only]), after a median follow-up of 58 months the 5-year disease-free and overall survival was 89% and 87% respectively in those patients who had achieved a pathological complete response and 64% and 58% in those who did not. Neither of these studies included patients with inflammatory breast cancer.

Primary chemotherapy in operable primary breast cancer

As the majority of patients in these series responded and achieved local control with chemotherapy the concept was extended to patients with large but operable primary breast cancer. The initial studies were concerned with the feasibility of this approach (Morrow et al., 1986; Schwartz et al., 1987). Subsequently, however, it was noted that as many patients achieved such good responses, including pathological complete responses, it was possible to offer conservative surgery for residual clinical or radiologically detected disease (Mansi et al., 1989; Bonadonna et al., 1990; Jacquillat et al., 1990; Bélembaogo et al., 1992; Smith et al., 1993). The knowledge that survival following conservative surgery was equivalent to mastectomy for patients who had their surgery at presentation (Fisher et al., 1985) further encouraged this approach.

A series of phase II and phase III studies were then set up and confirmed that mastectomy could be avoided in 75–94% of women (Table 10.1). Thus it was

Table 10.1. Response rate and breast conservation rate to primary chemotherapy in operable breast cancer

Study	No. of pts	Chemotherapy regimen (no. of courses)	Tamoxifen	Response rate (%)	Complete response (%)		Breast conservation rate (%)
					Clinical	Pathological	
Jacquillat et al., 1990	250	VTMF(A)	195	75	30	NA	94
Bélembaogo et al., 1992	126	AVCF (M) (6)	None	85	36	2	85
Smith et al., 1993	64	CMF/MMM (6/8)	After chemo	69	17	NA	76
Scholl et al., 1994	191	ACF (4)	None	65	30	NA	82
Botti et al., 1995	56	ECF/FEC	None	82	7	NA	75
Smith et al., 1995	50	ECF (8)	None	98	66	32	94
Veronesi et al., 1995	226	CMF/FAC/FEC/CMitoF	None	35	12	2.5	90
Chollet et al., 1997	50	TNCF (6)	None	88	51	22	78
Fisher et al., 1997	693	AC	After chemo	80	36	26% of 245 Total group = 693	67
Bonadonna et al., 1998	536	Various (3–4)	None	76	16	3	85
Makris et al., 1998	149	MM(M) (4)	Yes	83	22	7	46
Mauriac et al., 1999	134	EVMx3 + MMC, TP, Vix3	None	NA	NA	NA	63
Miller et al., 1999[a]	40	AT vs. A → T (4–6)	None	87	20	13	28
von Minckwitz et al., 1999[b]	42	AT (4)	None	93	33	5	70

[a]Breast conservation not primary aim of study.

[b]Includes a proportion who would have been able to have conservation surgery at presentation.

NA: Not available.

VTMF(A) vinblastine, thiotepa, methotrexate, 5-fluorouracil (adriamycin) (or epirubicin); AVCF(M) adriamycin, vincristine, cyclophosphamide, 5-fluorouracil (methotrexate); ACF or FAC or FEC adriamycin, cyclophosphamide, 5-fluorouracil; MM(M) mitoxantrone, methotrexate (Mitomycin C); ECF epirubicin, cisplatin, 5-fluorouracil; EC epirubicin, cyclophosphamide; CMF/CmitoF cyclophosphamide, methotrexate, mitoxantrone, 5-fluorouracil; TNCF adriamycin, vinorelbine, cyclophosphamide, 5-fluorouracil; AT adriamycin, doxetaxel; MMC, TP, Vi mitomycin C, thiotepa, vindesine.

concluded that the use of preoperative chemotherapy could be expanded, particularly for patients who otherwise would require a mastectomy for local control at presentation.

Furthermore, the risk of disease progression whilst receiving primary chemotherapy is very small (3%: Fisher et al., 1997; 1%: Makris et al., 1998).

Primary medical therapy in patients with small tumours

Having established that primary chemotherapy could be used to downstage large tumours and avoid mastectomy, this concept was extended to patients with smaller tumours. Both the NSABP-B18 (Fisher et al., 1997) and Makris et al. (1998) studies have included such patients, although it was recognized that some of these patients may have been over treated and could have been cured by surgery with or without radiotherapy. In particular, it is important to note that fine needle aspirate cytology cannot differentiate between carcinoma in situ and invasive carcinoma. In the study by Makris et al. (1998) 5 of 142 (3.5%) of patients in the adjuvant arm had noninvasive intraduct carcinoma, and Fisher et al. (NSABP-B18, 1997) reported an incidence of 12 of 693 (1.73%). Thus suitable patients for consideration of primary medical therapy should not receive this unless invasive cancer has been confirmed (usually by Trucut biopsy, or if necessary a diagnostic biopsy).

Chemotherapy regimens used in primary medical therapy

Over the years numerous chemotherapy regimens have been evaluated and some are summarized in Table 10.1. The majority of groups report response rates ranging from 65% up to as high as 98% (Jacquillat et al., 1990; Scholl et al., 1994; Smith et al., 1995; Veronesi et al., 1995; Fisher et al., 1997; Chollet et al., 1997; Bonadonna et al., 1998; Makris et al., 1998; von Minckwitz et al., 1999; Miller et al., 1999).

The recent aim has been to improve the response rate with specific emphasis on complete clinical and pathological response. The combination using low-dose infusional 5-fluorouracil combined with epirubicin and cisplatin (ECF) looked particularly interesting by virtue of increasing the complete clinical remission rate from between 15–28% to 66% with only 3 (6%) of the 49 patients requiring a mastectomy (Smith et al., 1995). This combination has been compared with adriamycin and cyclophosphamide in a randomized study to determine if the high complete remission rate translates into a survival advantage; early results, at a mediam follow-up of 30 months, suggest that this is the case (Smith et al., 2000). A further analysis of the NSABP B18 study also looked specifically at the relationship between outcome and response to preoperative chemotherapy; this confirmed that the disease-free survival at 5 years was better in patients who had a pathological complete response than in those who had a complete clinical response but still had invasive tumour at the time of surgery, and also for those patients who achieved a clinical partial response or no response (85.7%, 76.9%, 68.1% and 63.9% respectively, $p<0.0001$) (Fisher et al., 1998). Recent publications from groups with long follow-up also confirm this (Brain et al., 1997; Kuerer et al., 1999).

Traditional treatments include an anthracycline, as this group of drugs has been described as the most active single agents in the treatment of breast cancer. There are, however, a number of other agents that have significant activity. The taxanes have an established place in the management of metastatic breast cancer, particularly in patients who have relapsed after first-line therapy. Response rates of 50% have been achieved, and docetaxel, in particular, has been shown to be of value even in patients who are resistant to anthracyclines (Eisenhauer & Trudeau, 1995). These agents are now being evaluated in randomized studies as first line treatment in patients with metastatic breast cancer and in the adjuvant therapy setting. There have been a number of phase II studies evaluating their use as primary medical therapy in patients with large primary breast cancer. More recently, combinations of docetaxel with adriamycin given every 2 or 3 weeks (von Minckwitz et al., 1999) or the same combination compared with sequential adriamycin and docetaxel (Miller et al., 1999) have been evaluated with response rates of 93% (33% of 42 patients achieving a complete clinical remission) and 87% (22% of 40 patients achieving a complete clinical remission) respectively.

Hutcheon et al. have recently reported on a study involving 162 patients with large primary (≥ 3 cm) or locally advanced breast cancer who received four cycles of CVAP (cyclophosphamide, doxorubicin, vincristine, prednisolone) followed by either four further cycles of the same or four of taxotere if they achieved a partial or complete response; those with stabilization or progression received four cycles of taxotere. In the randomized patients the response rate was 66% in the CVAP arm and 94% in the taxotere arm ($p=0.001$). The response in the nonrandomized patients was 55%. The progression-free survival at a median follow-up of 104 weeks was significantly longer in the patients randomized to taxotere ($p=0.022$) (Hutcheon et al., 2000). The survival outcome is awaited with interest.

Current randomized studies include the NSABP-B27 in which patients with operable breast cancer (i.e. any size tumour) are randomly assigned to four cycles of adriamycin and cyclophosphamide followed by four cycles of docetaxel either before or after surgery compared with a control group of no further chemotherapy, and a study in which patients with large operable (i.e. requiring mastectomy), inoperable tumours and inflammatory tumours are randomized to receive a maximum of six courses of adriamycin with either docetaxel or cyclophospham-ide as part of the AngloCeltic 11 study.

Vinorelbine, a semisynthetic vinca alkaloid, has also proven efficacy in meta-static breast cancer, and more recently in combination as part of a phase II study of patients with high-risk primary breast cancer (Chollet et al., 1997, Table 10.1). It is now being evaluated in the United Kingdom in a randomized phase II trial with either epirubicin or mitozantrone compared with adriamycin and cyclophos-phamide (as the conventional standard).

Irrespective of the chemotherapy regimens used to date, the series of patients with the longest follow-up continue to confirm that the response rate to chemo-therapy decreases with increasing size of tumour and the presence of lymph nodes at presentation, and that this is also translated into a poorer outcome (Fisher et al., 1998; Makris et al., 1998; Bonadonna et al., 1998). Conversely, patients who have a complete pathological response to chemotherapy (both in the primary tumour and axillary lymph nodes) do better (Brain et al., 1997; Kuerer et al., 1999).

Duration of primary medical therapy

The majority of studies usually give a minimum of three courses and a maximum of six prior to surgery. This varies from study to study. Bélembaogo et al. (1992) looked specifically at this issue and concluded that the overall response rate was greater at the sixth cycle compared with the third as assessed clinically, mammo-graphically and on ultrasound (clinical response rate after three courses was 64.7% and 85.6% after six courses, $p < 0.0001$). Smith et al. (1995) prescribed eight courses of infusional ECF chemotherapy and reported that the median number of courses needed to achieve a complete response was four, but the range extended to the complete eight courses. Likewise, Scholl et al. (1994) reported an increase in response rate from 56% after two courses to 82% following four courses, with a concomitant increase in complete remission rate (4% to 30%).

These data indicate that a minimum of four courses should be given unless there is obvious evidence of progression, and that more could improve response rates in a proportion of patients.

Type of surgery

Conservative surgery has been one of the major endpoints of primary medical therapy as previously described. For patients who have a good partial response to treatment the decision is not complicated. Some groups advocate marking the original area with tattoos (Veronesi et al., 1995), whilst others place metallic markers under ultrasound guidance for subsequent intraoperative localization and specimen mammography (Kuerer et al., 1999). For those patients in whom a complete clinical and radiological response has been achieved the question arises as to whether these patients actually need surgery at all – however, Ellis et al. (1998) reported an increased rate of local recurrence in patients in clinical complete remission who electively did not have surgery. In the majority of reported studies most of the patients have undergone a surgical procedure as part of the planned treatment, and this has given important information regarding pathological complete response rates, in addition to helping design further studies. As long ago as 1986, Feldman et al. reported that a pathological complete response was one of the best prognostic factors.

Usually a mastectomy is performed in the following circumstances: for patients with a poor response in tumour reduction such that the tumour is still large compared with the breast size, tumour situated within 2 cm of the nipple, multifocal tumour, or where there is disseminated microcalcification on mammography. Immediate breast reconstruction can be discussed with these women.

The presence of positive excision margins is a well-recognized factor in the risk of local recurrence in patients who have undergone conservative surgery (Schnitt et al., 1994; DiBiase et al., 1998). The addition of radiotherapy to conservative surgery decreases the likelihood, but the risk is still greater than in those patients who have had their tumour completely excised (Fowble et al., 1991; Solin et al., 1991). Assersohn et al. (1999) addressed this issue, retrospectively, in patients taking part in a randomized clinical trial (Makris et al., 1998) of primary medical therapy compared with adjuvant chemotherapy in all patients presenting to a breast unit from 1991 to 1995. Of the 184 patients who had conservative surgery, 38% had unexcised microscopically involved margins (defined as positive if ductal carcinoma in situ or invasive carcinoma was present within 1 mm from the excision margin), but local relapse as the first site of relapse was only 1.9% after a median follow-up of 57 months. Most centres, however, advocate a policy of re-excision of involved margins (Veronesi et al., 1995).

One particular aspect of the surgical procedure includes axillary sampling or clearance. Again, is this technique performed to provide prognostic information or as a therapeutic procedure? Several workers have looked at lymph node status after primary medical therapy and found it to be the most important prognostic factor (McCready et al., 1989; Botti et al., 1995; Gardin et al., 1995; Cameron et al., 1997; Brain et al., 1997). In particular, the presence of positive lymph nodes confers a worse prognosis than initial tumour size and response to chemotherapy. The presence of involved nodes may therefore help to identify patients who require further therapy.

The timing of radiotherapy

For patients with locally advanced inoperable disease radiotherapy was one of the mainstays of treatment. Its position as front line treatment has largely been superseded by chemotherapy, and gives the added advantage of allowing clinicians to monitor the tumour response to the chemotherapy regimen. A few groups have looked at giving radiotherapy simultaneously with chemotherapy, however treatment toxicity was enhanced and delivery of full doses of chemotherapy was compromised (Piccart et al., 1988).

In general, if patients are to have surgery and axillary clearance then radiotherapy is usually given on completion in order to avoid problems with wound healing.

Another issue is the timing of radiotherapy if patients are to receive further chemotherapy on the basis of poor prognostic factors identified from the resected tumour. One study that addressed this issue, albeit retrospectively and nonrandomized, compared radiotherapy given concomitantly with adjuvant chemotherapy to that given on completion of chemotherapy. No significant difference in risk of local recurrence was shown ($p = 0.61$) (Bonadonna et al., 1998). Radiotherapy is particularly important for patients who have had conservative surgery to improve the rate of local control.

Local recurrence rates after combined modality treatment

One of the major concerns regarding conservative surgery after primary medical therapy is the risk of increasing the local recurrence rate. Table 10.2 summarizes the available data from the reported phase II and phase III studies. The incidence is variable with the majority of studies showing a relatively low rate of local recurrence when it is considered that this patient population with large primary tumours is at such high risk.

It is difficult to determine from these studies the reasons for the varied local recurrence rates. Factors that could be involved include the type and order of combined modality approach, the type of chemotherapy, and the type and extent of surgery (attention to detail regarding excision margins and microcalcification). Some groups include synchronous local and distant relapse in their figures, as well as contralateral breast cancer, and the reporting of in situ recurrence together with invasive recurrence. The studies with the longer follow-up are, however, the most meaningful. To date, on the basis of the small number of randomized studies, this does not appear to adversely affect survival.

Table 10.2. Relapse and overall survival in patients with large primary breast cancer

Study	Order of therapy	No. of pts	Median follow-up	Local recurrence (%)	Distant metastases (%)	Survival (%)
Bélembaogo et al., 1992	PMT	126	NA	4.7	10	NA
Smith et al., 1993	PMT	64	29 m	27	NA	NA
Scholl et al., 1994[a]	PMT	200	54 m	24	24	86
	Adj	190	54 m	18	32	78
Smith et al., 1995	PMT	50	15 m	4	8	NA
Brain et al., 1997	PMT	107	81 m	17.8	25.3	NA
Chollet et al., 1997	PMT	50	31 m	2	14	NA
Bonadonna et al., 1998	PMT	536	65 m	6.8	37	69
Makris et al., 1998	PMT	149	48 m	2.7	17	82
	Adj	144	48 m	3.5	19	82
Mauriac et al., 1999	PMT	134	124 m	23	NA	60
	Adj	138	124 m	9	NA	60

[a]Includes concomitant local and metastatic relapse; NA not available; PMT primary medical therapy.

The use of adjuvant therapy after surgery/radiotherapy

In some studies, patients were given maintenance tamoxifen after chemotherapy and local treatment. Although this was given to the majority of patients irrespective of oestrogen receptor status, the recent results from adjuvant studies indicate that tamoxifen is most beneficial in women in whom the receptor status is positive (Early Breast Cancer Trialists' Collaborative Group, 1998). Whether tamoxifen should be prescribed at the time of diagnosis or after induction chemotherapy requires further evaluation.

In other series patients have received three courses of induction chemotherapy followed by six courses of adjuvant chemotherapy (Gardin et al., 1995; Veronesi et al., 1995; Botti et al., 1995; Zambetti et al., 1999). There has been only one study in which patients have been randomized, and early results suggested an increase in the relapse-free survival for those who received adjuvant therapy, but this was in patients with locally advanced breast cancer (De Lena et al., 1978). In the study by Botti et al. (1995), those patients who had a good response to induction chemotherapy received the same chemotherapy in the adjuvant phase, whereas those who did not respond received alternative chemotherapy regimens; interestingly, although there were only small numbers involved, the patients with positive lymph nodes after surgery had a longer disease-free interval if they received alternative non-cross-resistant chemotherapy.

For patients presenting with primary breast cancer of any size the presence of involved axillary lymph nodes represents the single poorest prognostic factor. It is on the basis of this that the majority of women are offered adjuvant therapy. For those patients with a particularly poor prognosis (four or more involved nodes) high-dose therapy with peripheral stem cell rescue is currently being evaluated against conventional treatment, as well as the evaluation of some of the newer agents such as taxanes (Henderson et al., 1998).

For patients who still have involved nodes after primary medical therapy it is likely that the number of lymph nodes containing tumour would have been higher prior to the chemotherapy (Fisher et al., 1997). Thus, finding malignant lymph nodes after induction therapy is consistent with the reports of the poorer survival in these women (McCready et al., 1989; Botti et al., 1995; Gardin et al., 1995; Cameron et al., 1997; Bonadonna et al., 1998; Zambetti et al., 1999). This underpins the rationale for additional treatment which could include other non-cross-resistant cytotoxics or manipulation of the immune system with monoclonal antibody therapy, such as Herceptin (see Chapters 11, 12b) in selected patients who overexpress HER-2.

Moreover, as previously described, the outlook for those women who do not achieve a pathological complete remission is poorer than for those who do, and again, represents a subgroup who may benefit from additional treatment.

The recently launched NSABP B-27 study is recruiting three groups of patients all of whom receive preoperative chemotherapy and are then randomized to receive either an additional four courses of taxotere preoperatively, or post-operatively compared with a control group. This may help to answer some of these questions.

Endocrine therapy as primary medical therapy

The concept of giving tamoxifen as initial treatment for breast cancer was initially investigated in elderly patients who either had locally advanced inoperable cancer or were not fit for surgery. In the 1980s and early 1990s there was an increasing trend to give tamoxifen to elderly women with operable breast cancer, with the aim of avoiding surgery altogether (Preece et al., 1982; Allan et al., 1985). Randomized studies investigating this principle, however, confirmed that al-though tamoxifen was useful in stabilizing or reducing a large number of tumours the majority still required surgery because of local failure (Robertson et al., 1988). Unfortunately, the women were then older and thus represented a worse surgical risk than at the time of presentation. Primary tamoxifen is, therefore, usually reserved for elderly women with inoperable or metastatic disease or in those patients in whom surgery or chemotherapy is contraindicated.

Prognostic factors in primary medical therapy

Primary medical therapy offers the possibility of using the primary tumour as an indicator of treatment sensitivity as well as the opportunity to study biological changes during therapy (Soubeyran et al., 1996; Ellis et al., 1997; Makris et al., 1997; Chang et al., 1999; Colleoni et al., 1999). Tumour samples can either be compared pretreatment and then at the time of surgery, or serial fine needle aspirates or Trucut biopsies of the tumour can be analysed. Thus various biological parameters can then be correlated with response and survival (Bozzetti et al., 1994, Chang et al., 1999; Mackay et al., 2000). If these markers can be shown to predict for outcome then they may be useful in guiding therapy.

A variety of markers can be measured and include the steroid hormone receptor-related proteins (oestrogen and progesterone receptors), proliferation markers (Ki67, MIB1, PCNA), S-phase fraction, peptide hormone receptors (c-*erb*B2, epidermal growth factor receptor), p53 and proteins regulating apopto-sis such as Bcl-2 and a family of genes that share strong sequence homology with Bcl-2 (*Bax, Bcl-X1, Bcl-X8, Mcl*-1). In addition, mismatch repair deficiency in the development of drug resistance can also be investigated.

With the advent of the newer aromatase inhibitors, these alone or in conjunction with tamoxifen are being evaluated as induction treatment in post-menopausal women with oestrogen receptor-positive primary breast tumours. Endocrine treatment is given for 12 weeks prior to surgery with serial core biopsies taken pretreatment and at 2 weeks. Ki67 and apoptosis in these samples are being compared with the definitive surgically excised tumour to determine if serial measurements can predict for response and survival in patients receiving endocrine therapy (IMPACT study) (Boeddinghaus et al., 2000).

The influence of the presence, absence or changes of these markers with therapy as predictors of response or prognosis still requires clarification and is further addressed in Chapter 9a. Ongoing assessment of the newer molecular markers may provide additional information.

Impact of primary medical therapy on survival

The use of primary medical therapy clearly offers an opportunity of avoiding mastectomy without compromising local control. It also allows in vivo research into growth of and response to treatment for patients with primary carcinoma of the breast. But does this approach actually compromise or improve survival? A series of randomized studies were established to address this question (Table 10.3).

Scholl et al. (1994) initially published on 414 premenopausal patients and demonstrated a statistically significant survival advantage ($p = 0.039$) after a median follow-up of 54 months, but with only a trend in favour of delaying metastatic disease; further follow-up did not confirm this trend (Scholl et al., 1995). The long-awaited results of the NSABP-18 were initially published in 1997; here 1523 patients were randomized to either pre- or postoperative chemotherapy and at 5 years the disease-free survival was 67% and overall survival was 80% in both groups (Fisher et al., 1997, 1998). Likewise, Makris et al. (1998), have reported similar results with a median follow-up of 48 months (Table 10.3).

Clearly, the giving of primary medical therapy does not compromise survival. Thus, although the optimal treatment has not yet been identified the emphasis should be on determining this, as well as identifying patients who are at a particular risk and may require more intensive treatment or change in therapy to non-cross-resistant regimens.

Conclusion

The last decade has seen a considerable change in the way that we approach and manage women who present with locally advanced (both inoperable and

Table 10.3. Randomized studies in operable breast cancer

Study	No. of pts	Tumour size	PMT (no. of courses)	*AT	Median follow-up	PMT DFI (%)	AT DFI (%)	p	PMT OS (%)	AT OS (%)	p
Scholl et al., 1994	390	3–7 cm	4	4	54 m	59	55	0.4	86	78	0.04
Semiglazov et al., 1994	271	0–>5 cm	1–2 (+4–5 adj)	6	60 m	81	72	0.4	86	78	NS
Fisher et al., 1998	1523	0–5 cm	4	4	60 m	66.7	67.3		79.6	80	NS
Makris et al., 1998	309	0–>5 cm	4 (+4 adj)	8	48 m	80	80		82	82	NS
Mauriac et al., 1999	272	3–8 cm	6	6	124 m	NA	NA		60	60	NS

*Received primary radiotherapy; NA not available; NS not significant; PMT primary medical therapy; AT Adjuvant therapy; DFI disease-free interval; OS overall survival.

operable) breast cancer. Mastectomy can be avoided in the majority of women without a deleterious effect on survival. Numerous prognostic factors (clinical and pathological) have been identified which can help to define the poorer prognostic subgroups of women who may benefit from more intensive treatment. The advent of new drugs, including biological agents, may provide additional means of making an impact on survival. Further refinements of this, together with improved assessment and attention to locoregional treatment modalities will hopefully improve outcome.

REFERENCES

Allan, S.G., Rodger, A., Smyth, J.F. et al. (1985). Tamoxifen as primary treatment of breast cancer in elderly or frail patients: a practical management. *British Medical Journal*, 358.

Assersohn, L., Powles, T.J., Ashley, S. et al. (1999). Local relapse in primary breast cancer patients with unexcised positive surgical markings after lumpectomy, radiotherapy and chemoendocrine therapy. *Annals of Oncology*, 10, 1451–5.

Baclesse, F. (1949). Roentgen therapy alone as the method of treatment of cancer of the breast. *American Journal of Roentgenology*, 62, 311–19.

Balawajder, I., Antich, P.P. & Boland, J. (1983). An analysis of the role of radiotherapy alone in combination with chemotherapy and surgery in the management of advanced breast carcinoma. *Cancer*, 51, 574–80.

Bedwinek, J., Rao, D.V., Perez, C. et al. (1982). Stage III and localized stage IV breast cancer: irradiation alone versus irradiation plus surgery. *International Journal of Radiation Oncology, Biology, Physics*, 8, 31–6.

Bélembaogo, E., Feillel, V., Chollet, P. et al. (1992). Neoadjuvant chemotherapy in 126 operable breast cancer. *European Journal of Cancer*, 28A, 896–900.

Boeddinghaus, I.M., Dowsett, M., Smith, I.E. et al. (2000). Neoadjuvant 'Arimidex' or Tamoxifen, alone or combined, for breast cancer (IMPACT): PgR-related reductions in proliferation marker Ki67. *Proceedings of the American Society of Clinical Oncology*, 19, Abstract 360, 94a.

Bonadonna, G., Valagussa, P., Brambilla, C. et al. (1998). Primary chemotherapy in operable breast cancer: eight-year experience at the Milan Cancer Institute. *Journal of Clinical Oncology*, 16(1), 93–100.

Bonadonna, G., Veronesi, U., Brambilla, C. et al. (1990). Primary chemotherapy to avoid mastectomy in tumours with diameters of three centimeters or more. *Journal of the National Cancer Institute*, 82, 1539–45.

Bouchard, J. (1965). Advanced cancer of the breast treated primarily by irradiation. *Radiology*, 84, 823–42.

Botti, C., Vici, P., Lopez, M. et al. (1995). Prognostic value of lymph node metastases after neoadjuvant chemotherapy for large-sized operable carcinoma of the breast. *Journal of the American College of Surgeons*, 181, 202–8.

Bozzetti, C., Nizzoli, R., Naldi, N. et al. (1994). Fine-needle aspiration technique for the concurrent immunocytochemical evaluation of multiple biologic parameters in primary breast carcinoma. *Breast Cancer Research and Treatment*, 32, 221–8.

Brain, E., Garrino, C., Misset, J.-L. et al. (1997). Long-term prognostic and predictive factors in 107 stage II/III breast cancer patients treated with anthracycline-based neoadjuvant chemotherapy. *British Journal of Cancer*, 75(9), 1360–7.

Bruckman, J.E., Harris, J.R., Levene, M.B. et al. (1979). Results of treating stage III carcinoma of the breast by primary radiation therapy. *Cancer*, 43, 985–93.

Cameron, D.A., Anderson, E.D.C., Levack, P. et al. (1997). Primary systemic therapy for operable breast cancer: 10 year survival data after chemotherapy and hormone therapy. *British Journal of Cancer*, 76, 1099–105.

Chang, J., Powles, T.J., Allred, D.C. et al. (1999). Biologic markers as predictors of clinical outcome from systemic therapy for primary operable breast cancer. *Journal of Clinical Oncology*, 17(10), 3058–63.

Chollet, P., Charrier, S., Brain, E. et al. (1997). Clinical and pathological response to primary chemotherapy in operable breast cancer. *European Journal of Cancer*, 33, 862–6.

Colleoni, M., Orvieto, E., Nolé, F. et al. (1999). Prediction of response to primary chemotherapy for operable breast cancer. *European Journal of Cancer*, 35(4), 574–9.

De Lena, M., Varini, M., Zucali, R. et al. (1981). Multinodal treatment for locally advanced breast cancer. *Cancer Clinical Trials*, 4, 229–36.

De Lena, M., Zucali, R., Vigarott, G. et al. (1978). Combined chemotherapy–radiotherapy approach to locally advanced (T3b-4) breast cancer. *Cancer Chemotherapy Pharmacology*, 1(1), 53–9.

DiBiase, S., Korarnicky, L., Schwartz, G. et al. (1998). The number of positive margins influences the outcome of women treated with breast preservation for early stage breast carcinoma. *Cancer*, 82, 2212–20.

Early Breast Cancer Trialists' Collaborative Group (1998). Tamoxifen for early breast cancer: an overview of the randomised trials. *Lancet*, 351, 1451–67.

Eisenhauer, E.A. & Trudeau, M. (1995). An overview of phase II studies of docetaxel in patients with metastatic breast cancer. *European Journal of Cancer*, 31A (Suppl. 4), S11–S13.

Ellis, P., Smith, I., Ashley, S. et al. (1998). Clinical prognostic and predictive factors for primary chemotherapy in operable breast cancer. *Journal of Clinical Oncology*, 16(1), 107–14.

Ellis, P.A., Smith, I.E., McCarthy, K. et al. (1997). Preoperative chemotherapy induces apoptosis in early breast cancer. *Lancet*, 349, 849.

Feldman, L.D., Hortobagyi, G.N., Buzdar, A.U. et al. (1986). Pathological assessment of response to induction chemotherapy in breast cancer. *Cancer Research*, 46, 2578–81.

Fisher, B., Brown, A., Mamounas, E. et al. (1997). Effect of preoperative chemotherapy on local-regional disease in women with operable breast cancer: findings from National Surgical Adjuvant Breast and Bowel Project B-18. *Journal of Clinical Oncology*, 15(7), 2483–93.

Fisher, B., Bryant, J., Wolmark, N. et al. (1998). Effect of preoperative chemotherapy on the outcome of women with operable breast cancer. *Journal of Clinical Oncology*, 16(80), 2672–85.

Fisher, B., Redmond, C., Fisher, E.R. et al. (1985). Ten-year results of a randomised clinical trial comparing radical mastectomy and total mastectomy with or without radiation. *New England Journal of Medicine*, 312, 674–81.

Fletcher, G.H. (1972). Local results of irradiation in the primary management of localized breast cancer. *Cancer*, 29, 545–51.

Fowble, B.L., Solin, L.J., Schultz, D.J. (1991). Ten-year results of conservative surgery and irradiation for stage I and II breast cancer. *International Journal of Radiation Oncology, Biology, Physics*, 21, 269–77.

Gardin, G., Rosso, R., Campora, E. et al. (1995). Locally advanced non-metastatic breast cancer: analysis of prognostic factors in 125 patients homogenously treated with a combined modality approach. *European Journal of Cancer*, 31A(9), 1428–33.

Haagensen, C.D. (1971). *Diseases of the Breast*. 2nd edn, pp. 629. Philadelphia: Saunders.

Haagensen, C.D. & Stout, A.P. (1943). Carcinoma of the breast. II Criteria of Operability. *Annals of Surgery*, 118, 859–70, 1032–51.

Henderson, I.C., Berry, D., Demetri, G. et al. (1998). Improved disease free (DFS) and overall survival (OS) from the addition of sequential paclitaxel (T) but not from the escalation of doxorubicin (A) dose level in the adjuvant chemotherapy of patients (PTS) with node-positive breast cancer (BC). *Proceedings of the American Society of Clinical Oncology*, 17, Abstract 390, 101a.

Hobar, P.C., Jones, R.C., Schouten, J. et al. (1988). Multimodality treatment of locally advanced breast carcinoma. *Archives of Surgery*, 123, 951–5.

Hutcheon, A.W., Ogston, K.N., Heys, S.D. et al. (2000). Primary chemotherapy in the treatment of breast cancer: significantly enhanced clinical and pathological response with docetaxel. *Proceedings of the American Society of Clinical Oncology*, 19, Abstract 317, 83a.

Jacquillat, C., Weil, M., Baillet, F. et al. (1990). Results of neoadjuvant chemotherapy and radiation therapy in the breast-conserving treatment of 250 patients with all stages of infiltrative breast cancer. *Cancer*, 66, 119–29.

Kuerer, H.M., Newman, L.A., Smith, T.L. et al. (1999). Clinical course of breast cancer patients with complete pathologic primary tumor and axillary lymph node response to doxorubicin-based neoadjuvant chemotherapy. *Journal of Clinical Oncology*, 17(2), 460–9.

Langlands, A.O., Kerr, G.R. & Shaw, S. (1976). The management of locally advanced breast cancer by x-ray therapy. *Clinical Oncology*, 2, 365–71.

Lippman, M.E., Sorace, R.A., Bagley, C.S. et al. (1986). Treatment of locally advanced breast cancer using primary induction chemotherapy with hormonal synchronization followed by radiation therapy with or without debulking surgery. *NCI Monographs*, 1, 153–9.

Mackay, H.J., Cameron, D., Rahilly, M. et al. (2000). Reduced MLH1 expression in breast tumors after primary chemotherapy predicts disease-free survival. *Journal of Clinical Oncology*, 18(1), 87–93.

Makris, A., Powles, T.J., Ashley, S.E. et al. (1998). A reduction in the requirements for mastectomy in a randomized trial of neoadjuvant chemoendocrine therapy in primary breast cancer. *Annals of Oncology*, 9, 1179–84.

Makris, A., Powles, T.J., Dowsett, M. et al. (1997). Prediction of response to neoadjuvant chemoendocrine therapy in primary breast carcinomas. *Clinical Cancer Research*, 3, 593–600.

Mansi, J.L., Smith, I.E., Walsh, G. et al. (1989). Primary medical therapy for operable breast cancer. *European Journal of Cancer & Clinical Oncology*, 25(11), 1623–7.

Mauriac, L., MacGrogan, G., Avril, A. et al. (1999). Neoadjuvant chemotherapy for operable breast carcinoma larger than 3 cm: A unicentre randomized trial with a 124-month median follow-up. *Annals of Oncology*, 10, 47–52.

McCready, D.R., Hortobagyi, G.N., Kau, S.W. et al. (1989). The prognostic significance of lymph node metastases after preoperative chemotherapy for locally advanced breast cancer. *Archives of Surgery*, 124, 21–5.

Miller, K.D., McCaskill-Stevens, W., Sisk, J. et al. (1999). Combination versus sequential doxorubicin and docetaxel as primary chemotherapy for breast cancer: a randomized pilot trial of the Hoosier Oncology Group. *Journal of Clinical Oncology*, 17(10), 3033–7.

Morrow, M., Braverman, A., Thelmo, W. et al. (1986). Multimodal therapy for locally advanced breast cancer. *Archives of Surgery*, 121, 1291–6.

Perloff, M., Lesnick, G.J., Korzun, A., Chu, F. et al. (1988). Combination chemotherapy with mastectomy or radiotherapy for stage III breast carcinoma: A Cancer and Leukaemia Group B study. *Journal of Clinical Oncology*, 6(2), 261–9.

Piccart, M.J., De Valeriola, D., Paridaens, R. et al. (1988). Six-year results of a multimodality treatment strategy for locally advanced breast cancer. *Cancer*, 62, 2501–6.

Preece, P.E., Wood, R.A.B., Macbie, C.R. et al. (1982). Tamoxifen as initial sole treatment of localised breast cancer in elderly women: a pilot study. *British Medical Journal*, 284, 869–70.

Robertson, J.F.R., Todd, J.H., Ellis, I.O. et al. (1988). Comparison of mastectomy with tamoxifen for treating elderly patients with operable breast cancer. *British Medical Journal*, 297, 55–4.

Rubens, R.D., Bartelink, H., Engelsman, E. et al. (1989). Locally advanced breast cancer: the contribution of cytotoxic and endocrine treatment to radiotherapy. *European Journal of Cancer Clinical & Oncology*, 25, 667–78.

Schnitt, S.J., Abner, A., Gelman, R. et al. (1994). The relationship between microscopic margins of resection and the risk of local recurrence in patients with breast cancer treated with breast-conserving surgery and radiation therapy. *Cancer*, 74, 1746–51.

Scholl, S.M., Asselain, B., Bouzeboc, P. et al. (1995). Neoadjuvant versus adjuvant chemotherapy in premenopausal patients with tumours considered too large for conserving surgery: an update. *Anti-cancer drugs*, 6 (Suppl. 2), 69, Abstract 48.

Scholl, S.M., Fourquet, A., Asselain, B. et al. (1994). Neoadjuvant versus adjuvant chemotherapy in premenopausal patients with tumours considered too large for breast conserving surgery: preliminary results of a randomised trial: S6. *European Journal of Cancer*, 30A(5), 645–52.

Schwartz, G.F., Cantor, R.I. & Biermann, W.A. (1987). Neoadjuvant chemotherapy before definitive treatment for Stage III carcinoma of the breast. *Archives of Surgery*, 122, 1430–4.

Semiglazov, V.F., Topuzov, E.E., Bavli, J.L. et al (1994). Primary (neoadjuvant) chemotherapy and radiotherapy compared with primary radiotherapy alone in stage IIb–IIIa breast cancer. *Annals of Oncology*, 5, 591–5.

Smith, I.E., A'Hern, R.P., Howell, A. et al. (2000). Preoperative continuous infusional EcisF (epirubicin, cisplatin and infusional 5FU) vs conventional AC chemotherapy for early breast cancer: a Phase III multicentre randomised trial by the Topic Trial Group. *Proceedings of the American Society of Clinical Oncology*, 19, Abstract 320, 84a.

Smith, I.E., Jones, A.L., O'Brien, M.E.R. et al. (1993). Primary medical therapy (neo-adjuvant) chemotherapy for operable breast cancer. *European Journal of Cancer*, 29A, 1796–9.

Smith, I.E., Walsh, G., Jones, A. et al. (1995). High complete remission rates with primary neoadjuvant infusional chemotherapy for large early breast cancer. *Journal of Clinical Oncology*, 13(2), 424–9.

Solin, L.J., Fowble, B.L., Schultz, D.J. et al. (1991). The significance of the pathology margins of the tumor excision on the outcome of patients treated with definitive irradiation for early stage breast cancer. *International Journal of Radiation Oncology, Biology, Physics*, 21, 279–87.

Soubeyran, I., Quénel, N., Coindre, J.-M. et al. (1996). pS2 protein: a marker improving prediction of response to neoadjuvant tamoxifen in post-menopausal breast cancer patients. *British Journal of Cancer*, 74, 1120–5.

Swain, S.M., Sorace, R.A., Bagley, C.S. et al. (1987). Neoadjuvant chemotherapy in the combined modality approach of locally advanced nonmetastatic breast cancer. *Cancer Research*, 47, 3889–95.

Treurniet-Donker, A.D., Hop, W.C.J. & Hoed-Sijtsema, S. (1980). Radiation treatment of stage III mammary carcinoma: a review of 129 patients. *International Journal of Radiation Oncology, Biology, Physics*, 6, 1477–82.

Veronesi, U., Bonadonna, G., Zurrida, S. et al. (1995). Conservation surgery after primary chemotherapy in large carcinomas of the breast. *Annals of Surgery*, 222, 612–18.

von Minckwitz, G., Costa, S.D., Eiermann, W. et al. (1999). Maximized reduction of primary breast tumour size using preoperative chemotherapy with doxorubicin and docetaxel. *Journal of Clinical Oncology*, 17(7), 1999–2005.

Zambetti, M., Oriana, S., Quattrone, P. et al. (1999). Combined sequential approach in locally advanced breast cancer. *Annals of Oncology*, 10, 305–10.

Zucali, R., Uslenghi, C., Kenda, R. et al. (1976). Natural history of survival of inoperable breast cancer treated with radiotherapy and radiotherapy followed by radical mastectomy. *Cancer*, 37, 1422–3.

11

Medical therapy of advanced disease

Alison Jones[a] and Karen McAdam[b]

[a]Royal Free Hospital, Pond Street, London
[b]Peterborough District Hospital, Peterborough, UK

Introduction

Despite advances in the diagnosis and treatment of early breast cancer, approximately a third of patients still die from advanced breast cancer following the development of metastatic disease. Median survival from the time of metastasis is approximately 3 years (Harris et al., 1997), but some patients may have a protracted clinical course over many years, partly because of biological diversity with the disease itself behaving in an indolent fashion, and also because of the sensitivity to endocrine manipulation for some women with advanced breast cancer. The management of advanced breast cancer is a major health problem for two reasons: first because of the relatively long survival, which results in a high prevalence at just over 100 000 cases per annum, and secondly because of the nature of metastatic disease, with problems such as bone metastases, which result in high use of health resources. Breast cancer is a major consumer of resources within any healthcare system. A recent Canadian study modelled the life time costs of treating breast cancer and indicated that while 8% of overall costs are associated with metastatic disease, 16% of costs were due to ongoing care, with the average cost per case of metastatic disease being $36 340 Canadian (£16 500 sterling). This is a Canadian study and therefore cannot be viewed as a direct proxy for the UK. However, a UK study (Richards et al., 1992) also indicated that care costs were the main component of cost rather than drug costs.

The management of advanced disease is complex and should be managed by a multidisciplinary team so that specific intervention, such as orthopaedic surgical procedures, stenting of biliary ducts or surgical control of local disease, are not forgotten during the process of deciding on systemic treatment. Current systemic treatment includes the use of specific endocrine therapy and chemotherapy and also bisphosphonates for metastatic bone disease (see Chapter 13). In addition, emerging biological therapy with antibody treatments such as trastuzumab

(Herceptin) are showing promise in clinical practice and other approaches involving specific immunotherapy and vaccines are also in clinical trial (see Chapter 12b).

Principles of treatment

Currently metastatic breast cancer is not regarded as curable. The aim, therefore, of treatment is to increase the duration of time without disease-related symptoms with the least toxicity possible, i.e. the main issue is one of quality of life for the majority of patients. As yet there has been limited formal assessment of these endpoints, however studies have suggested that endocrine therapy is better tolerated than chemotherapy and that quality of life is linked to treatment response (Carlson, 1998; Ramirez et al., 1998; Tannock et al., 1998). It is questionable whether medical management has any impact on survival overall, although two retrospective studies have shown that the introduction of combination cytotoxic chemotherapy in the 1970s for metastatic disease was associated with a modest 9–12 month gain in survival in most prognostic subgroups compared with untreated patients (Cold et al., 1993; Ross et al., 1985). Those patients with life-threatening visceral disease, who respond to cytotoxic chemotherapy, clearly have a survival benefit on an individual basis.

The modest role of chemotherapy to date means that all patients should be considered for clinical trials, either to evaluate new treatments in the Phase I/II setting or to help establish the role of active new drugs or regimens in routine practice in Phase III/IV comparative studies. Any assessment of the benefit of treatment depends on defining appropriate aims of treatment within a given clinical context. In clinical trials evaluating new drugs/regimens traditional endpoints, including objective response, time to tumour progression and survival are important, and indeed may be associated with subjective palliation.

The value of early detection and treatment of metastases in asymptomatic patients is controversial, highlighting uncertainties about the value of actively screening for metastases during follow-up. In the absence of curative treatment this merely results in a lead time bias without definite benefit to the patient (Mansi et al., 1988; Rutgers et al., 1989). For those patients who are aware of metastases, however, it may be difficult to defer treatment until symptoms occur, and indeed the recognition of metastatic disease means that symptoms will be inevitable at some stage.

The importance of stable disease beyond 6 months as a valuable measure of efficacy in breast cancer, particularly in relation to endocrine treatment, is increasingly recognized (Howell et al., 1988). In addition, the evaluation of symptom relief and quality of life is essential both in clinical trials and routine practice. The use of these parameters as primary endpoints means that only 20–30% of patients have a net benefit from first-line chemotherapy (Ramirez et al., 1998), although overall a higher number of patients may benefit from endocrine treatment because of the lower toxicity compared with chemotherapy.

Endocrine versus cytotoxic treatment?

The choice of treatment depends on a careful clinical evaluation, which will include appreciation of the patient's breast cancer history, previous treatment, current comorbid conditions, performance status and preferences. Patients should have a careful clinical examination to determine the extent of disease and appropriate blood tests and imaging. In general, a chest X-ray and bone scan will suffice, although a liver ultrasound or CT scan would be useful if liver metastases or pelvic disease is suspected. The role of serum tumour markers such as CA15-3 and CEA are questionable both in terms of diagnosis and certainly in terms of monitoring response. While elevated markers may provide useful corroborative evidence for relapse in patients with suspected metastases, their routine use to detect relapse or follow progress on treatment is not currently recommended (Hayes, 1996). At first relapse most patients only have one or two organ systems involved, but as the disease progresses, multiple sites will be involved. The most common initial sites of involvement are the skin, soft tissue, lymph nodes and bone, and the next most common sites are visceral organs such as lung and liver.

When possible, endocrine treatments are the treatment of first choice in metastatic disease because of low toxicity and relatively long times to progression in responding patients. The rationale underlying endocrine treatment is the reduction of oestrogenic stimulation to breast cancer cell growth. It is hence important to know, if possible, the steroid hormone receptor status of the primary tumour (oestrogen receptor (ER) and/or progestogen receptor (PgR)). This can be measured retrospectively using immunohistochemistry on primary paraffin blocks. If the steroid hormone receptor status is not known, there are a number of surrogate factors which can give an indication of potential hormone sensitivity (Table 11.1). These include a long disease-free interval, soft tissue disease only and postmenopausal status (as ER positivity increases with age). The presence of visceral disease *per se* is not a contraindication to endocrine treatment if the patient's performance status is good and organ function is well maintained. Treatment with endocrine therapy does not prejudice a subsequent response to chemotherapy (Taylor et al., 1986).

These clinical factors can be used to guide the choice of treatment and ER-negative patients with favourable clinical factors may be considered for endocrine treatment. Approximately 30% of an unselected population respond to endocrine therapy, with a response of 60% in ER-positive patients, falling to less than 5% for ER-negative patients. Those patients whose tumour is strongly positive for PgR as

Table 11.1. Factors determining response to endocrine therapy

Predictive factor	Good response	Poor response
Steroid hormone receptor (oestrogen receptor, progesterone receptor)	Positive	Negative
Disease-free interval since primary treatment	Longer (>2 years)	Shorter (<2 years)
Disease sites	Soft tissue (nodes, skin)	Visceral (lymphangitis, extensive liver)
Postmenopausal status	Higher (because of association with ER)	
HER2 status[a]	Negative	Positive

[a]Under evaluation.

well as ER have the highest likelihood of response (Ravdin et al., 1992). Approximately 20% of patients achieve stable disease which is of clinical benefit (Howell et al., 1988). The median response duration for first-line endocrine treatment is 12–15 months. Response to one endocrine treatment predicts a moderate chance of subsequent responses, although the response rate decreases by around 50% with each successive administration. Hormone treatment is therefore used sequentially in both pre and postmenopausal women (Figure 11.1).

After tamoxifen or progestin treatment, but not aromatase inhibitors, some patients may experience a 'flare' phenomenon, with increased bone pain, hypercalcaemia or rapid growth of soft tissue metastases within the first month. This may appear within a few days and last for a few weeks. The incidence is estimated at around 3% and is likely to be followed by an objective response to therapy. With sequential therapy a 'washout period' is usually allowed between different endocrine agents in clinical trials because of the small possibility of the so-called withdrawal response. This is rare in practice and is probably not indicated outside routine clinical trials.

Selective oestrogen receptor modulators (SERMS)

Tamoxifen is a nonsteroidal competitive ER agonist/antagonist and is traditionally the drug of first choice for most endocrine-sensitive breast cancer in postmenopausal women. Tamoxifen binds to the oestradiol receptor, leading to activation and dimerization and subsequent binding to specific oestrogen response elements on DNA, which cause transcription of oestrogen-responsive genes. The pattern of expression influences whether tamoxifen has agonist or

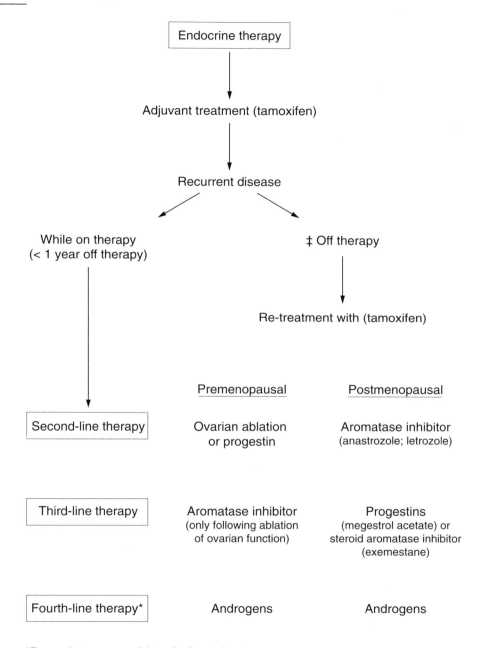

Figure 11.1 Sequential endocrine therapy in breast cancer

antagonist activity in a given tissue. The net result is reduction in proliferation in endocrine-sensitive breast cancer.

There is no dose-response curve for tamoxifen and the standard recommended dose is 20 mg a day, as higher doses incur a risk of increased oestrogen agonist activity in the endometrium and also the risk of retinopathy. The overall response rate is 30–35% as first-line therapy in advanced disease. Tamoxifen has a half-life exceeding 200 hours and it takes 6 weeks to reach steady state levels after continuous administration and also a further 6–12 weeks before blood levels become undetectable after cessation of treatment. Side-effects may be antioestrogenic including exacerbation of menopausal symptoms such as hot flushes and mood change and 10% of women experience a clear vaginal discharge, although any bloodstained discharge warrants a gynaecological referral. Venous thrombosis is more common than with placebo, but may be more common if tamoxifen is given concurrently with chemotherapy.

Despite clear clinical value, tamoxifen has limitations in terms of the inevitable development of resistance and possible long-term toxicity. Some ER-positive tumours show intrinsic resistance and do not respond to tamoxifen, and even in responding patients relapse eventually occurs due to acquired resistance (Johnston, 1997) (see Chapter 9b). The mechanisms underlying development of resistance are still under investigation, but are probably molecular rather than pharmacological (see Chapter 9b). In addition, tamoxifen is an oestrogen agonist/antagonist depending on coactivators and corepressors which modify the drug in the ER. There has been considerable interest in the development of alternative selective oestrogen receptor modulators, with the potential reduced agonist activity on the breast and endometrium, and possibly fewer long-term side-effects. These drugs include nonsteroidal compounds such as toremifene, droloxifene, idoxifene and raloxifene, all of which, other than toremifene, have improved antagonist/agonist activity in model systems. Toremifene has been studied in the most clinical trials and despite the benefit in animal models there is no clear clinical benefit over tamoxifen in terms of survival, time to progression or tolerability (Gershanovich et al., 1997; Pyrhonen et al., 1997). The steroidal antagonists, such as faslodex, are pure oestrogen antagonists with a relatively inactive complex of drug and ER; these agents are currently undergoing investigation in phase III trials.

Ovarian suppression

A theoretical concern regarding the use of tamoxifen in premenopausal women is the elevation of serum oestradiol in this age group. However, in clinical trials tamoxifen has similar activity to ovarian ablation and may be preferred to surgical ovarian ablation as any menopausal symptoms are reversible. The availability of luteinizing hormone-releasing hormone (LHRH) analogues which have equivalent activity to surgical ovarian ablation results in amenorrhoea after about 40 days. In younger women menses will resume approximately 80 days from cessation of therapy.

Aromatase inhibitors

There is a clear need for second-line endocrine treatment for women with breast cancer. This is due both to resistance to tamoxifen and also because increasing numbers of women are exposed to tamoxifen in the adjuvant setting. If patients relapse on, or within 12 months of, completing adjuvant tamoxifen, rechallenge with tamoxifen is inappropriate, but alternative endocrine treatment can be considered.

For postmenopausal women the class of drugs of choice is aromatase inhibitors. Circulating levels of oestradiol are approximately 10–20 pg/ml in postmenopausal women (Kirschner et al., 1982), but tumour levels of oestradiol are higher, possibly because of intratumoural oestrogen production by aromatization, and may be sufficient to achieve adequate levels of ER occupancy (Bradlow, 1982). The production of oestrogens in postmenopausal women depends on the presence of the aromatase enzyme in the endoplasmic reticulum of cells in adipose tissue, muscle and skin. The aromatase enzyme system catalyses the conversion of androgen to oestrone with subsequent conversion to oestradiol (Miller, 1989). Type II aromatase inhibitors (e.g. anastrozole, letrozole) are nonsteroidal competitive inhibitors of aromatase and bind reversibly to and inactivate the enzyme by interfering with the iron atom of the porphyrin of the cytochrome p-450 moiety of the enzyme. Continued presence of the drug is essential as blockade is reversible. Type I or suicide inhibitors (e.g. exemestane) are steroidal compounds, so called because they bind to the catalytic site of the aromatase enzyme and are metabolized, yielding a reactive alkylating intermediate which binds covalently with the active site and permanently inactivates the aromatase enzyme. This means new aromatase molecules must be synthesized before oestrogen production can resume (Miller, 1989). Both classes of aromatase inhibitor cause profound ($\geq 90\%$) suppression of oestradiol, oestrone and oestrone sulphate which is maintained over time.

Aminoglutethimide was the first aromatase inhibitor used in breast cancer, but is a nonspecific inhibitor of cytochrome p-450 and also causes inhibition of glucocorticoid biosynthesis and side-effects, including rash, lethargy and fever, which may result in treatment discontinuation in 10% of patients. The third generation of nonsteroidal aromatase inhibitors, anastrozole and letrozole, are extremely potent and highly selective inhibitors of cytochrome p-450 producing near maximal oestrogen suppression. Two randomized Phase III trials involving 764 patients, either treated with anastrozole or the progestin, megestrol acetate,

Table 11.2. Activity of main cytotoxic agents in phase II studies in breast cancer

Very active (>50% response rate)	Moderately active (20% to >50% response rate)	Weakly active (20% response rate)	
Navelbine	5-fluorouracil	Actinomycin-D	Gemcitabine
Doxorubicin	Cisplatin	Amonifide	Hexamethylmelam
Epirubicin	Cyclophosphamide	Amsacrine	Hydroxyurea
Docetaxel	Esorubicin	Bisantrene	Idarubicin
Paclitaxel	Estramustine	Carboplatin	Lomustine (CCNU)
	Ifosfamide	Carmustine (BCNU)	Lonidamine
	Losoxantrone	Chlorambucil	Melphalan
	Methotrexate	CPT-11	Menogaril
	Mitomycin	Cytarabine	6-Mercaptopurine
	Pirarubicin	Dacarbazine	Miltefosine
	Prednimustine	Elliptinium derivates	Mithramycin
	Thiotepa	Etoposide	Mitolactol
	Vinblastine	Fenretinide	Nitrogen mustard
	Vincristine	Fluoridine	Vindesine

after tamoxifen failure have been reported. There was no significant difference in terms of response rate (10.3% vs. 7.9%) or disease stabilization greater than 6 months (25.1% vs. 26.1%). However, tolerability was superior for anastrozole. At 31 months there was a significant survival advantage for anastrozole, with an absolute increase in 2-year survival from 46.3% to 56.1% and an improvement in median survival of approximately 4 months. There was no dose–response relationship and 1 mg anastrozole is the recommended dose (Buzdar et al., 1996b, 1997).

Two further trials have compared different dose levels of letrozole against either megestrol acetate (551 patients) (Dombernowsky et al., 1998) or the first-generation aromatase inhibitor, aminoglutethimide (555 patients) (Gershanovich et al., 1998). These studies established the optimal dose of letrozole to be 2.5 mg daily, which was superior in terms of objective response, duration of response and time to treatment failure compared with megestrol acetate and superior in terms of time to treatment progression and overall survival when compared with aminoglutethimide (Table 11.2). The main toxicities of this class of drugs include nausea, diarrhoea and arthralgia.

The Type I (steroidal) aromatase inhibitor, exemestane, at a dose of 25 mg/day was superior to megestrol acetate 40 mg qds after tamoxifen failure in a randomized trial involving 769 women with a higher overall response rate (15% vs.

12.4%), median survival (not reached with exemestane vs. 123.4 weeks) time to tumour progression (20.3 vs. 16.6 week) and time to treatment failure (16.3 vs. 15.7 weeks) (Kaufman et al., 2000). Previous work with formestane, another steroidal aromatase inhibitor, indicated tumour regression in patients with breast cancer resistant to the nonsteroidal drug, aminoglutethimide (Murray & Pitt, 1995). Exemestane has also shown objective response rates of 6.6% and 26% respectively in women who had progressed after a nonsteroidal aromatase inhibitor in two trials involving 80 and 241 patients, indicating a lack of cross-resistance between exemestane and nonsteroidal aromatase inhibitors (Thurliman et al., 1997; Lonning et al., 2000). In the latter study, exemestane was associated with responses in patients who had failed to respond to prior endocrine therapy.

While comparative data are available on the efficacy of aromatase inhibitors in terms of in vitro and in vivo suppression of aromatase, the clinical trials which may demonstrate the optimal drug(s) are still underway. Anastrozole, letrozole and exemestane have higher activity in patients with soft tissue disease only, but do have significant activity in visceral disease. Two recent trials have indicated that third-generation aromatase inhibitors such as anastrozole are at least as effective as tamoxifen as first-line therapy in metastatic breast cancer and may in fact be superior, especially in ER-positive women in terms of time to progression and with a favourable toxicity profile (Bonneterre et al., 2000; Nabholtz et al., 2000).

Progestins

Progestins have been regarded as third-line treatment in postmenopausal women with endocrine-sensitive disease, although the emerging data on the possible sequential use of nonsteroidal and steroidal aromatase inhibitors may relegate them to fourth-line treatment. They are also occasionally used as second-line treatment in women who are still premenopausal and have failed tamoxifen. However, most such women will have undergone ovarian ablation, or indeed be candidates for chemotherapy. The exact mechanism of action of progestins is uncertain but thought to be related to both a receptor-mediated mechanism and to interference with the pituitary ovarian and pituitary adrenal axis with suppression of circulating oestrogens (Lundgren, 1992). The drug most commonly used is megestrol acetate at a dose of 160 mg/day, but the side-effects, including weight gain (of more than 20% in 10% of patients), fluid retention, vaginal spotting and Cushingoid-like symptoms, can be considerable. These side-effects contribute to the superiority of aromatase inhibitors, which have a very favourable side-effect profile and superior quality of life in randomized studies with only minor gastrointestinal symptoms (Buzdar et al., 1996b, 1997; Lonning et al., 2000).

Combination endocrine treatment

A randomized trial of megestrol acetate together with tamoxifen versus megestrol acetate alone in 215 postmenopausal women with tamoxifen refractory disease showed no difference in response rate or survival (Byrne et al., 1997). In another trial of 288 patients randomized to receive either megestrol acetate, aminoglutethimide plus hydrocortisone, or a combination of the two, there was no difference in time to progression or survival (Russell et al., 1997). Corticosteroids themselves are sometimes used in combination treatment and two trials have shown an enhanced response with corticosteroids added to either ovarian ablation or tamoxifen (Rubens et al., 1988). Corticosteroids do have a low response in their own right, but long-term side-effects may outweigh any benefit.

Overall there is no advantage to be gained by combining endocrine agents, which are currently used sequentially on treatment failure. There may, however, be a rationale for planned sequential or stepwise approach and this is under investigation.

Chemotherapy

Cytotoxic chemotherapy in receptor-negative patients is used after failure of endocrine treatment with rapidly progressive visceral disease needing a rapid response. Response rates for most regimens range between 40–60% in clinical trials, but fall to 30% or less in routine practice (Gregory et al., 1993). This probably reflects both selection bias in trials which may exclude patients on the basis of age, performance status and nonevaluable disease such as bone or haematological and biochemical parameters, and a tendency to lower dose intensity outside trials possibly because of the above factors. Complete response rates are disappointingly low at 5–10% even with the most highly active regimens. The median time to response is approximately 7–14 weeks and the median duration of response around 6–12 months. Some patients become long-term survivors and chemotherapy may improve survival in some patients with visceral disease (Ross et al., 1985).

The most significant predictors of survival and quality of life are the responses to treatment. Complete or partial response is associated with relief of symptoms and improvement of quality of life (Baum et al., 1980). Factors predicting a good response and longer response duration include good performance status (WHO 1/2), limited disease burden and prior endocrine response. Menopausal status and steroid hormone receptor status do not affect response or the duration of the response. Age does not influence outcome with chemotherapy trials of CMF or doxorubicin-based regimens (Christman et al., 1992; Ibrahim et al., 1996), although older women are less likely to be offered chemotherapy possibly because of physician prejudices regarding tolerance and toxicity, but also because of a lower acceptance by older women because of concerns regarding subjective side-effects (Busch et al., 1996). Patients with extensive visceral disease, particularly with organ dysfunction, and extensive prior treatment, especially radiotherapy, will respond less well.

The issue of prior chemotherapy is important, particularly with the increased use of cytotoxic drugs in the adjuvant setting for node-negative as well as node-positive women. It has been suggested that adjuvant chemotherapy *per se* may lead to a poor response to cytotoxic therapy on relapse (Chlebowski et al., 1981), but this has been refuted by other investigators (Buzdar et al., 1981). Certainly the pattern of relapse in women after adjuvant chemotherapy was no different to that in women who did not receive adjuvant chemotherapy in the 20-year follow-up of the pivotal Milan adjuvant trial of chemotherapy with cyclophsophamide, methotrexate, 5-fluorouracil (CMF) versus control (Valagussa et al., 1989). In this trial, 40% of women relapsed with visceral disease irrespective of the initial treatment arm. This study also showed that if the disease-free interval after adjuvant treatment was less than 12 months there was no value in rechallenging patients with CMF because of the poor response rate. These patients might respond to an alternative regimen, such as doxorubicin. If a relapse occurred more than 12 months after completion of adjuvant treatment there was a similar response rate to doxorubicin and CMF. Other studies have confirmed the importance of a disease-free interval from adjuvant chemotherapy as a predictor of response and response duration (Kardinal et al., 1988; Falkson et al., 1991). The increasing use of anthracyclines in adjuvant therapy raises new problems in decisionmaking for chemotherapy in the metastatic patient setting. It may not be possible to rechallenge the patients with anthracyclines because of cardiotoxicity. This is discussed further in this section under anthracyclines and taxanes.

The response rate to second-line chemotherapy in unselected patients is around 20% and the median duration of response shorter than for first-line treatment at only 3–6 months (Gregory et al., 1993; Buzdar et al., 1996a) and further therapies confer an ever-decreasing benefit.

Duration of treatment

Chemotherapy is usually given for 4–6 months, provided the patient shows signs of response and symptom improvement within the first 6–8 weeks; chemotherapy is stopped if progression is observed. There is no clear advantage to prolonged maintenance chemotherapy in randomized trials comparing this approach with short-duration chemotherapy (Muss et al., 1991). Some patients, however, who have a partial response but are still symptomatic and continuing to respond, may benefit from continuing chemotherapy for longer than 6 months.

Single agent versus combination therapy

A number of drugs have single-agent activity. There is no consensus about single-agent chemotherapy used sequentially compared with combination treatment. The usual practice is to use combination regimens as it is felt that these are associated with higher response rates and possibly a longer duration response. In an overview of 106 randomized trials involving over 17 000 patients before the introduction of taxanes, there was a clinically small but significant advantage for polychemotherapy compared with single-agent chemotherapy. This overview also demonstrated no benefit from a combination of chemotherapy and endocrine treatment (Fossati et al., 1998). There is some evidence that anthracyclines, such as doxorubicin, and the taxanes given at optimal doses as single agents sequentially, may be as effective as combination treatment (Norton, 1997). In certain subgroups, such as patients with life-threatening visceral involvement of the liver or bone marrow, single-agent treatment may be preferable with the dose of individual drugs, such as anthracycline, titrated against changes in organ function (e.g. bilirubin) and responses to treatment.

Anthracyclines

Doxorubicin has been considered to be the most active drug in breast cancer. As a single agent there is a dose response curve with results at the maximum tolerated dose of 75 mg/m^2 equivalent to standard combinations such as CMF (Richards et al., 1992). The response rate to doxorubicin as a single agent is around 40% (Perez et al., 1991; Paridaens et al., 2000). Epirubicin has a similar response rate (Perez et al., 1991) and is sometimes preferred because of reduced potential for cardiotoxicity and more rapid hepatic elimination than doxorubicin, which may favour its use if liver function tests are deranged. Combination regimens with doxorubicin, such as doxorubicin and cyclophosphamide (AC), or doxorubicin, cyclophosphamide and 5-fluorouracil (CAF or FAC), are commonly used. However, two randomized trials have failed to show any actual advantage of CAF over nonanthracycline-based regimens such as CMF (Smalley et al., 1983; Cummings et al., 1985). The issue of hair loss may be important here in terms of determining the relative palliation of these treatments as although hair loss may be prevented by scalp cooling with anthracyclines, this is not always successful.

Cumulative cardiotoxicity is a concern for anthracycline-based chemotherapy. FEC (5-fluorouracil, epirubicin and cyclophosphamide) has been compared against the same regimen with doxorubicin instead of epirubicin in two randomized trials involving 263 and 497 patients. The response rates were equivalent (52% vs. 50% and 56% vs. 44%), but the toxicity was less in the FEC arm in terms of alopecia, emesis and cardiotoxicity (Stewart et al., 1997; Italian Multicentre Breast Study with Epirubicin, 1998). The anthraquinone, mitoxantrone, has less

haematological toxicity than doxorubicin or epirubicin, but is generally considered less effective and is mainly used as a palliative agent (French Epirubicin Study
Group, 1998). There has also been interest in improving the therapeutic ratio of
doxorubicin by using cardioprotective agents such as dexrazoxane, which chelates
iron, preventing free radical formation, and also some interest in liposomal
preparations of anthracyclines. Dexrazoxane has been evaluated in combination
regimens with doxorubicin (CAF) in two randomized placebo-controlled trials.
An initial report on 534 patients from both trials indicated that the risk of cardiac
events was 2.5-fold higher in patients not receiving dexrazoxane, but there was no
difference in time to treatment failure or survival. This still requires further
evaluation as in one trial there was a lower response rate in the dexrazoxane arm
(Swain et al., 1997a, b). The use of dexrazoxane in these trials, however, did allow a
median of 10 courses of therapy, equivalent to 750 mg/m^2 of doxorubicin. As the
trial was designed to allow crossover from placebo to dexrazoxane after six courses
of chemotherapy, this raised the issue of the possibility of using delayed cardiac
protection. This may be of interest in the adjuvant setting, but clearly requires
further evaluation.

Taxanes

The taxanes, docetaxel and paclitaxel, have at least equivalent activity to
doxorubicin as single agents. Taxanes stabilize polymerized microtubules thereby
disrupting mitoses and have significant activity in second- or third-line therapy in
patients resistant to anthracyclines with response rates of 16–21% for paclitaxel
(Seidman et al., 1995; Paridaens et al., 2000) and 42–51% for docetaxel (Ravdin et
al., 1995; Valero et al., 1995; Trudeau et al., 1996; Sjostrom et al., 1999). For
docetaxel the main side-effects included fluid retention syndrome with peripheral
oedema, skin and nail changes and febrile neutropenia in 10–20% of patients.
Fluid retention may be abrogated by pre and posttreatment with corticosteroids
and the subsequent use of diuretics. A compassionate use programme in 825
heavily pretreated patients (i.e. an unselected population), confirmed the activity
seen in trials even as third-line treatment with a response rate of 22.9% (95% CI:
20.2%–26.2%) (Alexandre et al., 2000). This study also highlighted the need for
dose reduction to 75 mg/m^2 or less in patients with liver dysfunction or heavy
pretreatment in whom toxicities such as leucopenia, oedema and fluid retention
are more frequent and severe, probably because hepatobiliary excretion is the
major elimination routine for docetaxel.

   These results in Phase II studies and a compassionate programme are encouraging as the options for women with anthracycline-resistant disease have been
limited. Mitomycin C and vinblastine is a commonly used palliative regimen with
a response rate of 16% in anthracycline-resistant breast cancer compared with

30% for docetaxel in a comparative study in 392 patients (Nabholtz et al., 1999). In this study, time to treatment progression was superior (19 vs. 11 weeks) for docetaxel as was survival (11.4 vs. 8.7 months). In comparison with 5-FU and methotrexate, docetaxel was again superior with a response rate of 42% compared with 21% (Sjostrom et al., 1999).

Paclitaxel is commonly given at doses of 175–200 mg/m^2 every three weeks. Higher doses (>250 mg/m^2 are not associated with improved response rates, but do incur a sensory neuropathy (Winer et al., 1998). The response rates in anthracycline-refractory patients between 16% and 21% appear lower than with docetaxel and similarly as a first-line agent the response rates with paclitaxel, 25–32%, are lower than with docetaxel (41–61%), although there are no direct comparative studies (Seidman, 1995; Vermoken & Ten Bokkel Huinick, 1996; Paridaens et al., 2000). Initial concerns about cardiotoxicity with paclitaxel have not resulted in clinical problems in single-agent studies, although asymptomatic arrythmias are seen. In first-line therapy doxorubicin was superior to paclitaxel with a response rate of 41% versus 25% and median progression-free survival (7.5 vs. 3.9 month) (Paridaens et al., 2000). In this study the crossover response to doxorubicin was 30% and to paclitaxel 16%, indicating non-cross resistance.

There is renewed interest in scheduling with both taxanes. For paclitaxel increased duration of infusion (24 h vs. 3 h) may have a slightly improved response rate, but is inconvenient and associated with more haematological and neurotoxicity. Weekly schedules have been used for both taxanes. Paclitaxel can be given at 80–90 mg/m^2 per week with response rates of around 30%, but a much lower incidence of neutropenia, neuropathy and alopecia than with the three-weekly scheduling possibly making this a useful schedule for patients requiring a taxane, but at risk of neutropenia (Seidman et al., 1998). Another potential use of weekly schedules may be with biological agents such as trastuzumab or cytotoxic drugs which are given weekly, e.g. vinorelbine, gemcitabine.

Both taxanes have been used in combination with anthracyclines (Gianni et al., 1995, 1997; Esposito et al., 1999; Sparano et al., 1999). There is no pharmacokinetic interaction between anthracyclines and paclitaxel, however docetaxel increases plasma concentration of doxorubicin (Gianni et al., 1997) leading to a need for dose reduction of docetaxel to 75 mg/m^2 in combination regimens. Despite high response rates in Phase II studies of up to 94% (Gianni et al., 1995) comparative studies have not demonstrated any superiority for anthracycline/taxane combinations over standard anthracycline/cyclophosphamide regimens to date. The lack of cross resistance demonstrated between paclitaxel and doxorubicin (Paridaens et al., 2000) makes sequential rather than combination studies attractive.

Vinorelbine

Vinorelbine is a semisynthetic vinca alkaloid which inhibits formation of the mitotic spindle (in contrast to taxanes which promote and stabilize assembly of microtubules after spindle formation). The response rate in phase II studies was 20–30% in previously treated patients, including those refractory to anthracyclines (Bertsch & Donaldson, 1995; Vermoken & Ten Bokkel Huinick, 1996). In a comparative study against melphalan the response rate was superior to melphalan at 46.5% compared with 28.2% with time to tumour progression of 12 weeks compared with 8 weeks (Jones et al., 1995). Haematological toxicity is dose-limiting with Grade 3 or 4 neutropenia in 75% of patients. Although this is not cumulative it may limit planned weekly administration. Vinorelbine also causes mild peripheral neuropathy and autonomic neuropathy but no alopecia. Vinorelbine is well tolerated with a symptomatic toxicity profile better than conventional regimens such as FEC or FAC in randomized trials, despite a higher incidence of neutropenia (Namer et al., 1997). Preclinical data indicate synergism between vinca alkaloids and taxanes and this has been confirmed in a trial of 49 patients (Romero Acna et al., 1999).

There have been no comparative trials as yet on the relative merits between vinorelbine and taxanes in terms of quality of life and health economics. One cost–utility analysis has demonstrated economic advantages for vinorelbine compared with taxanes with at least equivalent quality-adjusted progression-free survival despite lower absolute response rates and time to progression. (Leung et al., 1999).

Fluoropyrimidines

Capecitabine is a rationally designed selectively tumour-activated fluoropyrimidine carbamate which is effectively an oral 5-fluorouracil prodrug with intramoural activity. Interest in this arose because of the recognition that infusional 5-fluorouracil via central venous access, gave response rates of 20–30% in patients with end stage breast cancer even if they had received prior bolus 5-FU. However, continuous infusional treatment is inconvenient. Oral capecitabine has shown a response rate of 20% in 135 heavily pretreated paclitaxel-resistant patients, including patients who had received anthracyclines (Blum et al., 1999). This activity was confirmed in a randomized phase II trial against paclitaxel in anthracycline-resistant patients with response rates of 36% versus 21% and median time to disease progression of 92 versus 95 days (Moiseyenko et al., 1998). Toxicities are those expected with fluoropyramidines, with neutropenia, gastrointestinal problems (diarrhoea) and hand–foot syndrome.

A guiding principle in chemotherapy for breast cancer is to maximize response by using the best standard regimen first. This approach means that most new agents are evaluated in very advanced disease, the response rate is low in these resistant patients hence valuable drugs may be discarded. This approach can be challenged by a prospective randomized phase III trial in which the safety and efficacy of using a phase II drug before standard chemotherapy was evaluated (Constanza et al., 1999). This study in 365 women showed that the use of single-agent or phase II drugs (trimetrexate, melphalan, amonifide, carboplatin, elsamitrucin) for up to four cycles did not compromise response to a standard regimen (CAF) irrespective of the response to the experimental drug.

Dose intensification

Retrospective literature review had indicated that higher doses or dose intensity were associated with improved survival (Hryniuk & Bush, 1984). Certainly a moderate increase in dose of around twofold has been associated with increased response rate, but no improvement in time to progression or overall survival (Bastholt et al., 1996; Hortobagyi et al., 1987). These studies also confirmed that chemotherapy given at suboptimal doses resulted in an inferior outcome, emphasizing the need for standard doses when a decision to treat is made. These data led to renewed interest in dose intensification, with high-dose chemotherapy supported by growth factors and/or bone marrow transplantation or peripheral blood stem cell support. Phase II trials in the 1980s were promising and by 1995 breast cancer was the most common indication for high-dose chemotherapy and bone marrow transplant in the United States. Few patients were in clinical trials and any apparently superior results may have been due to selection bias in favour of younger age and good performance status (Antman et al., 1997). A retrospective analysis by Rahman et al. (1997) emphasized this issue. This group evaluated the results of 1581 patients with metastatic breast cancer who were treated with doxorubicin containing regimens with standard doses within clinical trials. Those who would have met the criteria for high-dose treatment, i.e. transplant candidates, had a better response rate, progression-free survival and overall survival although they only received standard chemotherapy. In a randomized trial comparing high-dose consolidation with maintenance chemotherapy in conventional doses after remission induction, there was no improvement in survival with the high-dose approach (Stadtmauer et al., 2000). There is, as yet, no evidence to support the routine use of high-dose chemotherapy outside clinical trials (see Chapter 12a).

Bisphosphonates

Bone metastases are common in breast cancer and are the first site of relapse in 35–40% of patients. Bone metastases are associated with considerable morbidity including pain, fractures and hypercalcaemia with impaired quality of life. Bisphosphonates have been used in metastatic cancer for treatment of hypercalcaemia for some time and are now established for use in patients with bone metastases to reduce the pain and the risk of fracture or skeletal events in combination with standard endocrine therapy or chemotherapy (Paterson et al., 1993; Conte et al., 1996; Hortobagyi et al., 1996, 1998). In these studies the use of bisphosphonates had no impact on survival (see Chapters 13 and 14).

There would appear to be a dose-response rate for bisphosphonates and currently newer more potent analogues for oral use, such as alendronate, ibandronate and zoledronate, are under development. Oral bisphosphonates tend to have poor bioavailability and intravenous treatment is currently the treatment of choice. The optimum duration for bisphosphonates is uncertain. Bisphosphonates are useful in patients with predominantly bone-only metastases, particularly if they have a good performance status, have had a skeletal event and/or bone pain and are oestrogen-receptor negative or have failed endocrine treatment and do not yet require chemotherapy. The role of radiotherapy and surgery in the management of solitary lesions or significant lesions in long bones should always be considered.

Trastuzumab

Conventional chemotherapy has the limitation of the inevitable development of drug resistance (see Chapter 9c). Biological therapy, including targeted therapy with antibodies or vaccine therapy, may offer new opportunities for treatment (see Chapter 12b). Trastuzumab (Herceptin®) is a humanized monoclonal antibody directed against HER2-*neu* oncogene which is located on chromosome 17 and encodes a tyrosine kinase with some homology to human epidermal growth factor. HER2 overexpression is seen in about 25% of women and is associated with gene amplification in 90% of cases (Dowsett et al., 2000) with breast cancer.

Some studies have indicated inferior response to hormonal therapy for cancers overexpressing HER2, although the number of ER-positive cancers which are also HER2 positive is small (5%). HER2 overexpression appears to confer increased sensitivity to doxorubicin, especially at higher dose levels (Paik et al., 1998; Thor et al., 1998). Certainly patients with HER2 overexpression have inferior prognosis with a shortened disease-free interval and survival.

Two pivotal trials have evaluated trastuzumab in metastatic breast cancer. Herceptin® monotherapy was used in a phase II trial in 222 women who had received one or two prior chemotherapy regimens for metastatic disease. In this study of poor prognosis patients a suitable comparator arm could not be identified. The overall response rate was 15% (95% CI: 11–21%) with median duration of response 9.1 months and median survival 12.8 months (Cobleigh et al., 1999). In those patients with strong overexpression of HER2 (3^+), the response rate was 18%, but only 6% in patients with moderate or 2^+ overexpression by immunohistochemistry. The drug is well tolerated without the side-effects of emesis, mucositis, alopecia, neuropathy and myelosuppression seen with cytotoxic drugs, although a symptom complex of fevers and chills is seen on the first infusion in 40% of patients, but rarely with subsequent infusions.

In combination with anthracyclines or paclitaxel, the addition of Herceptin® significantly improved response rate (62% vs. 36%) and prolonged time to progression (8.6 vs. 5.5 months) (Slamon et al., 1998). Herceptin is well tolerated with a symptom complex of fevers, chills and occasionally rigors with the first infusion, but few subsequent side-effects and no exacerbation of conventional cytotoxic drug toxicity. There appears to be an unexpected increase in the incidence of cardiotoxicity with Herceptin, which is apparently related to either current or past cumulative anthracycline exposure. This currently precludes the use of Herceptin with anthracyclines outside clinical trials. Current studies are evaluating the use of Herceptin in combination with other agents, such as vinorelbine or platinum.

Other biological approaches include antisense treatments and renewed interest in vaccines (see Chapter 12b). Although breast cancer cells are not inherently immunogenic, immune responses can be generated when synthetic peptides recognizing the MUC-1 glycoprotein, which is aberrantly glycosylated in breast cancer, are coupled to carrier proteins and an immunological adjuvant (Miles et al., 1996). Phase III trials are underway.

Specific problems
Liver metastases

About 25% of patients who die from breast cancer will have evidence of liver metastases before death. In general, the prognosis for these patients has been considered poor when compared with other sites, particularly when liver function is deranged. In this situation cytotoxic chemotherapy is the only treatment option, but as the active drugs, anthracyclines and taxanes, undergo hepatic metabolism, there can be increased toxicity. In general, epirubicin is preferred to doxorubicin because it is subject to glucuronidation and is metabolized more rapidly than doxorubicin. Certainly if the bilirubin is elevated the dose of doxorubicin should be reduced and in the presence of elevated transaminases (>2–3 times normal) the use of taxanes, in particular docetaxel, has to be cautious and dose reduction mandatory.

Bone marrow

Bone is the most prevalent site for metastatic disease and in some patients extensive infiltration of the bone marrow can cause leucoerythroblastic anaemia and pancytopenia. This problem may be exacerbated by previous treatment, in particular chemotherapy. Clearly these patients would be very sensitive to cytotoxic treatment and again monotherapy with anthracyclines at low dose, possibly supported by haematological growth factors, is the preferred treatment option. In both situations of liver and bone marrow infiltration the dose of drugs may need to be increased as the patient responds.

Brain metastases

Brain metastases may develop as an isolated site of disease in metastatic breast cancer or more commonly in association with advanced disease (see Chapter 14). The reported incidence is around 25%. With solitary metastasis, in the absence of significant metastatic disease at other sites, resection followed by radiotherapy should be considered as some patients become long-term survivors. With multiple metastases, the treatment is palliative and consists of whole brain radiotherapy, usually with short-term high-dose steroids to relieve oedema. There is no clear evidence that protracted radiotherapy schedules are superior compared to five or two fractions. A minority of patients will develop meningeal disease, which may present with impaired cranial or peripheral nerve function because of nerve root involvement. The diagnosis may be made by gadolinium-enhanced magnetic resonance imaging (MRI) and confirmed by examination of the cerebrospinal fluid to obtain a cytological diagnosis. Patients with meningeal disease can be considered for local radiotherapy to relieve nerve root pressure or intrathecal chemotherapy with methotrexate and cytosine arabinoside. This may be given via an ommaya reservoir twice-weekly for 2–3 weeks until clinical improvement is established, followed by maintenance treatment.

Serous effusion

Pleural effusions are common in patients with breast cancer either as an isolated site of disease or as part of the spectrum of metastatic disease (see Chapter 14). Isolated pleural effusions may be best managed by drainage, with consideration of a surgical pleurodesis, but patients will also require systemic management based on other factors such as performance status, other sites of disease and steroid hormone receptor status. If chemotherapy is used, care must be taken with methotrexate because of third space accumulation and excess toxicity.

Conclusion

Metastatic breast cancer is a complex disease requiring a multidisciplinary approach because of the protean manifestations and variable course. The availability of a wide range of treatments makes the disease a therapeutic challenge and the careful sequential use of endocrine treatment and chemotherapy may result in good quality of life and for some patients prolonged survival. The recent advances in breast cancer, in particular the introduction of taxanes and now of the monoclonal antibody, Herceptin, provide exciting avenues for further improvements in treatment of breast cancer. Results from studies in metastatic disease can, of course, be of use in the adjuvant setting.

REFERENCES

Alexandre, J., Bleuzen, P., Bonneterre, J. et al. (2000). Factors predicting for efficacy and safety of docetaxel and the compassionate-use cohort of 825 heavily pretreated advanced breast cancer patients. *Journal of Clinical Oncology*, 18, 562–73.

Antman, K.H., Rowlings, P.A., Vaughan, W.P. et al. (1997). High-dose chemotherapy with autologous hematopoietic stem-cell support for breast cancer in North America. *Journal of Clinical Oncology*, 15, 1870–9.

Bastholt, L., Dalmark, M., Gjedde, S.B. et al. (1996). Dose–response relationship of epirubicin in the treatment of postmenopausal patients with metastatic breast cancer: a randomised study of epirubicin at four different dose levels performed by the Danish Breast Cancer Cooperative Group. *Journal of Clinical Oncology*, 14, 1146–55.

Baum, M., Priestman, T., West, R.R. et al. (1980). A comparison of subjective responses in a trial comparing endocrine with cytotoxic treatment in advanced carcinoma of the breast. In: *Breast Cancer – Experimental and Clinical Methods*, ed. H.T. Mouridsen, D. Palshoft, pp. 223–8. London: Pergamon Press, *European Journal of Cancer* (Suppl. 1), 223–6).

Bertsch, L.A. & Donaldson, G. (1995). Quality-of-life analyses from vinorelbine (Navelbine) clinical trials of women with metastatic breast cancer. *Seminars in Oncology*, 22, 45–54.

Blum, J.L., Jones, S.G., Buzdar, A.U. et al. (1999). Multicenter phase II study of capecitabine in paclitaxel-refractory breast cancer. *Journal of Clinical Oncology*, 17, 485–93.

Bonneterre, J., Thurliman, B., Robertson, J.F.R. (2000). Anastrozole versus tamoxifen as first-line therapy for advanced breast cancer in 668 postmenopausal women: results of the tamoxifen or arimidex randomised group efficacy and tolerability study. *Journal of Clinical Oncology*, 18, 3748–57.

Bradlow, H.L. (1982). A reassessment of the role of breast tumor aromatization. *Cancer Research*, 42 (8 Suppl.), 3382s–86s.

Busch, E., Kemeny, M., Fremgen, A. et al. (1996). Patterns of breast cancer care in the elderly. *Cancer*, 78, 101–11.

Buzdar, A.U., Hortobagyi, G.N., Frye, D. et al. (1996a). Second-line chemotherapy for metastatic breast cancer including quality-of-life issues. *Breast Cancer*, 5, 312–17.

Buzdar, A., Jonat, W., Howell, A. et al. (1996b). Anastrozole, a potent and selective aromatase inhibitor, versus megestrol acetate in postmenopausal women with advanced breast cancer: results of overview analysis of two phase III trials. Arimidex Study Group. *Journal of Clinical Oncology*, 14(7), 2000–11.

Buzdar, A., Jonat, W., Howell, A. et al. (1997). Significant improved survival with Arimidex (Anastrozole) versus megestrol acetate in postmenopausal advanced breast cancer; update of results of two randomised trials. *Proceedings of American Society of Clinical Oncology*, 16, 854–5.

Buzdar, A.U., Legha, S.S., Hortobagyi, G.N. et al. (1981). Management of breast cancer patients failing adjuvant chemotherapy with adriamycin-containing regimens. *Cancer*, 47, 2798–802.

Byrne, M.J., Gebski, V., Forbes, J. et al. (1997). Medroxyprogesterone acetate addition or substitution for tamoxifen in advanced tamoxifen-resistant breast cancer: a phase III randomized trial. Australian–New Zealand Breast Cancer Trials Group. *Journal of Clinical Oncology*, 15(9), 3141–8.

Carlson, R.W. (1998). Quality of life issues in the treatment of metastatic breast cancer. *Oncology*, 12, 27–31.

Carmichael, J., Possinger, K., Phillip, P. et al. (1995). A phase II trial with gemcitabine. *Journal of Clinical Oncology*, 13, 2731–6.

Chlebowski, R.T., Weiner, J.M., Luce, J. et al. (1981). Significance of relapse after adjuvant treatment with combination chemotherapy or 5-fluorouracil alone in high-risk breast cancer. *Cancer Research*, 41, 4399–403.

Christman, K., Muss, H.B., Case, L.D. et al. (1992). Chemotherapy of metastatic breast cancer in the elderly: the Piedmont Oncology Association experience. *Journal of the American Medical Association*, 268, 57–62.

Cobleigh, M.A., Vogel, C.L., Tripathy, D. et al. (1999). Multinational study of the efficacy and safety of humanised anti-Her2 monoclonal antibody in women who have Her-2-overexpressing metastatic cancer that has progressed after chemotherapy for metastatic disease. *Journal of Clinical Oncology*, 17(9), 2639–48.

Cold, S., Jensen, N.V., Brincker et al. (1993). The influence of chemotherapy on survival after recurrence in breast cancer – a population-based study of patients treated in the 1950s, 1960s and 1970s. *European Journal of Cancer*, 29A(8), 1146–52.

Constanza, M.E., Weiss, R.B., Henderon, I.C. et al. (1999). Safety and efficacy of using a single agent or a phase II agent before instituting standard combination chemotherapy in previously untreated metastatic breast cancer: report of a randomised study. Cancer and Leukaemia Group B 8642. *Journal of Clinical Oncology*, 17(5), 1397–406.

Conte, P.F., Latreille, J., Mauriac, L. et al. (1996). Delay in progression of bone metastases in breast cancer patients treated with intravenous pamidronate: results from a multinational randomised controlled trial. The Aredia Multinational Cooperative Group. *Journal of Clinical Oncology*, 14(9), 2552–9.

Cummings, F.J., Gelman, R. & Horton, J. (1985). A comparison of CAF versus CMFVP in metastatic breast cancer: analysis of prognostic factors. *Journal of Clinical Oncology*, 3, 932–40.

Dombernowsky, P., Smith, I.E., Falkson, G. et al. (1998). Letrozole, a new oral aromatase inhibitor for advanced breast cancer: double-blind randomized trial showing a dose effect and improved efficacy and tolerability compared with megestrol acetate. *Journal of Clinical*

Oncology, 16(2), 453–61.

Dowsett, M., Cooke, T., Ellis, I. et al. (2000). Assessment of HER2 status in breast cancer: why, when and how? *European Journal of Cancer*, 36, 170–6.

Esposito, M., Venturini, M. & Vannozzi, M.O. (1999). Comparative effects of paclitaxel and docetaxel on the metabolism and pharmacokinetics of epirubicin in breast cancer patients. *Journal of Clinical Oncology*, 17, 1132–40.

Falkson, G., Gelman, R., Falkson, C.I. et al. (1991). Factors predicting for response, time to treatment failure and survival in women with metastatic breast cancer treated with DAVTH: a prospective Eastern Cooperative Oncology Group study. *Journal of Clinical Oncology*, 9, 2153–61.

Fossati, R., Confalonieri, C., Torri, V. et al. (1998). Cytotoxic and hormonal treatment for metastatic breast cancer: a systematic review of published randomized trials involving 31,510 women. *Journal of Clinical Oncology*, 16, 3439–60.

French Epirubicin Study Group (1998). A prospective randomized, phase III trial comparing combination chemotherapy with cyclophosphamide, fluorouracil and either doxorubicin or epirubicin. *Journal of Clinical Oncology*, 6, 679–88.

Gershanovich, M., Garin, A., Baltina, D. et al. (1997). A phase III comparison of two toremifene doses to tamoxifen in postmenopausal women with advanced breast cancer. Eastern European Study Group. *Breast Cancer Research and Treatment*, 45(3), 251–62.

Gershanovich, M., Chaudri, H.A., Campos, D. et al. (1998). Letrozole, a new oral aromatase inhibitor; randomised trial comparing 2.5 mg daily, 0.5 mg daily and aminoglutethimide in postmenopausal women with advanced breast cancer. Letrozole International Trial Group (ARBC3). *Annals of Oncology*, 9(6), 639–45.

Gianni, L., Munzone, E., Capri, D. et al. (1995). Paclitaxel by 3-hour infusion in combination with bolus doxorubicin in women with untreated metastatic breast cancer: high antitumour efficacy and cardiac effects in a dose-finding and sequence-finding study. *Journal of Clinical Oncology*, 13(11), 2688–99.

Gianni, L., Vigano, L., Locatelli, A. et al. (1997). Human pharmacokinetic/pharmacodynamics of docetaxel in phase II studies in patients with cancer. *Journal of Clinical Oncology*, 16, 187–96.

Gregory, W.M., Smith, P., Richards, M.A. et al. (1993). Chemotherapy of advanced breast cancer: outcome and prognostic factors. *British Journal of Cancer*, 68, 988–95.

Hainsworth, J.D., Burris, H.A., Erland, J.B. et al. (1998). Phase I trial of docetaxel administered by weekly infusion in patients with advanced refractory cancer. *Journal of Clinical Oncology*, 16(6), 2164–8.

Harris, J., Morrow, M. & Norton, L. (1997). Malignant tumours of the breast. In: *Cancer Principles and Practice of Oncology*, pp. 1557–602. Ed. V.T. De Vita, Jnr., S. Hellman, S.A. Rosenberg. Philadelphia: Lippincott-Raven.

Hayes, D.F. (1996). Serum (circulating) tumour markers for breast cancer. *Recent Results in Cancer Research*, 140, 101–13.

Hortobagyi, G.N., Bodey, G.P., Buzdar, A.U. et al. (1987). Evaluation of high-dose versus standard FAC chemotherapy for advanced breast cancer in protected-environment units: a prospective randomised study. *Journal of Clinical Oncology*, 5, 354–64.

Hortobagyi, G.N., Theriault, R.L., Porter, L. et al. (1996). Efficacy of pamidronate in reducing skeletal complications in patients with breast cancer and lytic bone metastases. *New England Journal of Medicine*, 335, 1785–91.

Hortobagyi, G.N., Theriault, R.L., Lipton, A. et al. (1998). Long-term prevention of skeletal complications of metastatic breast cancer with pamidronate. *Journal of Clinical Oncology*, 16, 2038–44.

Howell, A., Mackintosh, J., Jones, M. et al. (1988). The definition of the 'no change' category in patients treated with endocrine therapy and chemotherapy for advanced carcinoma of the breast. *European Journal of Cancer Clinical Oncology*, 24(10), 1567–72.

Hryniuk, W. & Bush, H. (1984). The importance of dose intensity in chemotherapy in metastatic breast cancer. *Journal of Clinical Oncology*, 2, 1281–8.

Ibrahim, N.K., Frye, D.K., Buzdar, A.U. et al. (1996). Doxorubicin-based chemotherapy in elderly patients with metastatic breast cancer. *Archives of Internal Medicine*, 156, 882–8.

Italian Multicentre Breast Study with Epirubicin (1998). A randomised phase III study of fluorouracil, epirubicin and cyclophosphamide versus fluorouracil, doxorubicin and cyclophosphamide in advanced breast cancer: an Italian multicenter trial. *Journal of Clinical Oncology*, 6, 976–82.

Johnston, S.R.D. (1997). Acquired tamoxifen resistance in human breast cancer – potential mechanisms and clinical implications. *Anticancer Drugs*, 8(10), 911–30.

Jones, S., Winer E., Vogel, C. et al. (1995). Randomised comparison of vinorelbine and melphalan in anthracycline-refractory advanced breast cancer. *Journal of Clinical Oncology*, 13(10), 2567–74.

Kardinal, C.G., Perry, M. C., Korzun, A. H. et al. (1988). Responses to chemotherapy or chemohormonal therapy in advanced breast cancer patients treated previously with adjuvant chemotherapy – a subset of CALGB Study 8081. *Cancer*, 61, 415–19.

Kaufman, M., Bajetta, E., Dinx, L.Y. et al. (2000). Exemestane is superior to megestrol acetate after taxoxifen failure in postmenopausal women with advanced breast cancer: results of a phase III randomised double-blind trial. *Journal of Clinical Oncology*, 18, 1399–411.

Kirschner, M.A., Schneider, G., Ertel, N.H. et al. (1982). Obesity, androgens and cancer risk. *Cancer Research*, 42(8), (Suppl.), 3281s–5s.

Leung, P.P., Tannock, I.F., Oza, A.M. et al. (1999). Cost-utility analysis using paclitaxel, docetaxel or vinorelbine for patients with anthracycline-resistant breast cancer. *Journal of Clinical Oncology*, 17(10), 3082–90.

Lonning, P.E., Bajetta, E., Murray, R. et al. (2000). Activity of exemestane in metastatic breast cancer after failure of nonsteroidal aromatase inhibitors: a phase II trial. *Journal of Clinical Oncology*, 2234–44.

Lundgren, S. (1992). Progestins in breast cancer treatment: a review. *Acta Oncology*, 31(7), 709–22.

Mansi, J.L., Earl, H.M, Powles, T.J. et al. (1988). Tests for detecting recurrent disease in the follow-up of patients with breast cancer. *Breast Cancer Research and Treatment*, 11(3), 249–54.

Miles, D.W., Towlson, K.E., Graham, R. et al. (1996). A randomised phase-II study of sialyl-Tn and DETOX-B adjuvant with or without cyclophosphamide pretreatment for the active specific immunotherapy of breast cancer. *British Journal of Cancer*, 74, 1292–6.

Miller, W.R. (1989). Aromatase inhibitors in the treatment of advanced breast cancer. *Cancer*

Treatment Reviews, 16(2), 83–93.

Moiseyenko, M., O'Reilly, S.M., Talbot, D.C. et al. (1998). A randomised, phase-II trial of Xeloda (capcitabine) versus paclitaxel in breast cancer patients failing previous anthracycline therapy. *Annals of Oncology*, 9, 620–4.

Murray, R. & Pitt, P. (1995). Aromatase inhibition with 4-OH androstenedione after prior aromatase inhibition with aminoglutethimide in women with advanced breast cancer. *Breast Cancer Research and Treatment*, 35, 249–53.

Muss, H.B., Case, L.D., Richards, F. et al. (1991). Interrupted versus continuous chemotherapy in patients with metastatic breast cancer. *New England Journal of Medicine*, 325, 1342–6.

Nabholtz, J.M., Senn, H.J. & Bezwoda, W.R. (1999). Prospective randomised trial of docetaxel versus mitomycin plus vinblastine in patients with metastatic breast cancer progressing despite previous anthracycline-containing chemotherapy. *Journal of Clinical Oncology*, 17, 1413–24.

Nabholtz, J.M., Buzdar, A., Pollak, M. et al. (2000). Anastrozole is superior to tamoxifen as first-line therapy for advanced breast cancer in postmenopausal women: results of a North American multicenter randomised trial. *Journal of Clinical Oncology*, 18, 3758–67.

Namer, M., Soler-Michelle, P., Mefti, F. et al. (1997). Is the combination of FAC/FEC always the best regimen in advanced breast cancer? Utility of mitoxantrone and vinorelbine combination as an alternative: results from a randomised trial. *Breast Cancer Research and Treatment*, 46, 94, Abstract 406.

Norton, L. (1997). Evolving concepts in systemic drug treatment of breast cancer. *Seminars in Oncology*, 24, S10 – 3–10.

Paik, S., Bryant, J., Paik, C. et al. (1998). ErbB-2 and response to doxorubicin in patients with axillary lymph node-positive, hormone receptor-negative breast cancer. *Journal of National Cancer Institute*, 90, 1361–70.

Paridaens, R., Biganzoli, L., Brunning, J.G.M. et al. (2000). Paclitaxel versus doxorubicin as first line single agent chemotherapy for metastatic breast cancer: a European Organisation for Research and Treatment of Cancer randomised study with crossover. *Journal of Clinical Oncology*, 18(4), 724–33.

Paterson, A.H.G., Powles, T.J., Kanis, J.A. et al. (1993). Double-blind, controlled trial of oral clodronate in patients with bone metastases from breast cancer. *Journal of Clinical Oncology*, 11, 59–65.

Perez, D.J., Harvey, V. J., Robinson, B.A. et al. (1991). A randomized comparison of single-agent doxorubicin and epirubicin as first-line cytotoxic chemotherapy in advanced breast cancer. *Journal of Clinical Oncology*, 9, 2148–52.

Pyrhonen, S., Valavaara, R., Modig H. et al. (1997). Comparison of toremifene and tamoxifen in post-menopausal patients with advanced breast cancer: a randomized double-blind, the 'nordic' phase III study. *British Journal of Cancer*, 76(2), 270–7.

Rahman, Z.U., Frye, D.K., Buzdar, A.U. et al. (1997). Impact of selection process on response rate and long-term survival of potential high-dose chemotherapy candidates treated with standard-dose doxorubicin-containing chemotherapy in patients with metastatic breast cancer. *Journal of Clinical Oncology*, 15, 3171–7.

Ramirez, A.J., Towlson, K.E., Leaning, M.S. et al. (1998). Do patients with advanced breast cancer benefit from chemotherapy? *British Journal of Cancer*, 78(11), 1488–94.

Ravdin, P.M., Green, S., Dorr, T.M. et al. (1992). Prognostic significance of progesterone receptor levels in estrogen receptor-positive patients with metastatic breast cancer treated with tamoxifen: results of a prospective Southwest Oncology Group study. *Journal of Clinical Oncology*, 10, 1284–91.

Ravdin, P.M., Burris, H.A., Cook, G. et al. (1995). A phase-II trial of docetaxel in advanced anthracycline-resistant or anthracenedione-resistant breast cancer. *Journal of Clinical Oncology*, 13, 2879–85.

Richards, M.A., Hopwood, P., Ramirez, A.J. et al. (1992). Doxorubicin in advanced breast cancer: influence of the schedule on response, survival and quality of life. *European Journal of Cancer*, 28, 1023–8.

Romero Acna, L., Langhi, M., Perez, J. et al. (1999). Vinorelbine and paclitaxel as first line therapy in metastatic breast cancer. *Journal of Clinical Oncology*, 17(1), 74–81.

Ross, M.B., Buzdar, A.U., Smith, T.L. et al. (1985). Improved survival of patients with metastatic breast cancer receiving combination chemotherapy. *Cancer*, 55(2), 341–6.

Rubens, R.D., Tinson, C.L., Coleman, R.E. et al. (1988). Prednisolone improves response to primary endocrine treatment for advanced breast cancer. *British Journal of Cancer*, 58(5), 626–30.

Russell, C.A., Green, S.J., O'Sullivan, J. et al. (1997). Megestrol acetate and aminoglutethimide/hydrocortisone in sequence or in combination as second-line endocrine therapy of estrogen receptor-positive metastatic breast cancer: a Southwest Oncology Group phase III trial. *Journal of Clinical Oncology*, 15(7), 2494–501.

Rutgers, E.J., van Slooten, E.A. & Kluck, H.M. (1989). Follow-up after treatment of primary breast cancer. *British Journal of Surgery*, 76(2), 187–90.

Seidman, A.D., Tierston, A., Hidis, C. et al. (1995). Phase II trial of paclitaxel by 3h infusion as initial and salvage chemotherapy for metastatic breast cancer. *Journal of Clinical Oncology*, 13, 2575–81.

Seidman, A.D., Hudis, C.A., Albanel, J. et al. (1998). Dose-dense therapy with weekly 1-hour paclitaxel infusion in the treatment of metastatic breast cancer. *Journal of Clinical Oncology*, 16(10), 3353–61.

Sjostrom, J., Blomqvist, C., Mouridson, H. et al. (1999). Docetaxel compared with sequential methotrexate and 5-fluorouracil in patients with advanced breast cancer after anthracycline failure: a randomised phase II study with crossover on progression by the Scandinavian Breast Group. *European Journal of Cancer*, 35, 1194–201.

Slamon, D., Leyland-Jones, B., Shak, S. et al. (1998). Addition of Herceptin (humanised anti-Her-2 antibody) to first-line chemotherapy for Her-2-overexpressing metastatic breast cancer markedly increases anti-cancer activity: a randomised, multinational, controlled, phase-III trial. *Proceedings of the American Society of Clinical Oncologists*, 17, 98, Abstract.

Smalley, R.V., Lefante, J., Bartolucci, A. et al. (1983). A comparison of cyclophosphamide, adriamycin and 5-fluorouracil (CAF) and cyclophosphamide, methotrexate, 5-fluorouracil, vincristine and prednisolone (CMFVP) in patients with advanced breast cancer. *Breast*

Cancer Research and Treatment, 3, 209–20.

Sparano, J.A., Hu, P., Rao, R.M. et al. (1999). Phase II trial of doxorubicin and paclitaxel plus granulocyte colony-stimulating factor in metastatic breast cancer: an Eastern Cooperative Group Study. *Journal of Clinical Oncology*, 17(12), 3828–34.

Stadtmauer, E.A., O'Neill, A., Goldstein, L.J. et al. (2000). Conventional-dose chemotherapy compared with high-dose chemotherapy plus autologous haematopoietic stem-cell transplantation for metastatic breast cancer. Philadelphia Bone Marrow Transplant Group. *New England Journal of Medicine*, 342(15), 1069–76.

Stewart, D.J., Evans, W.K., Shepherd, F.A. et al. (1997). Cyclophosphamide and fluorouracil combined with mitoxantrone versus doxorubicin for breast cancer: superiority of doxorubicin. *Journal of Clinical Oncology*, 15, 1897–905.

Swain, S.M., Whaley, F.S., Gerber, M.C. et al. (1997a). Delayed administration of dexrazoxane provides cardioprotection for patients with advanced breast cancer treated with doxorubicin-containing therapy. *Journal of Clinical Oncology*, 15, 1333–40.

Swain, S.M., Whaley, F.S., Gerber, M.C. et al. (1997b). Cardioprotection with dexrazoxane for doxorubicin-containing therapy in advanced breast cancer. *Journal of Clinical Oncology*, 15, 1318–32.

Tannock, I.F., Boyd, N.F., Deboer, G. et al. (1998). A randomised trial of two dose levels of cyclophosphamide, methotrexate and fluorouracil chemotherapy for patients with metastatic breast cancer. *Journal of Clinical Oncology*, 6, 1377–87.

Taylor, S.G., Gelman, R.S., Falkson, G. et al. (1986). Combination chemotherapy compared with tamoxifen as initial therapy for stage IV breast cancer in elderly women. *Annals of Internal Medicine*, 104(4), 455–61.

Thor, A., Berry, D., Budman, D. et al. (1998). *ErbB*-2 p53 and efficacy of adjuvant therapy in lymph node-positive breast cancer. *Journal of National Cancer Institute*, 90, 1346–60.

Thurlimann, B., Paridaens, R., Serin, D. et al. (1997). Third-line hormonal treatment with Exemestane in postmenopausal patients with advanced breast cancer progressing on aminoglutethimide: a phase II multicentre multinational study. Exemestane Study Group. *European Journal of Cancer*, 33(11), 1767–73.

Trudeau, M.E., Eisenhauer, E.A., Higgins, B.P. et al. (1996). Docetaxel in patients with metastatic breast cancer: a phase-II study of the National Cancer Institute of Canada – Clinical Trials Group. *Journal of Clinical Oncology*, 14, 422–8.

Valagussa, P., Brambilla, C., Zambetti, M. et al. (1989). Salvage treatments in relapsing resectable breast cancer. *Recent Results in Cancer Research*, 115, 69–76.

Valero, V., Holmes, F.A., Walters, R.S. et al. (1995). A phase-II trial of docetaxel: a new, highly effective antineoplastic agent in the management of patients with anthracycline-resistant metastatic breast cancer. *Journal of Clinical Oncology*, 13, 2886–94.

Vermoken, J.B. & Ten Bokkel Huinick, W.W. (1996). Chemotherapy for advanced breast cancer: the place of active new drugs. *Breast*, 5, 304–11.

Winer, E., Berry, D., Duggan, D. et al. (1998). Failure of higher-dose paclitaxel to improve outcome in patients with metastatic breast cancer: results from CALGB9342. *Proceedings of the American Society of Clinical Oncologists*, 17, 101, Abstract.

12

Experimental approaches

High-dose chemotherapy in breast cancer

John Crown[a] and R.C.F. Leonard [b]

[a]St Vincent's University Hospital, Elm Park, Dublin 4, Ireland
[b]University of Wales, Swansea

Background: chemotherapy of breast cancer – theory and practice

Breast cancer is a partially chemotherapy sensitive neoplasm. Patients with metastases will usually achieve a degree of tumour response, with amelioration of the distressing symptoms of cancer, and some degree of survival prolongation. Some patients who are close to death, with impending failure of crucial organ systems, will be restored to reasonably good health, and will go on to live for months, or in some cases for years. Most responses are partial, however, and in all but exceptional cases, are temporary. Durable complete remission is only anecdotally reported (Cold et al., 1993; Greenberg et al., 1996).

Chemotherapy given as an adjuvant treatment to patients with earlier stage disease has a greater survival impact, and may contribute to cure (Early Breast Cancer Trialists' Collaborative Group, 1992). This is consistent with the results of the classic experiments of Skipper and Schabel, which suggested that tumours grew exponentially with a constant growth rate, and that chemotherapy killed a constant proportion of cells. These investigators also found that there was an invariably inverse relationship between the size of a tumour and its curability by chemotherapy. Their model had profound implications for the concept of adjuvant systemic therapy, and appeared to be particularly relevant to breast cancer therapeutics (Skipper & Schabel, 1988). While several generations of studies have confirmed that adjuvant chemotherapy has a beneficial impact in patients with both node-positive and node-negative breast cancer, the impact is less than might have been expected on the basis of the Skipper–Schabel model (Norton & Simon, 1986).

Norton and Simon proposed an alternative model for tumour growth kinetics, and one which went some considerable distance to explaining why the impact of chemotherapy had not been more substantial. These researchers hypothesized that tumours grew and regressed according to Gompertzian kinetics. The essential feature of Gompertzian populations is that the rate of growth is not constant, as had been predicted in the exponential model, but, rather, varied inversely with the size of the tumour. Thus, large tumours had lower growth fractions than did smaller ones, and hence were less sensitive to cytotoxics. They also proposed that the cell kill induced by a chemotherapy drug was directly related to the size of the dose, and to the growth rate of the unperturbed tumour at that point in its growth curve (Norton et al., 1976). According to this model, patients with overt cancer should first be treated with chemotherapy to reduce their tumour burden, which would place them in the more sensitive phase of their growth curve. At this point tumour eradication might be attempted. Paradoxically, the same rapid regrowth that enhances cytotoxicity of smaller populations, could, in the case of very small amounts of residual cancer cells, also make tumour eradication more difficult, in that any minimal residual populations of cells which survive a given cycle of treatment would undergo rapid, but wholly clinically inapparent regrowth prior to the next cycle. Thus, the late phase of the treatment should be 'intensified'. Several randomized trials have tested this hypothesis. The CALGB randomized patients with node-positive breast cancer to receive either intensification (i.e. anthracycline-containing chemotherapy) or further CMF (cyclophosphamide, methotrexate and 5-fluorouracil) (Perloff et al., 1996) as crossover therapy following a phase of CMF induction. The Italian GOIRC group performed a similar study in patients with metastases (Cocconi et al., 1990). Both studies showed advantages for crossover late intensification therapy.

Further support for the Norton–Simon model came from the work of Buzzoni, Bonadonna and colleagues who tested alternating putatively non-cross-resistant chemotherapy (an approach based on the Goldie–Coldman hypothesis) (Goldie & Coldman, 1979) versus the sequential administration of the same regimens, in patients with node-positive breast cancer. Sequential chemotherapy was highly statistically significantly superior (Buzzoni et al., 1994).

Chemotherapy dose-response effect

This frustrating partial chemotherapy sensitivity has prompted a critical evaluation of dose escalation or intensification in the therapy of both early and late stage breast cancer. There is ample experimental evidence that a relationship exists between the concentration of a drug to which a cancer cell is exposed, and the likelihood that the cell will be killed. Skipper and Schabel (1998) and Teicher et al. (1988) demonstrated that there was a relationship between dose and cell kill. In these studies, the degree of dose escalation which was required to fully eradicate cancers was in general, substantial, typically of a log order of magnitude. It would obviously be very difficult to replicate this degree of escalation in routine clinical practice, due to toxicity. It is thus, scarcely surprising, that in the clinic (as will be discussed), minor degrees of dose escalation within the 'conventional' range (i.e. to levels which do not require haematopoietic autograft support), have had a modest and inconsistent effect on antitumour endpoints. The concept of dose intensity relates to dose per unit time. Some but not all retrospective studies have suggested that there is a relationship between dose intensity and survival in breast cancer (Hryniuk & Bush, 1984). The colony stimulating factors (CSFs) facilitate somewhat more substantial increases in dose and intensity, although for most drugs and combinations it does not approximate to the level which the preclinical models predicted to be sufficient (O'Dwyer et al., 1992). For the purposes of this section, we will define moderate dose escalation or intensification as increases in dose and/or dose intensity which do not require autograft support, and will include both agents and combinations which are given with, and those which are given without, CSFs.

Retrospective studies which have suggested the existence of a relationship between dose and anticancer effect, do not prove causality. Similarly, single-arm studies of moderately intensified therapy in both early and late stage breast cancer raised the possibility that this strategy might produce superior outcomes compared to standard dose therapy (Bronchud et al., 1989).

A number of prospective random assignment trials have now addressed the issue of moderate dose escalation or intensification in the clinical treatment of either metastatic or early stage breast cancer. These studies have produced inconsistent results, with generally higher response rates reported for higher-dose therapy in metastatic disease, but limited survival impact in either this setting or in patients with early stage disease (Bastholt et al., 1996; Hortobagyi et al, 1987; Ardizzoni et al., 1994; Henderson et al., 1998; Fisher et al., 1997; Levine et al., 1990; Bonneterre et al., 1998; Tannock et al., 1988). One conclusion which can be reached on the basis of these studies, however, is that arbitrary reductions below standard dose should be avoided.

Haematopoietic support of high-dose chemotherapy

It has long been known that it is possible to harvest bone marrow, and to cryopreserve it for subsequent reinfusion following intensive chemotherapy or radiotherapy (Lazarus et al., 1987). This technology allowed for a degree of clinical dose escalation which approximated those which were necessary for cure in experimental systems. In early studies, very-high-dose chemotherapy with bone marrow autograft support was reported to produce exceptionally high rates of complete remission in patients with relapsed metastatic breast cancer (Eder et al., 1986). However, treatment-related mortality was as high as 20% in some series.

The introduction of the haematopoietic CSFs had a powerful impact on the field of autograft-supported high-dose chemotherapy. The administration of these CSFs following marrow reinfusion resulted in a dramatic abbreviation of the period of neutropenia, and a consequent fall in mortality (Peters et al., 1993). It was also discovered that the administration of CSFs to patients, either at steady state or following myelosuppressive chemotherapy resulted in the mobilization of large numbers of haematopoietic progenitors into the peripheral blood (Socinski et al., 1988). These progenitors (PBP) could in turn be harvested by leukapheresis, and used as a substitute for autologous bone marrow (ABM). PBP were demonstrated to be superior to growth factors alone, or to marrow in prospective random assignment trials (Beyer et al., 1993; Kritz et al., 1993). The dramatic improvement in the toxicity profile of high-dose chemotherapy now allowed a more sytematic investigation of this modality in a number of clinical settings, including high-risk early stage disease, and in metastatic breast cancer. In studying the reported literature on single-arm studies, Eder et al. (1986) reported that high-dose chemotherapy with autograft support produced complete remission more than four times more frequently than did conventionally dosed therapy. There is fairly general agreement that high-dose therapy is indeed more active than low-dose therapy, i.e. it produces more frequent and more complete responses. The controversies surrounding this modality relate to claims that it improves survival, or indeed that it is curative. Investigators have attempted to harness this activity using one or other of a number of different high-dose strategies. Before studying the history of high-dose chemotherapy in this disease, we will first discuss these strategies.

High-dose chemotherapy strategies

Primary high-dose chemotherapy

In this strategy, high-dose chemotherapy is administered as one (or uncommonly, two or more), definitive cycles of 'stand alone' treatment to patients with cancer. This approach predominated in early studies. Toxicity in these early programmes was substantial. High rates of usually short-lived response were reported in several of these studies, especially in metastatic breast cancer. It was noted that patients who underwent this treatment for cancer which had been resistant to prior conventionally dosed therapy, had very poor outcomes (Eder et al., 1986). Primary high-dose chemotherapy has had rather little investigation, due primarily to the fact that late intensification rapidly became the dominant strategy for high-dose chemotherapy (Peters et al., 1988).

Late intensification

This model is an adaptation of the work of Norton and Simon. As has been outlined above, these researchers suggested that curative chemotherapy should consist of a phase of induction treatment, which would induce response, and thus 'shift' the tumour to the left along its Gompertzian growth curve. The smaller tumour would have a higher growth fraction and would hence be more sensitive to chemotherapy. It would, however, have a propensity for rapid regrowth according to the principles of Gompertzian mechanics. In order to ensure eradication of the 'left-shifted' tumour, it should then be treated with a 'clinically tolerable dose intensification'. As has been mentioned, the types of intensification which were available in the 1970s, when the Norton–Simon model was first formulated, were not in fact very intensive. Obviously, marrow or peripheral blood progenitor autografting allowed a much more substantial degree of dose escalation, and during the 1980s, late intensification became the most widespread application of high-dose chemotherapy.

In addition to the kinetic rationale, several other clinical arguments were advanced in support of using high-dose chemotherapy as a form of late intensification. It was proposed that the cytoreduction which was achieved by conventional chemotherapy might increase the ability of the subsequent high-dose cycle to eradicate the cancer, by presenting it with a smaller tumour burden. In addition, as early studies of high-dose chemotherapy in a variety of disease types had indicated that it seldom produced cures in patients with disease that was resistant to conventional chemotherapy, the early, conventionally dosed induction phase of the programme would allow the identification of those patients whose cancer was resistant. These women could then be spared the rigours of therapy which was toxic and expensive, and which would be ultimately futile. Thus, according to this interpretation, conventional chemotherapy acted as an in vivo chemosensitivity assay, which determined which patients would proceed to high-dose chemotherapy. Conventional chemotherapy might also improve the performance status of patients with advanced cancer prior to their being subjected to high-dose treatment.

The only precise validation for the use of high-dose chemotherapy as a form of late intensification would come from a random assignment trial in which primary high-dose chemotherapy was compared to the use of the same regimen as intensification following conventional therapy. None have as yet been carried out, but a historical comparison using identical high-dose chemotherapy regimens did not suggest a major benefit for the induction component of a late intensification regimen (Peters et al., 1988; Jones et al., 1990).

High-dose sequential

The innovative high-dose sequential approach devised by Gianni and colleagues in Milan enabled very high doses of drugs to be delivered in a fashion which does not predispose to overlapping toxicity, and which also attempts to deal with the clonal heterogeneity predicted by Goldie and Coldman. In this approach, patients are treated with a number of different drugs and regimens given at, or close to, maximum dose. High-dose sequential therapy has produced highly promising results in the treatment of aggressive lymphoma (Gianni et al., 1997) and high-risk stage II breast cancer (Gianni et al., 1992). It is the subject of a number of randomized trials in these diseases. High-dose sequential therapy has also been studied in metastatic breast cancer. A principal theoretical argument against the high-dose sequential approach is that single cycles of therapy have not been shown to be an efficient means of eradicating cells which are sensitive to those agents, i.e. in curing cancer in the clinic.

Multicycle high-dose chemotherapy

The multicycle high-dose chemotherapy model represents another attempt to improve on the promising but somewhat marginal clinical results which were reported in early trials of high-dose chemotherapy. It has its origins both in a critical analysis of the general development of clinical chemotherapy theory and practice, and in an alternative interpretation of the Norton–Simon model, which was proposed by Crown and Norton (Crown & Norton, 1995).

It will be apparent, that viewed in the context of the curative therapy programmes which have evolved for the treatment of lymphoma, Hodgkin's disease, early-stage breast cancer and testicular germ cell cancer, the induction/consolidation and high-dose sequential programmes look very odd. Curative chemotherapy has generally involved the identification of highly active regimens, and then the application of a sufficient number of cycles of those regimens to achieve tumour eradication. Thus, in the early MOPP (mustine, vincristine, procarbazine, prednisolone) programme of chemotherapy for Hodgkin's disease from the United States National Cancer Institute, patients achieved remission after, on average, three cycles of therapy. It is thus reasonable to assume that the cure rate in this series would have been low if only a single cycle of MOPP had been administered. Similarly, is it not possible that single applications of high-dose chemotherapy would not represent the optimal use for this technology in patients with breast cancer? Should we not instead try to administer multiple high-dose cycles?

Another observation that emerged in early chemotherapy studies in Hodgkin's disease was the finding that pretreatment with largely ineffective single-agent therapy compromised the ability of subsequent active combination regimens to effect cure. In short, it would appear that the application of relatively ineffective therapy might compromise the ability of subsequent potentially curative therapy to effect cure. This flawed strategy is exactly what the late intensification model of high-dose chemotherapy does.

It can thus be argued that primary single-cycle high-dose chemotherapy, late intensification high-dose chemotherapy and high-dose sequential therapy all represent substantial departures from classic chemotherapy theory and practice. Multicycle high-dose chemotherapy on the other hand, appears to be more consistent with successful precedents.

The original Norton–Simon interpretations of the kinetics of tumour growth and chemotherapy-induced regression were that tumour regression was directly related both to the dose of drug administered, and to the growth rate of the unperturbed tumour at the time of treatment. It was nowhere stated that the dose response relationship only existed for the late, intensified part of therapy. Rather, the greatest curative impact of intensified therapy might be at a time of minimal residual disease. As has been discussed, at the time of the formulation of these recommendations, it would not have been feasible to administer multiple cycles of highly intensive therapy.

Another consideration is that the Norton–Simon model emphasizes the potential for accelerated regrowth of surviving cells in between cycles of effective therapy. This acceleration would, according to the model, have its greatest impact in patients who harboured very small, subclinical populations of cells. Thus, according to this interpretation of tumour kinetics, the intercycle interval between such high-dose treatments might be of crucial importance. The essential difference between multicycle high-dose chemotherapy and high-dose sequential chemotherapy is that the latter attempts to overcome drug resistance by introducing a number of different drugs and regimens, whereas multicycle high-dose chemotherapy is designed to ensure that the therapeutic effects of 'effective' therapy are maximized by administering an optimum number of cycles.

Investigators in New York demonstrated the feasibility of accelerated, progenitor-supported, multicycle high-dose chemotherapy in breast and ovarian cancer (Crown et al., 1992). Conventional dose induction therapy might in theory allow the proliferation of those cells which are resistant to conventional doses, and sensitive only to high doses. Thus, the later application of high-dose chemotherapy might result in the high-dose therapy 'confronting' a higher burden of cancer than it would have done had it been applied at the outset.

Single-arm trials of high-dose chemotherapy with autograft support in breast cancer

Metastatic disease

Only a small number of trials explored primary high-dose therapy as initial treatment for metastatic disease. The group at Duke University treated newly diagnosed patients with metastatic disease with a single cycle of high-dose cyclophosphamide, BCNU and cisplatin. The rate of complete remission was 54%, and one quarter of these remissions were durable at 5 years. It was in an attempt to improve on these promising results that most investigators turned to the late intensification model, and the overwhelming majority of trials which were conducted over the next 10 years used this model.

Typically, patients in such studies were treated with four to six cycles of anthracycline-containing induction therapy, and those patients who had achieved either a partial or complete response were then 'consolidated' with single (or in a few cases) tandem cycles of high-dose therapy. Patients with highly resistant disease were thus spared the rigours of high-dose therapy, and the cytoreduction achieved with conventional therapy might contribute to ultimate cure by presenting the high-dose therapy with a smaller tumour burden to eradicate. Typically, approximately 50–70% of patients responded to induction therapy, and proceeded to 'transplant'. Some patients in partial response following induction were 'converted' to complete remission, and of course patients were consolidated while already in complete remission from induction. In most of these studies, approximately 50–70% of patients achieved complete remission overall following both phases of therapy. The great majority of these remissions ended in relapse, but a proportion, generally 10–15% of patients subjected to the induction-consolidation approach remained in complete response for 5 years. It must be stated that while there were no direct randomized comparisons of late intensification versus primary high-dose therapy, that it is not immediately obvious that the results of the former were superior.

The 'high-dose sequential' model has also had little study in metastatic breast cancer. Patrone and colleagues treated patients with stage IV disease with a regimen which was similar to that employed by Gianni et al. (1992). Again, a small proportion of patients achieved durable remissions (Patrone et al., 1995).

The approach of accelerated multicycle high-dose chemotherapy was studied by investigators at Memorial Sloan-Kettering Cancer Center in New York. Patients in a state of ongoing response following conventional chemotherapy were treated with a sequence of high-dose single alkylating agents. In the first trial, 42 patients received tandem cycles of cyclophosphamide followed by tandem cycles of autograft supported thiotepa. There were no treatment-related deaths, and overall, 20% of patients achieved prolonged remission (Vahdat et al., 1995). In a second trial, the therapy was further intensified, by substituting autograft supported high-dose melphalan for one of the cyclophosphamide cycles. The regimen was active but toxic, and three of 17 patients died from an unanticipated syndrome of fulminant interstitial pneumonitis. A fourth patient developed late leukaemia. Five patients however remain alive and in continued remission at up to 5 years from treatment (Crown et al., 1994).

While historical comparisons seem to suggest a substantial survival advantage compared to conventional chemotherapy (Antman et al., 1992), the possibility that case selection bias might be an important contributory factor to the apparent success of high-dose chemotherapy in this setting mandated prospective random assignment trials (Rahman et al., 1997).

Adjuvant treatment of high-risk early stage disease

Peters and colleagues treated patients with breast cancer involving at least 10 axillary lymph nodes with an aggressive doxorubicin-based regimen followed by a single cycle of high-dose late intensification chemotherapy supported by an autograft of bone marrow or peripheral blood. These authors reported that 70% of patients remained free of relapse at 5 years. Interestingly, many of the relapses which did occur in this study were locoregional recurrences before the routine introduction of radiotherapy consolidation (Peters et al., 1993). Gianni and colleagues studied 'high-dose sequential chemotherapy' (see below) in patients with stage II breast cancer involving 10 or more axillary lymph nodes. In their study, 65% of patients remained free of relapse (Gianni et al., 1992).

Randomized trials of high-dose chemotherapy with autograft support in breast cancer

Metastatic disease

Four randomized trials comparing high-dose chemotherapy to conventional dose chemotherapy have been carried out in patients with overtly metastatic breast cancer (Table 12a.1). Three utilized the late intensification approach and were all either negative or ambiguous (Stadtmauer et al., 2000). Peters and colleagues (1996) treated patients with metastatic disease using four cycles of an aggressive doxorubicin-based regimen. Patients who achieved complete remission were randomized to receive high-dose chemotherapy as intensification, or to observation. Patients who were randomized to observation were treated with the same high-dose regimen at the time of relapse. Those patients who achieved partial response or stable disease following induction proceeded automatically to high-dose chemotherapy. Interestingly, 15% of this latter group were converted to long-term remission. Of the randomized patients, those who received the consolidative 'transplant' had significantly prolonged disease-free survival compared to those who were observed. Paradoxically, those who received the salvage high-dose regimen had superior survival which was significant at the initial analysis but is no longer so at further follow-up. Interestingly, somewhat similar results have recently been reported by the same investigators in patients with bone only metastases (Madan et al., 2000). In this study, patients whose cancer did not

Table 12a.1. Metastatic randomized controlled trials including high-dose consolidation

	Number randomized	Median FU (years)	3 yr DFS % HD/Control	p value	3 yr OS % HD/Control	p value
Stadtmauer et al., 2000	199	3.1	6/12	NS	32/38	NS
Peters et al., 1996	98	6.3	25/10	<0.01	33/38	NS
Lotz et al., 1999 (Pegase)	61	4.4	49/21	0.05	55/28	NS

Bezwoda trial discontinued.

Adapted from Antman, 2001.

FU – follow-up; DFS – disease-free survival; HD – high dose; OS – overall survival; NS – not significant.

progress following induction chemotherapy were randomized to consolidative or salvage high-dose chemotherapy. Again, late intensification resulted in a significant improvement in disease-free survival.

The French PEGASE cooperative group randomized patients who were in an ongoing state of response to induction therapy to receive either further conventional therapy or a single high-dose cycle of mitoxantrone, cyclophosphamide and melphalan. There were more patients with pulmonary metastases in the high-dose arm (15/32 versus 4/29 conventional) and two of the high-dose patients had had central nervous system metastases. Patients who received the high-dose chemotherapy had a statistically significantly prolonged duration of response (35.3 versus 20 months) in favour of high dose, but only a trend at the time of reporting for survival at 43 versus 20 months, 5-year survivals being 30 versus 18 months. At 5 years of follow-up, however, the difference in relapse-free survival had disappeared (Peters et al., 1996).

In a similar but larger study, Stadtmauer and colleagues (2000) randomized patients who were in an ongoing state of response to conventional therapy after four to six cycles of CAF or CMF to receive either further conventional therapy for up to 24 cycles or a single high-dose cycle of cyclophosphamide, thiotepa and carboplatin. Although 553 patients entered the trial, only 199 were actually randomized after initial partial or complete response. Only 164, however, received their assigned treatment. Some patients who were assigned to conventional chemotherapy received high-dose chemotherapy as salvage treatment after relapse. No advantage for high-dose was demonstrated in either disease-free or overall survival. It should be noted that only 7% of patients who were in partial

Table 12a.2. Adjuvant randomized controlled trials including high-dose consolidation

	Number randomized	Median FU (years)	3 yr DFS % HD/Control	p value	3 yr OS % HD/Control	p value
Rodenhuis et al., 1998 1	81	4.1	70/65	NS	82/75	NS
Rodenhuis et al., 2000 2	885	3.5	72/65	0.057	84/80	NS
Subset from above	*284*	*7.0*	*77/62*	*0.009*	*89/79*	*0.039*
Peters et al., 1999	783	3.6	71/64	NS	79/79	NS
Hortobagyi et al., 1998	78	6.5	48/62	NS	58/77	NS
Bergh, 2000	525	2.0	68/62	NS	79/76	NS

Bezwoda trial discounted; NS not significant.
Adapted from Antman, 2001.

remission after induction chemotherapy, were 'converted' to complete remission by high-dose consolidation therapy, suggesting that the particular high-dose regimen used may have been less than optimal.

The sole study of primary multicycle HDC was conducted by Bezwoda and colleagues. In this trial patients were randomly assigned to receive either tandem cycles of autograft-supported high-dose mitoxantrone, cyclophosphamide and etoposide, or standard doses of mitoxantrone, cyclophosphamide and vincristine. This study showed striking advantages for the high-dose arm, both in terms of disease-free and overall survival (Bezwoda et al., 1995). The trial has been criticized on several accounts. First, it was relatively small, including only 90 patients. Secondly, the control group is alleged to have had an unusually poor outcome. Thirdly, there was a disproportionate use of tamoxifen post-chemotherapy, which favoured the high-dose arm. The results of the Bezwoda study are currently the subject of an audit, following the discovery of substantial research irregularities in the conduct of another high-dose randomized trial by the same investigator.

Adjuvant treatment of high-risk early stage disease

Currently, the results of five randomized trials in which the role of high-dose chemotherapy in the treatment of high-risk early stage breast cancer were studied have been reported. In four of these studies, the strategy of late intensification was studied (Rodenhuis et al., 1998; Bergh et al., 2000; Peters et al., 1999; Hortobagyi et al., 1998) (Table 12a.2).

In the Scandinavian study of Bergh et al. (2000) patients with high-risk disease were randomly assigned to receive either FEC chemotherapy followed by a single high-dose cycle, or in the comparator arm, six further cycles with individually tailored doses to maximum tolerance of FEC chemotherapy. Patients on the tailored dose arm in fact received substantially higher cumulative doses of anthracycline, cyclophosphamide and 5-fluorouracil than patients on the high-dose arm. This study shows 60% survival in both arms at median follow-up of 2 years. The intensive anthracycline dosing in the comparator arm was associated with 8% incidence of topoisomerase-associated acute leukaemia or myelodysplasia against none in the high-dose arm. The negative trial was in fact a comparison between two intensive dose strategies, and as such contributes little to the debate concerning the merits of high-dose therapy.

The CALGB (Peters et al., 1999) attempted to validate the earlier cited Peters adjuvant single-arm study in a large randomized trial. Patients received aggressive doxorubicin-based induction, followed by either high-dose cisplatin, BCNU, cyclophosphamide with an autograft, or, lower, but still aggressive doses of the same triplet with filgrastim support. At 3.6 years median follow-up there are significantly fewer relapses for the high-dose treatment. Patients on the high-dose arm of this study, however, had an unusually high (7.4%) rate of treatment-related mortality due to the variable outcome from pulmonary and hepatic toxicity at different participating centres. Two other very small studies in which late-intensification high-dose chemotherapy was compared to conventionally dosed therapy were also negative. The MD Anderson trial randomized 78 patients to eight cycles of cyclophosphamide, adriamycin and 5-fluorouracil and half of the patients received consolidation cyclophosphamide, etoposide and cisplatin. Six patients did not actually receive the high-dose therapy allocated and three who were allocated no consolidation received high-dose chemotherapy. The small size of the trial was not powered to detect smaller than a 30% difference between the two arms. In the first of two studies reported by Rodenhuis et al. (1998), 81 patients with a positive apical lymph node were randomly assigned to receive FEC chemotherapy with or without a single cycle of high-dose consolidation. This pilot trial, powered to detect only a 30% or greater difference showed no differences at 4.1 years follow-up.

In the subsequent Dutch national study, 885 patients were enrolled. Patients received four cycles of cyclophosphamide, epirubicin and 5-fluorouracil and were then randomly allocated to either one further cycle of FEC or high-dose cyclophosphamide, carboplatin and thiotepa (CTCb). At 3 years median follow-up the disease-free survival trend in favour of high-dose therapy just fails to reach statistical significance at $p = 0.057$. In a protocol planned assessment of the first 284 patients (with 7 years median follow-up) both disease-free survival and overall survival showed a significant benefit for the high-dose chemotherapy. One of 443 patients in the control arm and 4 of the 442 in the high-dose arm died of treatment-associated toxicity.

The results of a fifth study by Bezwoda and colleagues are now considered unsafe, as an independent audit has revealed major flaws in the conduct of the trial.

Critical analysis of the literature of randomized trials of high-dose chemotherapy in breast cancer

The sceptic may be inclined to the view that the highly promising results of the initial historically controlled studies of high-dose chemotherapy have not been confirmed in random assignment trials, and were thus, likely artifacts of case selection. This position may be correct. It must be admitted that the evidence to date does not support the use of single-cycle late intensification high-dose chemotherapy as an evidence-based standard treatment for patients with metastatic or multinode positive breast cancer.

However, all of the 'negative' studies that have been conducted to date, can be criticized on the grounds of their design or execution. The principal objection to many of these studies relates to their size. For instance, none of the metastatic trials has included more than 200 patients. Excluding Bezwoda's trial, only 427 patients have been randomized in aggregate. It is impossible, in the light of available evidence therefore to draw any firm conclusions about high-dose chemotherapy for metastatic disease. The apparently compelling trends in favour of high-dose therapy in the PEGASE trial make it particularly regrettable that it did not achieve higher accrual. The Stadtmauer study, though relatively small, would appear to represent a reasonably fair (and wholly negative) trial of late intensification therapy in metastatic breast cancer. The fact that patients on the control arm had very prolonged maintenance chemotherapy (up to 2 years) may affect its significance.

Two of the adjuvant studies recruited fewer than 90 patients each, and as such would have to be considered grossly underpowered. Other aspects of the design of some of these studies limits their contribution to the debate regarding the benefits if any, of high-dose therapy. The Peters metastatic trial, was in fact a comparison between early and late high-dose therapy, albeit at different phases of the natural history of the disease. In addition, as has been mentioned above, patients on the low-dose arm of the Scandinavian adjuvant trial received higher doses of three of the four study drugs than did patients on the high-dose arm.

The situation with regard to adjuvant high-dose therapy is particularly ambiguous given the apparently positive preliminary data from the still maturing Dutch National study.

Table 12a.3. Current unpublished trials

Group	Setting	Target number	Status
Belgian (Piccart)	Metastatic	400	Open
German (Kanz)	Metastatic	350	Open
NCIC (Crump)	Metastatic	300	Open
IBDIS (Crown)	Metastatic	264	Open
GITMO (Rosti)	Metastatic	240	Open
PEGASE3 (Biron)	Metastatic	180	Closed
ECOG (Tallman)	Adjuvant >9 nodes	550	Closed
IBCSG (Basser)	Adjuvant >9 nodes	340	Closed
German (Zander)	Adjuvant >9 nodes	NA	Open
German (Seeber)	Adjuvant >9 nodes	NA	Open
PEGASE 1 (Roche)	Adjuvant >7 nodes	314	Closed
BCIRG (Russell)	Adjuvant >4 nodes	460	Open
Intergroup (Bearman)	Adjuvant >4 nodes	1000	Open
ACCOG (Authors)	Adjuvant >3 nodes	604	Closed
Milan (Gianni)	Adjuvant >3 nodes	350	Closed

Adapted from Antman, 2001.

Research priorities and future directions

When one considered the still dismal prognosis of metastatic and early stage high-risk breast cancer, together with the (as yet, wholly unproven but, *not disproven)* reports which suggested that high-dose therapy may result in improved rates of durable remission, then the current situation with regard to high-dose therapy can be regarded as nothing less than a potential tragedy for breast cancer sufferers.

It seems entirely possible that a potentially beneficial treatment may be discarded on the basis of incomplete data. The results of current, ongoing randomized trials will be key determinants of the direction of future investigative efforts in the field of dose intensive chemotherapy. In the event that these studies demonstrate meaningful clinical benefits for the high-dose approach, two broad strategies will need to be addressed in successor trials.

(1) Attempts will have to be made attempting to improve on this treatment. The impact of new high-dose regimens versus existing programmes, engineered versus unmanipulated autograft products (Brugger et al., 1995; Shpall et al., 1994), adjuvant immunotherapy (Kennedy et al., 1993), gene therapy (Hesdorffer et al., 1998) multiple versus single high-dose cycles, and of late

intensification versus high-dose sequential and primary high-dose chemotherapy strategies could all be studied. Antiangiogenesis factors might usefully
be employed to maintain high-dose chemotherapy-induced remissions
(O'Reilly et al., 1996). Allogeneic transplantation is also under investigation
(Ueno et al., 1998).

(2) There have also been substantial advances in conventionally dosed therapy in
recent years. Thus, some current control groups may be considered suboptimal by the time that current random assignment trials might produce positive
results (Chan et al., 1999).

Even if the current studies are negative (Table 12a.3) the possibility would still
have to be entertained that the high-dose arms of current studies could be
improved on. In the case of breast cancer, will these trials confirm an emerging
suspicion that late intensification, the dominant strategy in the current studies, is
not the optimal use of this technology after all?

REFERENCES

Antman, K.H. (2001). A critique of the eleven randomised trials of high dose chemotherapy for
breast cancer. *European Journal of Cancer*, 37, 173–9.

Antman, K., Ayash, L., Elias, A. et al. (1992). A phase II study of high-dose cyclophosphamide,
thiotepa, and carboplatin with autologous marrow support in women with measurable
advanced breast cancer responding to standard-dose therapy. *Journal of Clinical Oncology*, 10,
102–10.

Ardizzoni, A., Venturini, M., Sertoli, M.R. et al. (1994). Granulocyte-macrophage colony-
stimulating factor (GM-CSF) allows acceleration and dose-intensity increase of CEF chemotherapy: a randomized study in patients with advanced breast cancer. *British Journal of
Cancer*, 69, 385–91.

Bastholt, L., Dalmark, M. & Gjedde, S. (1996). Dose-response relationship of epirubicin in the
treatment of postmenopausal patients with metastatic breast cancer: a randomized study of
epirubicin at four different dose levels performed by the Danish Breast Cancer Cooperative
Group. *Journal of Clinical Oncology*, 14, 1146–55.

Bergh, J., Wiklund, T., Erikstein, B. et al. (2000). Tailored fluorouracil, epirubicin, and
cyclophosphamide compared with marrow-supported high-dose chemotherapy as adjuvant
treatment for high-risk breast cancer: a randomised trial. Scandinavian Breast Group 9401
study. *Lancet*, 356(9239), 1384–91.

Beyer, J., Schwella, N., Zingsem, J. et al. (1993). Bone marrow versus peripheral blood stem cells
as rescue after high-dose chemotherapy. *Blood*, 82 (Suppl. 1), 454a.

Bezwoda, W.R. (1999). Randomised, controlled trial of high dose chemotherapy (HD-CNVp)
vs. standard dose (CAF) chemotherapy for high risk, surgically treated, primary breast cancer.
Proceedings of the American Society of Clinical Oncology, 18, 2a.

Bezwoda, W.R., Seymour, L. & Dansey, R.D. (1995). High-dose chemotherapy with hematopoietic rescue as primary treatment for metastatic breast cancer: a randomised trial. *Journal of Clinical Oncology*, 13, 2483–9.

Bonneterre, J., Roché, H. & Bremond, A. (1998). Results of a randomised trial of adjuvant chemotherapy with FEC 50 vs FEC 100 in high-risk node positive breast cancer patients. *Proceedings of the American Society of Clinical Oncology*, 17, 124a.

Bronchud, M.H., Howell, A., Crowther, D. et al. (1989). The use of granulocyte colony-stimulating factor to increase the intensity of treatment with doxorubicin in patients with advanced breast and ovarian cancer. *British Journal of Cancer*, 60, 121–5.

Brugger, W., Heimfeld, S., Berenson, R.J. et al. (1995). Reconstitution of hematopoiesis after high-dose chemotherapy by autologous progenitor cells generated ex vivo. *New England Journal of Medicine*, 333, 283–7.

Buzzoni, R., Bonnadonna, G., Vallagussa, P. et al. (1994). Adjuvant chemotherapy with doxorubicin plus cyclophosphamide, methotrexate, and flurouracil in the treatment of resectable breast cancer with more than 3 positive axillary nodes. *Journal of Clinical Oncology*, 9, 2134–40.

Chan, S., Friedrichs, K., Noel, D. et al. (1999). Prospective randomized trial of docetaxel versus doxorubicin in patients with metastatic breast cancer. *Journal of Clinical Oncology*, 17(8), 2341–54.

Cocconi, G., Bisagni, G., Bacchi, M. et al. (1990). A comparison of continuation versus late intensification followed by discontinuation of chemotherapy in advanced breast cancer: a prospective randomized trial of the Italian Oncology Group for Clinical Research. (G.O.I.R.C.). *Annals of Oncology*, 1(1), 36–44.

Cold, S., Jensen, N.V., Brincker, H. et al. (1993). The influence of chemotherapy on survival after recurrence in breast cancer – a population-based study of patients treated in the 1950s, 1960s and the 1970s. *European Journal of Cancer*, 29A, 1146–52.

Crown, J. & Norton, L. (1995). Potential strategies for improving the results of high-dose chemotherapy in patients with metastatic breast cancer. *Annals of Oncology*, 6 (Suppl. 4), s21–s26.

Crown, J., Raptis, G., Vahdat, L. et al. (1994). Rapid administration of sequential high-dose cyclophosphamide, melphalan, thiotepa supported by filgrastim and peripheral blood progenitors in patients with metastatic breast cancer: a novel and very active treatment strategy. *Proceedings of the American Society of Clinical Oncology*, 13, 110, Abstract.

Crown, J., Wasserheit, C. & Hakes, T. et al. (1992). Rapid delivery of multiple high-dose chemotherapy courses with G-CSF and peripheral blood-derived haemopoietic progenitor cells. *Journal of the National Cancer Institute*, 84, 1935–6.

Early Breast Cancer Trialist's Collaborative Group (1992). Systemic treatment of early breast cancer by hormonal, cytotoxic or immune therapy: 133 randomized trials involving 31,000 recurrences and 24,000 deaths among 75,000 women. *Lancet*, 339, 1–15.

Eder, J.P., Antman, K., Peters, W.P. et al. (1986). High-dose combination alkylating agent chemotherapy with autologous marrow support for metastatic breast cancer. *Journal of Clinical Oncology*, 4, 1592–7.

Fisher, B., Anderson, S., Wickerham, D.L. et al. (1997). Increased intensification and total dose of cyclophosphamide in a doxorubicin-cyclophosphamide regimen for the treatment of primary breast cancer: findings from National Surgical Adjuvant Breast and Bowel Project B-22. *Journal of Clinical Oncology*, 15, 1858–69.

Gianni, A.M., Bregni, M., Siena, S. et al. (1997). High-dose chemotherapy and autologous bone marrow transplantation compared with MACOP-B in aggressive B-cell lymphoma. *New England Journal of Medicine*, 336(18), 1290–7.

Gianni, A.M., Siena, S., Bregni, M. et al. (1992). Growth factor supported high-dose sequential adjuvant chemotherapy in breast cancer with > 10 positive nodes. *Proceedings of the American Society of Clinical Oncology*, 11, 60.

Goldie, J. & Coldman, A.J. (1979). A mathematical model for relating the drug sensitivity of tumors to their spontaneous mutation rate. *Cancer Treatment Reports*, 63, 1727–73.

Greenberg, P.A.C., Hortobagyi, G.N., Smith, T.L. et al. (1996). Long-term follow-up of patients with complete remission following combination chemotherapy for metastatic breast cancer. *Journal of Clinical Oncology*, 14, 2197–205.

Henderson, I.C., Berry, D., Demetri, G. et al. (1998). Improved disease-free survival and overall survival from the addition of sequential Paclitaxel but not from the escalation of doxorubicin dose in the adjuvant chemotherapy of patients with node-positive primary breast cancer. *Proceedings of the American Society of Clinical Oncology*, 17, 101a.

Hesdorffer, C., Ayello, J., Ward, M. et al. (1998). Phase I Trial of retroviral-mediated transfer of the human MDR1 gene as marrow chemoprotection in patients undergoing high-dose chemotherapy and autologous stem-cell transplantation. *Journal of Clinical Oncology*, 16, 165–72.

Hortobagyi, G.N., Buzdar, A.U., Bodey, G.P. et al. (1987). High-dose induction chemotherapy of metastatic breast cancer in protected environment units: a prospective randomized study. *Journal of Clinical Oncology*, 5, 178–84.

Hortobagyi, G.N., Buzdar, A.U. & Champlin, R. (1998). Lack of efficacy of adjuvant high-dose tandem combination chemotherapy for high-risk primary breast cancer a randomised trial. *Proceedings of the American Society of Clinical Oncology*, 17, 123a.

Hryniuk, W. & Bush, H. (1984). The importance of dose intensity in chemotherapy of metastatic breast cancer. *Journal of Clinical Oncology*, 2, 81–8.

Jones, R.B., Shpall, E.J., Ross, M. et al. (1990). AFM induction chemotherapy followed by intensive alkylating agent consolidation with autologous bone marrow support for advanced breast cancer: current results. *Proceedings of the American Society of Clinical Oncology*, 9(9).

Kennedy, M.J., Vogelzang, G., Beveridge, R. et al. (1993). Phase I trial of intravenous cyclosporine to induce graft versus host disease in women undergoing autologous bone marrow transplantation for breast cancer. *Journal of Clinical Oncology*, 11, 478–84.

Kritz, A., Crown, J. & Motzer, R. (1993). Beneficial impact of peripheral blood progenitor cells in patients with metastatic breast cancer treated with high-dose chemotherapy plus GM-CSF: a randomized trial. *Cancer*, 71, 2515–21.

Lazarus, H., Reed, M.D., Spitzer, T.R. et al. (1987). High-dose iv thiotepa and cryopreserved autologous bone marrow transplantation for therapy of refractory cancer. *Cancer Treatment Reports*, 71, 689–95.

Levine, M.N., Gent, M., Hryniuk, W.M. et al. (1990). A randomized trial comparing 12 weeks versus 36 weeks ofadjuvant chemotherapy in stage II breast cancer. *Journal of Clinical Oncology*, 8(7), 1217–25.

Lotz, J.-P., Cure, H., Janvier, M. et al. and the PEGASE Group (1999). High-dose chemotherapy (HD-CT) with hematopoietic stem cells transplantation (HSCT) for metastatic breast cancer: results of the French Protocol Pegase 04. *Proceedings of the American Society of Clinical Oncology*, 18, 43a.

Madan, B., Broadwater, G., Rubin, P. et al. (2000). Improved survival with consolidation high dose cyclophosphamide, cisplatin and carmustine (Hd-Cpb) compared with observation in women with metastatic breast cancer (Mbc) and only bone metastases treated with induction adriamycin, 5-fluorouracil and methotrexate. *Proceedings of the American Society of Clinical Oncology*, 19, 48a, Abstract 184.

Norton, L. & Simon, R. (1986). The Norton–Simon hypothesis revisited. *Cancer Treatment Reports*, 70, 163–9.

Norton, L., Simon, R., Brereton, H.D. et al. (1976). Predicting the course of Gompertzian growth. *Nature* (London), 264, 542–5.

O'Dwyer, P.J., LaCreta, F.P., Schilder, R. et al. (1992). Phase I trial of thiotepa in combination with recombinant human granulocyte-macrophage colony-stimulating factor. *Journal of Clinical Oncology*, 10, 1352–8.

O'Reilly, M.S., Holmgren, L., Chen, C. et al. (1996). Angiostatin induces and sustains dormancy of human primary tumors in mice. *Nature Medicine*, 2(6), 689–92.

Patrone, F., Ballestrero, A., Ferrando, F. et al. (1995). Four-step high-dose sequential chemotherapy with double hematopoietic progenitor-cell rescue for metastatic breast cancer. *Journal of Clinical Oncology*, 13, 840–6.

Perloff, M., Norton, L., Korzun, A.H. et al. (1996). Post surgical adjuvant chemotherapy of stage II breast carcinoma with or without crossover to a non-cross-resistant regimen: a Cancer and Leukemia Group B Study. *Journal of Clinical Oncology*, 14, 1589–98.

Peters, W.P., Jones, R.B., Vredenburgh, J. et al. (1996). A large, prospective, randomized trial of high-dose combination alkylating agents (CBP) with autologous cellular support as consolidation for patients with metastatic breast cancer achieving complete remission after intensive doxorubicin-based induction therapy (AFM). *Proceedings of the American Society of Clinical Oncology*, 15, 121.

Peters, W.P., Rosner, G., Ross, M. et al. (1993a). Comparative effects of granulocyte-macrophage colony-stimulating factor (GM-CSF) and granulocyte colony-stimulating factor (G-CSF) on priming peripheral blood progenitor cells for use with autologous bone marrow after high-dose chemotherapy. *Blood*, 81, 1709–19.

Peters, W., Rosner, G., Vredenburgh, J. et al. for CALGB, SWOG and NCIC (1999). A prospective, randomized comparison of two doses of combination alkylating agents as consolidation after CAF in high-risk primary breast cancer involving ten or more axillary lymph nodes: preliminary results of CALGB 9082/SWOG 9114/NCIC MA-13. *Proceedings of the American Society of Clinical Oncology*, 18, 1a.

Peters, W.P., Ross, M., Vredenburgh, J.J. et al. (1993b). High-dose chemotherapy and autologous bone marrow support as consolidation after standard-dose adjuvant therapy for high risk primary breast cancer. *Journal of Clinical Oncology*, 11, 1132–44.

Peters, W.P., Shpall, E.J., Jones, R.B. et al. (1988) High-dose combination alkylating agents with bone marrow support as initial treatment for metastatic breast cancer. *Journal of Clinical Oncology*, 6, 1368–76.

Rahman, Z.U., Frye, D.K. & Buzdar, A.U. (1997). Impact of selection process on response rate and long-term survival of potential high-dose chemotherapy candidates treated with standard-dose doxorubicin-containing chemotherapy in patients with metastatic breast cancer. *Journal of Clinical Oncology*, 15, 3171–7.

Rodenhuis, S., Richel, D.J., van der Wall, E. et al. (1998). Randomised trial of high-dose chemotherapy and haemopoietic progenitor-cell support in operable breast cancer with extensive axillary lymph-node involvement. *Lancet*, 352, 515–21.

Rodenhuis, S., Bontenbal, M., van der Wall, E. et al. (2000). Randomized phase III study of high-dose chemotherapy with cyclophosphamide, thiotepa and carboplatin in operable breast cancer with 4 or more axillary lymph nodes. *Proceedings of the American Society of Clinical Oncology*, 19, 74, Abstract 286.

The Scandinavian Breast Cancer Study Group 9401 (1999). Results from a randomized adjuvant breast cancer study with high-dose chemotherapy with CTC$_b$ supported by autologous bone marrow stem cells versus dose escalated and tailored FEC therapy. *Proceedings of the American Society of Clinical Oncology*, 2a.

Shpall, E.J., Jones, R.B., Bearman, S.I. et al. (1994). Transplantation of enriched CD34-positive autologous marrow into breast cancer patients following high-dose chemotherapy: influence of CD34-positive peripheral-blood progenitors and growth factors on engraftment. *Journal of Clinical Oncology*, 12, 28–36.

Skipper, H.E. & Schabel, F.M. (1988). Quantitative and cytokinetic studies in experimental tumor systems. In: J. Holland and F.E. Frei (eds.), *Cancer Medicine*. Philadelphia: Lea and Febiger, pp. 663–84.

Socinski, M.A., Elias, A., Schnipper, L. et al. (1988). Granulocyte-macrophage colony-stimulating factor expands the circulating haemopoietic progenitor cell compartment in man. *Lancet*, i, 1194–8.

Stadtmauer, E.A., O'Neill, A., Goldstein, L.J. et al. (2000). Conventional-dose chemotherapy compared with high-dose chemotherapy plus autologous hematopoietic stem-cell transplantation for metastatic breast cancer. *The New England Journal of Medicine*, 342(15), 1069–76.

Tannock, I.F., Boyd, N.F., Deborer, G. et al. (1988). A randomized trial of two dose levels of CMF chemotherapy for patients with metastatic breast cancer. *Journal of Clinical Oncology*, 6, 1377–87.

Teicher, B.A., Holden, S.A., Cucchi, C.A. et al. (1988). Combination thiotepa and cyclophosphamide in vivo and in vitro. *Cancer Research*, 48, 94–100.

Ueno, N., Rondón, G. & Mirza, N.Q. (1998). Allogeneic peripheral-blood progenitor-cell transplantation for poor-risk patients with metastatic breast cancer. *Journal of Clinical Oncology*, 16, 986–93.

Vahdat, L., Raptis, G., Fennelly, D. et al. (1995). Rapidly cycled courses of high-dose alkylating agents supported by filgrastim and peripheral blood progenitor cells in patients with metastatic breast cancer. *Clinical Cancer Research*, 1, 1267–73.

New immunological approaches to treatment for breast cancer

A.G. Dalgleish

Department of Oncology, St George's Hospital Medical School, Cranmer Terrace, London

Introduction

In spite of numerous advances that have been made in the screening and management of patients with breast cancer, an unacceptable number of patients die of this disease even though they may have had optimal therapy and management. It is therefore necessary to assess the possible impact of different treatment modalities currently used more in other tumour types and consider this application to the treatment of breast cancer. These include immunotherapy (active: vaccines, and passive: antibodies), gene therapy, antisense technology and antiangiogenic agents.

Cancer and the immune system

Macfarlane Burnet (1970) postulated that the immune system kept potential cancer cells under surveillance and could detect and kill thousands of emerging cancer cells every day. This concept had gradually fallen out of favour as regards the common solid tumours as they do not appear to be increased in conditions where the immune system is compromised, such as autoimmune deficiency syndrome (AIDS) and renal transplant patients. However, both of these conditions have an increased incidence of viral driven cancers such as Epstein–Barr Virus (EBV) associated lymphomas and HHV-8-associated Kaposi's sarcoma. In these conditions there is a foreign viral antigen(s) which can be detected and contained by a healthy immune system and the failure to do so leads to viral-driven proliferation and oncogenesis. The absence of increased breast, lung and bowel cancer in HIV infection however, does not mean that the immune system has no role in containment of tumour progression.

Table 12b.1. Cancer and chronic inflammation

Site	Infection	Chronic inflammation	Cancer
Lung	Chronic bronchitis	Inflammation of bronchial tunica in asymptomatic cases	Bronchi Lung
Oesophagus		Reflux oesophagitis	Lower oesophagus
Stomach	? *Helicobacter pylorii*	Gastritis	Stomach
Colon		Colitis	Colon
Liver	Hepatitis B Hepatitis C	Chronic hepatitis Cirrhosis	Liver
Cervix	Chronic inflammation ? cause	+HPV	Cervix
Prostate	Prostatitis ? cause	(often histologically)	Prostate
Breast	Mastitis ? cause	(often histologically)	Breast

O'Byrne et al., 2000.

Solid tumour oncogenesis

It is well established that cancer cells do not suddenly appear but evolve slowly, acquiring a number of 'oncogenic' events until the cell is autonomous and no longer under normal cell cycle control. These events include mutated normal oncogenes such as ras mutations, mutated suppressor genes, for example p53, as well as loss of heterozygosity with chromosome deletions, presumably containing further suppressor genes. Since these genes are often mutated in the early stages of oncogenesis they will be non-self and appear foreign and rejected by the immune system exactly as proposed by Macfarlane Burnet (1970). It is likely that cancer can only be initiated in an environment where cell-mediated immunity is suppressed for long periods of time, thus allowing a ras or p53 mutations to confer survival advantage to a cell in order to develop a second 'hit' without being killed by a killer T cell (for reviews see Dalgleish & Browning, 1996; Maraveyas et al., 1999; O'Byrne et al., 2000).

It has been noted that cancers often arise in areas of chronic inflammation (O'Byrne et al., 2000) which may or may not be due to chronic infection (see Table 12b.1). Areas of chronic inflammation are associated with cell-mediated suppression and increased angiogenesis (both features associated with wound healing). It is therefore likely that oncogene changes occur in this immunologically altered environment and that these changes may take decades to initiate and progress. This could explain the lack of solid tumours seen in AIDS and transplant patients, i.e. because of their poor prognosis. Another possible additional explanation is that the immune system in AIDS patients is pan activated (which paradoxically invokes antigen-specific T cell deletion) and similar to chronic graft-versus-host (GVH) disease which can include graft-versus leukaemia/tumour activity. We have previously suggested that HIV induces AIDS because of its HLA-like sequences inducing alloactivation (Westby et al., 1996).

The association between inflammation or chronic infection with prostate and breast cancer is less absolute than with the other cancers listed. Both cancers, however, have the compounding sensitivity to their endocrinological environment which may have complex interplay with immune surveillance, for example steroids, which are well-known suppressers of inflammation and cell-mediated surveillance. However, different steroid environments have markedly different effects in the immune response.

Potential for therapy

If solid tumours do arise in immunologically compromised sites then they should be susceptible to immunological therapies. Tumours such as melanoma, renal cancer and sarcoma are known to be relatively resistant to chemotherapy and radiotherapy and have been treated with a number of immunotherapeutic approaches for several decades. Most approaches are greeted with much initial enthusiasm followed by objective gloom in a pattern which has repeated itself every 10–15 years using nonspecific stimulants, for example bacillus Calmette–Guérin (BCG), autologous and allogeneic cells, interferons, interleukin-2 (1L-2) and other cytokines, and monoclonal antibodies. The *raison d'être* of this approach was the observation by William Coley, a New York surgeon at the turn of the last century (1890s), who noted occasional spontaneous remissions in patients who survived severe postoperative infections, such as erysipelas. He spent several years identifying the active components of known bacteria involved in these infections, and was able to put together a preparation of these bacterial products which became known as 'Coley's toxins'. Over the next two decades, Coley was subjected to considerable cynicism when many were unable to repeat his clinical responses. However, he noted that minor details in preparation dose and administration were paramount in determining success. Unfortunately, the advent of radiotherapy and latterly chemotherapy meant a general loss of interest in his approach as the new treatments were seen as more understandable and practical.

Over the years, immunotherapy in the shape of BCG, autologous and allogeneic cells (with or without BCG), interferons, interleukins and more recently antibodies have been tried mainly on leukaemia, lymphoma, renal cell, bladder cancer and malignant melanoma. In spite of the fact that intravesical BCG is remarkably

Table 12b.2. Tumour antigens (examples not exhaustive)

Viral antigens	Antigen	Tumour
HPV	E6.E7	Cervix, anal
EBV	EBNA.1	Hodgkind/Burkitt's lymphomas
HBV	HB Ags	Hepatoma
HHV-8	?	Kaposi's sarcoma
Self-antigens (nonmutated)		
Oncofetal/differentation/cancer-testes		
	CEA	Gastrointestinal tract
		Lung
		Breast
	MUC-1	Breast
	MAGE	Breast, Melanoma
	BAGE	Breast, Melanoma
	GAGE	Melanoma/Sarcoma
	MART-1/Melan	Melanoma
	Tyrosinase	Melanoma
Mutated, self-antigens		
Oncogenes and suppressor genes e.g. Ras, p53, p210, E50-1, Catenin, TRP-1 tk	Wide variety of tumours (if not all)	

HPV human papilloma virus; EBV Epstein–Barr virus; HBV hepatitis B virus; HHV human herpes virus type 8; MUC mucin antigen; CEA carcinoma embryonic antigen.
Dalgleish, 2000.

effective in the treatment of bladder cancer, the erratic nature of responses to most of these treatments in other conditions, coupled with a failure to understand the relevant immune responses, has frustrated any significant clinical progress. However, the last few years have seen a number of new developments in our understanding of the immune response to cancer. These principles can apply to breast cancer and include the following:

- tumour cells express a number of unique antigens or common or differentiation antigens inappropriately (see Table 12b.2);
- tumour cells avoid presenting these antigens (many of which are self and hence tolerant) to the immune system by down-regulating various components of their antigen presenting machinery and by actively secreting immunosuppressive factors/cytokines.

The therapeutic implications of this are as follows:

- there is no shortage of tumour-specific or tumour-associated antigens to target.

Many are shared by tumours of different origins;

- the immune system's 'blind eye' or tolerance to these antigens needs to be broken and a strategy employed to prevent the immunosuppressive factors from being produced.

Experience with a number of mainly cell-based vaccines in the treatment of malignant melanoma has shown that vaccination strategies are more likely to be effective against residual disease (small volume) than against bulky disease and that vaccination needs to be administered regularly (therapeutically, unlike protective vaccines against infectious diseases). These observations make sense in the light of the immunosuppressive, evasive and potentially tolerating properties of tumour cells.

Evidence of an immune response to breast cancer

Numerous studies note a general trend between general immune responsiveness as measured by delayed type hypersensitivity (DTH) and leukocyte adherence inhibition assays and the presence of, and stage of, breast cancer (Boeva et al., 1978; Sanner et al., 1983; Lopez et al., 1998; Remedi et al., 1998). More recently, a number of tumour antigens have been described as good therapeutic targets for immunotherapy; namely the mutated C-*erb*B-2, oncogene receptor HER-2/*neu* and the Sialy1 Tn epitope of a mucin carbohydrate associated with the MUC-1 antigen. Antibody and vaccine strategies against these antigens are already being tested in the clinical setting.

The concept that immune responses could be relevant to human breast cancer came from the murine parallel which is caused by a retrovirus, namely, mouse mammary tumour virus (MMTV) which naturally presents viral epitopes as good foreign antigens. The immune response to this virus, especially with regard to the way it activates the immune system, determines the clinical outcome (Luther & Acha-Orbea, 1996). This model would be of little relevance for human breast cancer if it were not for the recent discovery of a similar retrovirus (probably endogenous) in human cancer (Pogo et al., 1999). This was first suspected over a decade ago and not readily detected by other investigators (Al-Sumidaie et al., 1988). Now supersensitive and specific polymerase chain reaction (PCR) assays can be used to see if this is a local (contamination!) or a general real phenomenon (Magrath & Bhatia, 1999).

The use of IL-2 and activated lymphocytes in the early eighties led to the observation that some patients given IL-2 had a partial response, although this was associated with severe toxicity. IL-2 acts indirectly by activating T cells (it was formally known as T cell growth factor, TCGF). We have injected IL-2 in low doses locally into the tumour and draining lymph nodes in locally advanced, inoperable nonresectable breast cancers. Marked softening of the tumours was detected in all cases with an objective response in one case (Dalgleish et al., 1990). Patients were subsequently treated with radiotherapy or chemotherapy to which they appeared to be very sensitive. A synergy between IL-2 treatment and radiotherapy has been demonstrated in murine models and needs to be studied formally in humans. The logic for local IL-2 is to expand those tumour-infiltrating T-cells that have already 'seen' the tumour antigens, as the help that IL-2 can provide would normally be available if the tumour was a foreign invader and not an immunosuppressive tumour trying to turn off any IL-2 production (Vaage, 1991; Fiszer-Maliszewska et al., 1999). A logical consequence of this strategy is to try to make tumour cells make IL-2 themselves in situ by gene transfer (gene therapy) (Dalgleish, 1994).

Current immunotherapeutic clinical studies

IL-2 continues to be studied in breast cancer as part of the induction regimen as well as being administered as maintenance treatment (Toh et al., 2000). In addition, its delivery by viral vectors is currently under development (Stewart et al., 1999).

Vaccines

Theratope (STh-KLH) is an antigen-specific vaccine construct consisting of the sialylated carbohydrate mucin antigen coupled to KLH. This is currently being evaluated in a multicentre randomized phase III study after chemotherapy in patients with metastatic breast cancer on the basis of an encouraging phase II study (Sandmaier et al., 1999). It is thought that a strong anti-STh immune response correlates with a better outcome and survival. A large number of similar studies using MUC-1, anti-idiotype antibodies to the dominant epitope as well as MUC-I DNA presented in a variety of viral vectors as a vaccine, are undergoing early clinical analysis (Miles, 1997).

Antibodies (Herceptin)

The major immunotherapy to be currently used in breast cancer is the antibody against the new oncogene receptor, 'Herceptin' (Yarbro & Mastrangelo, 1999). Herceptin is a humanized antibody to an epitope on the extracellular domain of the c-erbB-2 receptor, which is overexpressed in 20–40% of breast tumours. Following a number of encouraging studies showing a survival advantage over standard therapies it has been licensed for use in patients in the USA with metastatic breast cancer who overexpress the c-erbB-2 protein. This is further discussed in Chapter 11.

The clinical effectiveness of Herceptin will allow more sophisticated targeting of this receptor and the p185 receptor tyrosine kinase that it encodes (Zhang et al., 1999). It is currently being evaluated in the adjuvant setting as mainline treatment with or after taxanes or after anthracyclines (Lebwohl & Canetta, 1999; Hortobagyi, 1999). A vaccine against this receptor either as a protein or its anti-idiotype or as a DNA construct may allow prolonged targeting of c-erbB-2 to be achieved in early disease. Moreover, viral vectors targeting the promoter may allow more aggressive inhibition of c-erbB-2 positive cells in advanced bulky disease.

Future approaches

Apart from more sophisticated approaches to targeting c-erbB-2, a number of other breast cancer-associated antigens could also be targeted in a similar manner. Other technologies being considered are antisense oligonucleotide therapy or antisense gene delivery by a variety of viral vectors. Other ligands to consider include other members of the HER family of which there are four, transforming growth factors, insulin-like growth factors I and II, platelet-derived growth factor and heparin-binding growth factor(s). Furthermore, specific compounds targeting the relevant signalling pathways may also be effective such as targeting ras activation with farnesyl transferase inhibitors.

Suicide gene therapy

A number of studies have now reported the marked bystander killing ability of HSV-tk when transduced into cells in the presence of ganciclovir. Although cell to cell transmission of the toxic phosphorylated ganciclovir has been demonstrated there is also a significant immune response component as the effect is only transient in nude mice, implying that immune recognition is necessary for control. This means that only 20–30% of tumour cells need to be infected with a viral vector carrying HSV-tk in order to be able to kill 100% of its cells. c-erbB-2 is one of several targets that may be suitable for this approach (Freeman, 2000).

Angiogenesis and telomerase inhibitors

Other new approaches which may be relevant to breast cancer include angiogenesis inhibitors such as the somatostatins and endostatins. It is of interest that many currently used agents such as tamoxifen, interferons and thalidomide all have weak antiangiogenic activity, and hence any new agent would need to have considerably greater and more specific activity to make a clinical impact.

Telomeres are the ends of the chromosome which gradually shorten with each replication hence ensuring senescense. Telomerase inhibits this process, hence continued activity, which is a feature of many tumours, implies immortality.

Table 12b.3. Possible approaches to the treatment of breast cancer alone or in combination

Surgery	
Chemotherapy	
Radiotherapy	
Endocrine/hormone therapy	
Biological therapy	1L-2 γ-IFN, GM-CSF
	Antibodies (alone or coagulated) as therapy or vaccines, e.g. HER/2, MUC-I, MAGE etc.
	Cellular therapy and cytokines
Signal transduction inhibition	Tyrosine kinase inhibitors
	Farnesyl transferase inhibitors
	Antisense therapy
Angiogenesis inhibitors	
Telomerase inhibitors	
Matrix metalloprotease inhibitors	
Gene therapy	Transcriptional downregulation
	Antisense
	Suicide gene

Therefore, a telomerase inhibitor should be effective against cancer cells which have high telomerase activity. Although possible in vitro there is considerable doubt about the ability to translate this to an effective in vivo product.

The immediate future

Biological and gene therapy will continue to be evaluated in breast cancer given the success of current trials. The considerable benefit of adding Herceptin to standard chemotherapy, as well as similar improved outcomes seen with other combinations in other tumour types, will add further impetus to investigate combined modality therapy with these agents (Table 12b.3). Other epitopes on breast cancer, some of which are on other tumours, are the subject of clinical trials, such as MUC-1, gangliosides, ras and p53 mutants. These may be used in addition to, or in combination with, each other and/or chemotherapy.

Limited response rates of monoclonal antibodies given alone may be increased by conjugation with cytotoxic agents, natural or synthetic toxins or with radioactive agents, all of which can amplify activity.

Vaccine approaches will constantly evolve to consider better adjuvant(s) schedules, cell-based vaccines transfected with immunostimulatory cytokines (e.g. IL-

12, GM-CSF) and dendritic cell therapy and/or combinations thereof. Dendritic cells are professional antigen-presenting cells with all the necessary costimulatory molecules. They can be harvested from peripheral blood cells and expanded in vitro using GM-CSF and 1L-4 or TNFα following which they can be pulsed with tumour antigens (proteins, peptides, cells, for example) and then reinfused back into the patient inducing an enhanced immune response against tumour antigens. Encouraging clinical responses have been reported in a wide variety of tumours with this approach, although striking tumour regression is still anecdotal (Holtl et al., 1998; Dallal & Lotze, 2000; Geiger et al., 2000).

Gene therapy will be employed to deliver HSV-tk, and other suicide genes to convert non-toxic therapy into localized toxic molecules. Other likely targets include antisense oligonucleotides to genes which are known to drive *ras* genes of some tumours, as well as substitution of mutated genes, e.g. suppressor genes.

In addition, a number of small molecules targeting signal transduction pathways as well as, or alone, will be actively researched and developed. Matrix-metalloproteinase inhibitors (which also have an antiangiogenic role) are already in clinical trials and nontoxic versions could find a place in addition to other therapies (Schoof et al., 1998; Hortobagyi et al., 1998; Patterson & Harris, 1999; Pegram et al., 1999).

In the meantime there is an urgent need to reconsider both animal and human studies showing the potential benefit of simple 1L-2 based regimens (intratumoral and low, rather than high, dose) in addition to other therapies.

REFERENCES

Al-Sumidaie, A.M., Leinster, S.J., Hart, C.A. et al. (1988). Particles with properties of retro-viruses in monocytes from patients with breast cancer [see comments]. *Lancet*, 1, 5–9.

Boeva, M., Donchev, T., Markova, R. et al. (1978). Delayed hypersensitivity reactions in patients with breast cancer. *Neoplasma*, 25(6), 733–6.

Burnet, F.M. (1970). The concept of immunological surveillance. *Progress in Experimental Tumor Research*, 13, 1–27.

Dalgleish, A.G. (1994). The role of IL-2 in gene therapy. *Gene Therapy*, 1, 83–7.

Dalgleish, A.G. (2000). Cancer vaccines. *British Journal of Cancer*, 82(10), 1619–24.

Dalgleish, A. & Browning, M. (1996). Tumour immunology: Immunotherapy and cancer vaccines. In: *Cancer: Clinical Science in Practice* (Edited K.S.). Cambridge University Press.

Dalgleish, A.G., Sauven, P., Fermont, D. et al. (1990). Local IL-2 in locally advanced breast cancer. *Journal of Experimental Clinical Cancer Research*, 9, 237–8.

Dallal, R.M. & Lotze, M.T. (2000). The dendritic cell and human cancer vaccines. *Current Opinion in Immunology*, 12(5), 583–8.

Fiszer-Maliszewska, L., Den Otter, W. & Mordarski, M. (1999). Effect of local interleukin-2 treatment on spontaneous tumours of different immunogenic strength. *Cancer Immunology Immunotherapy*, 47, 307–14.

Freeman, S.M. (2000). Suicide gene therapy. *Advances in Experimental Medicine and Biology*, 465, 411–22.

Geiger, J., Hutchinson, R., Hohenkirk, L. et al., (2000). Treatment of solid tumours in children with tumour-lysate-pulsed dendritic cells. *Lancet*, 356(9236), 1163–5.

Holtl, L., Rieser, C., Papesh, C. et al. (1998). CD83+ blood dendritic cells as a vaccine for immunotherapy of metastatic renal-cell cancer. *Lancet*, 352(9137), 1358.

Hortobagyi, G.N. (1999). Recent progress in the clinical development of docetaxel (Taxotere). *Seminars in Oncology*, 26 (3 Suppl. 9), 32–6.

Hortobagyi, G.N., Hung, M.C. & Lopez-Berenstein, G. (1998). A Phase I multicenter study of E1A gene therapy for patients with metastatic breast cancer and epithelial ovarian cancer that overexpresses HER-2/neu or epithelial ovarian cancer. *Human Gene Therapy*, 9, 1775–98.

Lebwohl, D.E. & Canetta, R. (1999). New developments in chemotherapy of advanced breast cancer. *Annols of Oncology*, 10 Suppl. 6, 139–46.

Lopez, C.B., Roa, T.D., Feiner, H. et al. (1998). Repression of interleukin-2 mRNA translation in primary human breast carcinoma tumor-infiltrating lymphocytes. *Cell Immunology*, 190(2), 141–55.

Luther, A.A. & Acha-Orbea, H. (1996). Immune response to mouse mammary tumour virus. *Current Opinion Immunology*, 8(4), 498–502.

Magrath, I. & Bhatia, K. (1999). Breast cancer: a new Epstein-Barr virus-associated disease? (Editorial; comment). *Journal of National Cancer Institute*, 91, 1349–50.

Maraveyas, A., Baban, B., Kennard, D. et al. (1999). Possible improved survival of patients with stage IV AJCC melanoma receiving SRL 172 immunotherapy: correlation with induction of increased levels of intracellular interluekin-2 in peripheral blood lymphocytes. *Annals of Oncology*, 10, 817–24.

Miles, D. (1997). Breast cancer tumour vaccines. *Cancer Treatment Reviews*, 23, Suppl. 1, S77–85.

O'Byrne, K.J., Dalgleish, A.G., Browning, M.J. et al. (2000). The relationship between angiogenesis and the immune response in carcinogenesis and the progression of malignant disease. *European Journal of Cancer*, 36, 151–69.

Patterson, A. & Harris, A.L. (1999). Molecular chemotherapy for breast cancer. *Drugs Aging*, 14, 75–90.

Pegram, M., Hsu, S., Lewis, G. et al. (1999). Inhibitory effects of combinations of HER-2/neu antibody and chemotherapeutic agents used for treatment of human breast cancers. *Oncogene*, 18, 2241–51.

Pogo, B.G., Melana, S.M., Holland, J.F. et al. (1999). Sequences homologous to the mouse mammary tumor virus env gene in human breast carcinoma correlate with overexpression of laminin receptor. *Clinical Cancer Research*, 5, 2108–11.

Remedi, M.M., Hliba, E., Demarchi, M. et al. (1998). Relationship between immune state and tumor growth rate in rats bearing progressive and non-progressive mammary tumors. *Cancer Immunology and Immunotherapy*, 46(6), 350–4.

Sandmaier, B.M., Oparin, D.V., Holmberg, L.A. et al. (1999). Evidence of a cellular immune response against sialyl-Tn in breast and ovarian cancer patients after high-dose chemotherapy, stem cell rescue, and immunization with Theratope STn-KLH cancer vaccine. *Journal of Immunotherapy*, 22(1), 54–66.

Sanner, T., Kotlar, H.K., Eker, P. et al. (1983). Early detection of breast cancer by leukocyte adherence inhibition assay. *Cancer Detection and Prevention*, 6(4–5), 443–50.

Schoof, D.D., Smith, J.W., Disis, M.L. et al. (1998). Immunization of metastatic breast cancer patients with CD80-modified breast cancer cells and GM-CSF. *Advances in Experimental Medical Biology*, 451, 511–18.

Stewart, A.K., Lassam, N.J., Quirt, I.C. et al. (1999). Adenovector-mediated gene delivery of interleukin-2 in metastatic breast cancer and melanoma: results of a phase I clinical trial. *Gene Therapy*, 6(3), 350–63.

Toh, H.C., McAfee, S.L., Sackstein, R. et al. (2000). High-dose cyclophosphamide + carboplatin and interleukin-2 (IL-2) activated autologous stem cell transplantation followed by maintenance IL-2 therapy in metastatic breast carcinoma – a phase II study. *Bone Marrow Transplant*, 25(1), 19–24.

Vaage, J. (1991). Peri-tumor interleukin-2 causes systemic therapeutic effect via interferon-gamma induction. *International Journal of Cancer*, 49, 598–600.

Westby, M., Manca, F. & Dalgleish, A.G. (1996). The role of host immune responses in determining the outcome of HIV infection. *Immunology Today*, 17, 120–6.

Yarbro, J.B.R. & Mastrangelo, M. (eds.) (1999). M.D. Anderson Conference on Trastuzumab (Herceptin). *Seminars in Oncology*, 26, Suppl. 12 (Aug.).

Zhang, H., Wang, Q., Montone, K.T. et al. (1999). Shared antigenic epitopes and pathobiological functions of anti-p185 (her2/neu) monoclonal antibodies. *Experimental and Molecular Pathology*, 67(1), 15–25.

13

The place of bisphosphonates in the management of breast cancer

A.H.G. Paterson

Tom Baker Cancer Centre and University of Calgary

Introduction

Bone pain, fractures and hypercalcaemia are important causes of morbidity in patients with metastatic breast cancer despite recent advances in endocrine and cytotoxic therapy. These skeletal complications arise because of progressive focal or generalized osteolysis. Osteolysis occurs because of osteoclast activation, either directly by tumour products or by products secreted by nearby host cells in response to tumour cell products (Mundy et al., 1984). Since the osteoclast plays a central role in focal or generalized osteolysis, inhibitors of osteoclast function may lead to palliation and, in some cases, to prevention of osteolytic destruction and its complications (Taube et al., 1994). It is also possible that the growth and development of bone metastases may be inhibited in a proportion of patients and the bone loss associated with premature menopause induced by adjuvant chemotherapy may be prevented.

The clinical problem

Skeletal pain, fracture and hypercalcaemia are well recognized by oncologists as major causes of morbidity in patients with breast cancer. Vertebral fractures not only cause pain and disability, but may lead to spinal cord compression. In women, the problems of bone metastases are compounded by the propensity to osteoporosis. Women have a lower total bone mass than men and the threshold for developing fractures tends to be reached at an earlier age than in men. In addition, in premenopausal women with breast cancer, the increasing use of adjuvant cytotoxic chemotherapy or adjuvant LHRH analogues leads to earlier menopause with subsequent earlier accelerated loss of bone.

Normal and abnormal bone remodelling

Bone remodelling is a dynamic process occurring in response to poorly under-stood physical and chemical forces along lines of stress (Kaplan, 1987). Remodell-ing may result from initial stimulation by osteoblastic cells which are derived from bone marrow stromal cells (Mundy, 1987). Osteoclasts which are derived from haematopoietic precursor cells are recruited to an area of damaged or worn bone which is then broken down to form a bone resorption bay by the action of lytic substances secreted by the osteoclast. Osteoblasts then move into the bone resorp-tion bay (Howship's lacuna), and new bone precursor substances, largely consist-ing of type I collagen, are laid down in layers which, over time, become min-eralized. The formation of new bone following orderly resorption in the resorption cavities is termed 'coupling'. Bone remodelling normally occurs, there-fore, as the result of a balance between bone destruction and new bone formation.

When malignant cells infiltrate bone spaces, the balance of new bone formation and bone destruction is perturbed and bone remodelling and turnover becomes abnormal. Under these circumstances, three mechanisms contribute to abnormal-ities of bone remodelling (Kanis & McCloskey, 1997). The first occurs when a wave of bone resorption is initiated, usually focally, but sometimes generally, leading to increased bone turnover; loss of bone occurs because the resorption phase precedes the formation phase. A second mechanism comes into play when the normal connection between bone resorption and formation is disrupted and new bone is formed at sites other than where resorption has recently taken place, and erosion cavities are never subsequently repaired. A third mechanism occurs when the amount of new bone formed in the resorption bays does not match quantitatively the amount of bone resorbed.

Carcinoma cells can secrete a variety of substances, such as parathormone related peptide (PTHrP), prostaglandin E and transforming growth factors, which might stimulate tumour growth by autocrine or paracrine mechanisms, but which also have stimulatory effects on osteoclast function. Most of these effects occur locally, but these substances can also be secreted into the circulation, and have a generalized effect on bone metabolism (Mundy, 1988). In prostate cancer, where osteoblastic metastases predominate, the excessive, deranged and uncoupled new bone formation can lead to the 'bone hunger syndrome', a situation where Ca^{2+} entrapment in bone leads to lower than normal plasma Ca^{2+} levels, with subse-quent elevation of parathormone. This secondary hyperparathyroidism can lead to further generalized bone loss (Berruti et al., 1997). In breast cancer, PTHrP release also leads to increased proximal tubular reabsorption of Ca^{2+} within the kidney, and this is an important mechanism for the appearance of hypercalcaemia in breast and other cancers (Kanis et al., 1986).

'Seed and soil' theories

The concept of malignant cell-matrix interaction is an old one, and hypotheses have been developed to explain the appearance of metastases at specific sites. These have been termed 'seed and soil' theories. Experiments designed to investigate the relationship between malignant cells and their surrounding tissues at sites of metastases suggest that chemical interactions form the basis of the association (Kamenor et al., 1984).

The association of breast cancer with the development of bone metastases was first expressed in print by Sir James Paget in 1889 when he wrote: 'The evidence seems to be irresistible that in cancer of the breast, the bones suffer in a special way, which cannot be explained by any theory of embolism alone' (Paget, 1889). The notion that there might be a local reason for the development of metastases at specific sites beyond a chance colonization following embolism was further developed by Batson (1940), who described the connection between the vertebral venous plexus and the bone marrow spaces, hypothesizing a retrograde spread that would allow metastases from a primary prostate cancer to lodge preferentially in the lower vertebrae. Once within the marrow space, metastases have a blood supply for further growth. Mundy has taken the seed and soil idea one step further by adding the concept of a 'vicious cycle', with products from tumour-induced breakdown of bone leading to stimulation and further growth of malignant cells (Mundy, 1997).

Bone metastases

Incidence and morbidity

The association of osteolytic, osteosclerotic and mixed lytic/sclerotic bone metastases with breast cancer is well known to clinicians. In the experience of a major clinical trials group, the National Surgical Adjuvant Breast and Bowel Project (NSABP) in the United States, bone metastases account for the highest proportion of first sites of distant relapse in breast cancer patients suffering recurrence of their disease after adjuvant therapy with hormones and/or chemotherapy. Approximately one-third of patients who develop distant metastases do so in bone either as the sole site of recurrence or simultaneously with other sites of disease (Smith et al., 1999). As the disease progresses, the majority of patients will develop bone metastases; their median survival from diagnosis of bone metastases is between 18 and 20 months (Paterson, 1987). Recently, we have shown that patients presenting with breast cancer have a four to five times higher rate of vertebral fracture than an age-matched group of well women (Kanis et al., 1999). This is most likely related to chemotherapy-induced premature menopause with accelerated bone loss.

Bone pain

When malignant cells invade the intertrabecular spaces, the malignant cells may form a mass to a size where secreted substances have an impact on local physiology. It is too simplistic to explain bone pain on purely mechanistic grounds by suggesting that a bone metastasis causes pain because trabecular fractures occur and bone collapses, leading to compression and distortion of the periosteum, a site known to be innervated by pain fibres. It is difficult to understand how bone pain can occur in the absence of fracture, but this does happen commonly. Bone marrow spaces are innervated by nociceptive C-fibres sensitive to changes in pressure, and it is probable that the malignant cells secrete pain-provoking factors such as substance P, bradykinins, prostaglandins and other cytokines, which lead to stimulation of C-type fibres within bone. Prostaglandins may also play a role by sensitizing free nerve endings to release vasoactive amines and kinins (Ferreira, 1983). The precise interaction between tumour and bone microenvironment is unknown. The subject of bone pain due to metastases has been well reviewed (Ernst, 1997).

General principles of management

While this review focuses on the place of bisphosphonates on bone metastases in breast cancer, mainly because this area has provided some of the most exciting research in recent years, other modalities continue to provide the mainstay of therapy.

Bone pain management includes a thorough history and physical examination, full discussion with the patient about a plan of action, and attempts to modify the pathological process. These attempts include external beam radiotherapy (still the most effective remedy for alleviation of localized bone pain) and palliative chemotherapy. A good response to chemotherapy includes subjective relief of symptoms, including pain. Hormone therapy in breast cancer can provide a high quality remission in patients with bone metastases. Radionuclide therapy with strontium-89 can be effective in alleviating the bone pain of breast cancer. Patients may require sequential therapy with bisphosphonates and strontium-89. Trials of both modalities used together are overdue.

Elevation of the pain threshold with the use of nonpharmacological methods as well as analgesics, interruption of pain pathways by local or regional anaesthesia or neurolysis, and modification of lifestyles are all helpful, but invariably opiate and other adjuvant analgesic management will be required.

Prophylactic surgery and radiation therapy for patients with cortical erosion caused by metastasis in the femur and humerus may prevent the distress of a pathological fracture.

Bisphosphonates

Many bisphosphonates have been assessed in the management of malignant hypercalcaemia. These include etidronate, pamidronate, clodronate, residronate, mildronate, neridronate, alendronate, ibandronate and zoledronate. Etidronate, pamidronate and clodronate have been the most extensively tested bisphosphonates and are widely available for the treatment of hypercalcaemia and Paget's disease of bone. We have previously demonstrated the action of etidronate in the treatment of hypercalcaemia (Ryzon et al., 1985). Pamidronate, clodronate and etidronate lead to an effective lowering of serum calcium which is attributable to decreased bone resorption, but etidronate appears to impair the mineralization of bone and must be given intermittently to allow normal bone formation to occur (Kanis et al., 1984). Pamidronate, an aminobisphosphonate, may not be ideal for oral use because of dose-related gastrointestinal toxicity. There is some evidence that long-term pamidronate administered orally may also induce osteomalacia (Adamson et al., 1993). Clodronate is effective when given intravenously for hypercalcaemia and bone pain and can be used orally. Its long-term administration is not associated with a defect in the mineralization of bone (Taube et al., 1993).

The geminal bisphosphonates are analogues of pyrophosphate characterized by a stable P–C–P bond. They bind with high affinity to hydroxyapatite crystals in bone, and are potent inhibitors of normal and pathological bone resorption (Fleisch, 2000). Several mechanisms of action seem to operate, the dominant mechanism differing in different compounds, but all appear to have a final common effect of inhibition of osteoclast function. The osteoblast might be the initial target cell for bisphosphonates, exerting an effect on the osteoclast by modulation of stimulating and inhibiting factors which control osteoclast function (Sahni et al., 1993). Transforming growth factor β (TGF-β) is known to induce osteoclast apoptosis and its production by bone surface osteoblasts as a result of bisphosphonate stimulation may partly explain this phenomenon.

These agents appear to promote apoptosis in murine osteoclasts both in vivo and in vitro, the more potent bisphosphonates exhibiting the greatest apoptotic action (Hughes et al., 1995). In the absence of apoptosis, inhibition of osteoclast function appears to be mediated by osteoblasts, which produce a factor that inhibits osteoclastic function (Siwek et al., 1997). This action does not interfere with the ability of cells of the monocyte-macrophage lineage to produce colonies (Nishikawa et al., 1996). Bisphosphonates can also inhibit the proliferation and promote the cell death of macrophages (Rogers et al., 1996; Selander et al., 1996). Again, the process is one of apoptosis rather than necrosis and may, in part, explain the pain-relieving properties of bisphosphonates. More recently, Shipman et al. (1997) have described the induction of apoptosis by bisphosphonates in human myeloma cell lines.

Recent discoveries regarding the molecular mechanism of action in osteoclasts have suggested that amino bisphosphonates (e.g. pamidronate, clendronate, ibandronate and zoledronate) inhibit the mevalonate pathway in osteoclasts thereby interrupting prenylation of signalling proteins required for osteoclast function (Rogers et al., 2000). Moreover, nonnitrogen-containing bisphosphonates (e.g. etidro-nate, clodronate, tiludronate) are incorporated into the phosphate chains of ATP forming nonhydrolyase analogues which inhibit osteoclast function (Monkkonen et al., 2000).

Clinical trials of bisphosphonates in breast cancer

Hypercalcaemia

As a result of secretion of factors from infiltrating malignant ductal cells acting focally and humorally, osteoclast activity is markedly increased, with a reduction in osteoblast activity, leading to 'uncoupling' of bone resorption and formation (Body & Delmas, 1992). PTHrP appears to play a central role in malignant hypercalcaemia (Grill et al., 1991).

We have recently reviewed the evidence for the treatment of hypercalcaemia and offered some broad guidelines (Body et al., 1998). Saline rehydration will usually effect a median reduction of 0.25 mM/l but its effect is transient (Singer et al., 1991). Rehydration is useful for treating mild degrees of hypercalcaemia but usually should be accompanied by bisphosphonate therapy. Symptomatic hypercalcaemia, especially with levels of Ca^{2+} greater than 3.0 mM/l, requires vigorous rehydration (normal saline 150–200 ml/hr with KCl 20–40 mEq/l added, and the administration of clodronate 1500 mg in 500 cc normal saline over 2–3 hours or pamidronate 60–90 mg in 500 ml normal saline over 2–3 hours. Pamidronate may give a longer duration of maintenance of normocalcaemia (Purohit et al., 1995) action than clodronate (28 days median vs. 14 days) but in many countries is significantly more expensive. Newer bisphosphonates, such as ibandronate and zoledronate, are currently being studied. Ibandronate at doses of 4–6 mg i.v. (Ralston et al., 1997) and zoledronate at 4 mg i.v. (Major et al., 2000) appear to be at least as efficacious and may be superior to pamidronate 60–90 mg i.v. in terms of duration of response and may have the added advantage of a shorter infusion time. These studies are notoriously difficult to assess, since results are heavily dependent on the clinical case mix.

Skeletal complications

Early clinical investigations of bisphosphonates were performed in uncontrolled trials of patients with advanced disease or small non-placebo-controlled, open studies (Elomaa et al., 1987). Although it has been shown that these investigators were correct in their conclusions, it is difficult to determine the extent to which patient selection and the placebo effect influenced the positive results of the investigations.

One of the first randomized, controlled studies to be published was an open trial of the aminobisphosphonate, pamidronate, given orally for 2 years at 300 mg/day in patients with bone metastases from breast cancer (van Holten-Verzanvoort et al., 1987). The investigators demonstrated a reduction in the skeletal complications of hypercalcaemia and vertebral fractures. Radiation treatments for bone pain were also reduced, but there was difficulty in patient compliance with gastrointestinal side-effects.

In a double-blind, randomized, placebo-controlled trial of oral clodronate, 1600 mg given daily for 2 years, we confirmed this beneficial effect on skeletal morbidity in patients with bone metastases from breast cancer (Paterson et al., 1993). The number of patients suffering from episodes of hypercalcaemia and the total number of episodes were reduced; the number of major vertebral fractures and the vertebral deformity rate were also reduced; and the number of radiation therapy treatments was lower in the clodronate-treated patients. No survival benefit was evident. McCloskey et al. (1993) reviewed the pre-entry and follow-up vertebral fracture prevalence in 163 of the 173 patients in this trial and found that 46% of the patients had evidence of vertebral fracture at trial entry. The patients deriving the greatest benefit from the oral clodronate were those who had already sustained vertebral fractures and were therefore at greatest risk for sustaining further fractures.

Pamidronate, which can occasionally induce sclerosis in osteolytic lesions when used as the only therapy (Coleman et al., 1988) has been investigated in several trials. Measurement of response in bone can be a difficult process and unless differences in the arms of a trial are large, small but significant differences can be missed. Tumour response in bone and duration of response were assessed in a double-blind, randomized trial, which showed similar response rates in bone but a significantly ($p = 0.02$) increased duration of response for patients receiving pamidronate 45 mg given intravenously every three weeks (249 days median time to progression compared to 168 days in controls) (Conte et al., 1996). Hortobagyi et al. (1996) have reported a randomized trial of 380 patients with recurrent breast cancer in bone and demonstrated a convincing reduction in the skeletal complications of vertebral fracture, pain and hypercalcaemia with intravenous pamidronate 90 mg given monthly for two years. No survival benefit was apparent.

As a result of these well-controlled trials, we currently recommend the use of either oral clodronate 1600 mg/day orally (preferably taken 0.5 to 1 hour before breakfast or, less preferably, at least 2 hours before food) or intravenous pamidronate 90 mg every 4 weeks in patients with radiologically established bone metastases from breast cancer. The length of treatment with oral clodronate is continuous and life-long; with i.v. pamidronate, treatment should continue for as long as is practical, with conversion to an oral bisphosphonate, if available, after 18 months.

Bone pain

The idea that bisphosphonates might decrease bone pain in some patients with bone metastases arose from clinical observations of patients receiving bisphosphonates for hypercalcaemia. Patients experienced not only normalization of serum Ca^{2+} and relief of the symptoms of hypercalcaemia, but also reported relief of pain.

Ernst et al. (1992) demonstrated in a double-blind, crossover trial of intravenous clodronate in patients with bone pain caused by a variety of malignancies that clodronate had useful analgesic properties. This was confirmed in a larger randomized, double-blind, controlled trial of intravenous clodronate in patients with metastatic bone pain (Ernst et al., 1997). No dose-response relationship was seen. Improvement in pain and mobility scores had been described in a previously reported trial of oral pamidronate, although these patients had not been selected specifically because of bone pain but because they had osteolytic metastases (van Holten-Verzanvoort et al., 1991); however, the modest effect, coupled with its poor oral tolerability as demonstrated by Coleman et al. (1998), make oral pamidronate unlikely to supersede its intravenous counterpart. Pain relief has also been described with intravenous pamidronate in a placebo-controlled trial in patients with bone metastases from breast cancer (Hortobagyi et al., 1996). The mechanism of pain relief is unknown but may be related to the previously described mechanisms of action on osteoclast and macrophage apoptosis or an inhibition of pain-provoking cellular and humoral factors.

Trials of adjuvant bisphosphonates

Patients with recurrent disease but no bone metastases

Some intriguing pioneer data were generated in a small, randomized, placebo-controlled clinical trial of continuous oral clodronate in patients who had recurrent breast cancer but with no evidence of bone metastases on bone scanning and conventional radiology (Kanis et al., 1996). Although overall survival in the two arms was similar, there was an expected significant reduction in skeletal complications. When the incidence of new bone metastases was assessed, a significant reduction in the number of new bone metastases in the clodronate treated group was found. However, the number of patients developing bone metastases, although lower in the clodronate-treated group, was not significantly different from the control group. This study is one of the first of its kind to suggest that the intervention of a bisphosphonate, which primarily acts on osteoclasts, can have an impact on the behaviour of bone metastases.

One other trial has assessed oral pamidronate in a similar group of patients with advanced or recurrent disease but no bone metastases. The trial was randomized but not placebo controlled, and was also relatively small, with an accrual of 124 patients. A large number of patients withdrew from the trial because of the gastrointestinal side-effects of oral pamidronate and compliance was a problem. Results showed no effect on rate of development of skeletal metastases, quality of life or survival (van Holten-Verzanvoort et al., 1996).

Patients with operable breast cancer

As Goldhirsch has pointed out in reviewing the trials of the International Breast Cancer Study Group, the main effect of the adjuvant therapy used in the group's trials has been to reduce local, regional and distant soft-tissue recurrences. First recurrences in bone and viscera have been minimally affected (Goldhirsch et al., 1994).

At menopause, bone resorption accelerates in women and they reach the fracture threshold at an earlier mean age than men, largely because of their lower peak bone mass. Combination chemotherapy is now used in premenopausal women with all stages of breast cancer. Many women with multiple positive lymph nodes receive high-dose chemotherapy with stem cell rescue. One of the effects of these treatments, particularly when high-dose chemotherapy is used, or when the protocol contains alkylating agents, is to cause ovarian ablation leading to premature menopause. The skeletal effects of oophorectomy in rats are predictable, and consist of an early acceleration of bone turnover with loss of bone substance, especially cancellous bone. This accelerated bone turnover can be reduced by oestrogen or the bisphosphonate, residronate. The effect of oestrogen is lost 90 days after cessation of oestrogen therapy. In contrast, the bisphosphonate is still effective 180 days after withdrawal (Wronski et al., 1993). The bone loss following premature menopause in patients can be substantial, reaching as much as 7% in the first year in some women, but can be prevented by clodronate (Powles et al., 1997) and residronate (Delmas et al., 1997).

The results of adjuvant chemotherapy and hormone therapy show that there is room for improvement in dealing with bone metastasis as a site of recurrence of disease. Tamoxifen does appear to reduce the incidence of new bone metastases as well as metastases at other sites (Fisher et al., 1989). This reduction of the incidence of bone metastases as site of first recurrence is not seen with chemotherapy. Tamoxifen is also known to have a beneficial effect on reducing bone resorption in postmenopausal women (Turken et al., 1989). Early attempts to reduce the incidence of bone metastases in patients with operable breast cancer using prostaglandin inhibitors, such as aspirin and indomethacin, were unsuccessful. This was despite in vitro data from the Walker carcinoma and in vivo data in the osteolytic rabbit VX2 tumour, which suggested that osteolysis and bone metastases could be inhibited by early treatment with prostaglandin inhibitors (Powles et al., 1982). These agents, although useful for the relief of pain, have little effect on the skeletal complications of established bone metastases. Bisphosphonates, which have an established record in reducing the skeletal complications of bone metastases, are a more promising group of compounds for prevention trials.

If clodronate and pamidronate can reduce the skeletal complications of patients with breast cancer, myeloma and possibly other malignancies, do they achieve this by means of a protective 'antiosteolytic' mechanism, as is implied by their known mechanisms of action, or is it possible that their final pathway mode of action, the inhibition of osteoclast function, has a feedback effect leading to inhibition of the growth of bone metastases? Can we, by affecting the 'soil' of the microenvironment in which deposits of tumour cells grow, influence the behaviour of the 'seeds', the tumour micrometastases, themselves? Production of PTHrP by breast carcinoma cells in bone is enhanced by growth factors such as activated TGF-β, produced as a result of both normal bone remodelling and accelerated osteolysis; this sets up a vicious cycle. It is also known that breast cancer cells secrete low molecular weight factors that specifically affect human osteoblast cell lines, inhibiting their proliferation and increasing their cAMP response to parathormone.

Is it possible that we are merely interfering with the mechanisms of diagnosis, for example, by inhibiting the uptake of radiolabelled technetium pertechnetate in the bone reaction surrounding a metastasis, thereby reducing the tumour:background ratio of radionuclide uptake? This is unlikely, given the extensive experience of bone scanning in patients with bone metastases who have received oral or intravenous bisphosphonates. There have been no reports of inhibition of uptake of bone-seeking radionuclides by bisphosphonates. Pecherstorfer et al. (1993) have demonstrated that there was no effect on bone scintigraphy in 11 patients with breast cancer scanned after receiving daily intravenous clodronate for three weeks. Similarly, there was no inhibition of uptake documented in post-bisphosphonate scans compared with baseline scans after intravenous pamidronate had been administered as little as 24 hours previously (Macro et al., 1995).

A body of animal experimental data suggests that bisphosphonates have an inhibitory effect on the development of bone metastases. Pretreatment with bisphosphonates protects against the development of bone metastases in rats. When the Walker 256B carcinosarcoma is implanted intraosseously into Wistar–

Lewis rats, pretreatment with clodronate inhibits the development of bone metastases compared with controls (Krempien, 1994). Shorter intervals between the bisphosphonate therapy and the inoculation of tumour cells gave the best results, suggesting that, in the human setting, early therapy might give better results. This protective effect diminished with time after inoculation. Low-dose, continuous therapy also provided protection against metastatic growth.

Cell adhesion molecules are likely to be involved in the growth and invasion of breast cancer cells in bone (Yoneda et al., 1994). Van der Pluijm et al. (1996) have demonstrated that the more potent bisphosphonates can inhibit the adhesion of breast cancer cells to neonatal murine bone matrices (cortical bone slices and trabecular bone cryostat sections), although no effect was seen with etidronate or clodronate in this system. This antiadhesion effect has been confirmed by Boissier et al. (1997), who examined both prostate and breast cancer cells. No direct cytotoxicity on tumour cells was seen.

These animal studies suggest that it is possible to use bisphosphonates not only as a treatment for skeletal complications of cancer in humans but also as a 'protectant' against the development of metastases in bone. However, the effects of bisphosphonates may last only as long as medication is continued or for a few months after stopping, unlike chemotherapy which acts by cytotoxicity. Patients with operable breast cancer, although at risk for recurrence in bone, are essentially well women. It seems impractical to ask these patients to continue intravenous medications much past the period of their intravenous chemotherapy. Quite apart from the patient inconvenience, the utilization of resources is considerable. Either an intravenous medication with a long duration of action or a continuous oral medication would be preferred. Oral clodronate, which is reasonably well tolerated, has been the most studied. Another interesting possibility is oral ibandronate, a potent nitrogen-containing bisphosphonate, which seems to be well tolerated at doses of 25–50 mg/day (Coleman et al., 1999).

Trials have shown that bisphosphonates can prevent the accelerated bone loss following the menopause and that this might prevent the development of osteoporosis. Saarto et al. (1997) demonstrated that two years of clodronate therapy reduced bone loss compared with controls in all groups of patients, including those receiving chemotherapy, although the effect was greatest in those women receiving tamoxifen, some of whom gained bone density.

The ideal setting for testing whether bisphosphonates can have a beneficial effect on the rate of development of bone metastases is in the setting of the adjuvant therapy of operable breast cancer. The diagnosis of new bone metastases and differentiation from vertebral osteopenic fractures is manageable in patients who are relatively fit, and the development of metastasis can be correlated with measurements of bone density and other parameters. One interesting trial of adjuvant bisphosphonates has been reported (Diel et al., 1998). In this study, 142 patients with primary breast cancer and no evidence of distant metastases were randomized to receive 1600 mg daily of oral clodronate, and a further 142 were randomized into a non-placebo control group. These patients all had bone marrow involvement (micrometastases), with tumour cells detectable using the technique described by this group (Diel et al., 1996). After a median follow-up of 3 years, 21 patients in the clodronate group had developed distant metastases, compared with 42 patients in the control group. There were 10 patients relapsing in bone, with an average of 3.1 metastases per patient in the clodronate group, compared with 19 patients relapsing in bone, with an average of 6.3 metastases per patient in the control group. The relapse-free interval for bone was 23 months for the clodronate group, compared with 16 months for the control patients. Not only was there a reduction in new bone metastases but there was also a significant reduction in new visceral metastases and a survival advantage in the clodronate-treated group.

In a similarly sized trial, Saarto et al. (1999) showed no benefit for oral clodronate compared to untreated control patients who had operable breast cancer with positive nodes; indeed, in this trial, the rate of development of extraosseous metastases was higher and survival was poorer than in control patients.

In an interim analysis of a larger, randomized placebo-controlled trial, we have been unable to confirm the effect of oral clodronate on the incidence of visceral metastases; there does appear to be an effect, however, on the incidence of bone metastases, at least during the period of medication (Powles et al., 1998). These conflicting data require further assessment in larger placebo-controlled, randomized trials.

Conclusions

The following suggestions are submitted for consideration by physicians treating patients with breast cancer:

(1) Hypercalcaemia: pamidronate intravenously or clodronate intravenously with rehydration as described in the text. Newer, more potent drugs, such as ibandronate or zoledronate may offer some advantages, but are more expensive;

(2) presence of bone metastases (symptomatic or asymptomatic): oral clodronate 1600 mg/day orally or pamidronate 90 mg every 4 weeks i.v.;

(3) bone pain: pamidronate 90 mg i.v. every 4 weeks, clodronate 1500 mg i.v. every 2 weeks;

(4) postchemotherapy bone loss: oral clodronate 1600 mg/day orally if, on bone

densitometry, the T-score is > 2.5, annual rate of bone loss $> 10\%$, or fragility fractures are documented;

(5) operable breast cancer: further controlled trials are required, preferably with oral bisphosphonates.

REFERENCES

Adamson, B.B., Gallacher, S.J., Byars, J. et al. (1993). Mineralization defects with pamidronate therapy for Paget's disease. *Lancet*, 342, 1459–60.

Batson, O.V. (1940). The function of the vertebral veins and their role in the spread of metastases. *Annals of Surgery*, 112, 138.

Berruti, A., Sperone, P., Fasolis, G. et al. (1997). Pamidronate administration improves the secondary hyperparathyroidism due to 'bone hunger syndrome' in a patient with osteoblastic metastases from prostate cancer. *Prostate*, 1, 252–5.

Body, J.J., Bartl, R., Burckhardt, P. et al. (1998). Current use of bisphosphonates in oncology. International Bone and Cancer Study Group. *Journal of Clinical Oncology*, 16(12), 3890–9.

Body, J.J. & Delmas, P.D. (1992). Urinary pyridinium cross-links as markers of bone resorption in tumour-associated hypercalcemia. *Journal of Clinical Endocrinology and Metabolism*, 74, 471–5.

Boissier, S., Magnetto, S., Frappart, L. et al. (1997). Bisphosphonates inhibit prostate and breast cancer cell adhesion to unmineralized and mineralized bone extracellular matrices. *Cancer Research*, 57, 3890–4.

Coleman, R.E., Houston, S., Purohit, O.P. et al. (1998). A randomized Phase II evaluation of oral pamidronate for advanced bone metastases from breast cancer. *European Journal of Cancer*, 34, 820–4.

Coleman, R.E., Purohit, O.P., Black, C. et al. (1999). Double-blind, randomised, placebo-controlled, dose-finding study of oral ibandronate in patients with metastatic bone disease. *Annals of Oncology*, 10(3), 311–16.

Coleman, R.E., Woll, P.J., Miles, M. et al. (1988). Treatment of bone metastases from breast cancer with (3-amino-1-hydroxy-propylidene)-1, 1-bisphosphonate (APD). *British Journal of Cancer*, 58, 621–5.

Conte, P.F., Latreillie, J., Mauriac, L. et al. (1996). Delay in progression of bone metastases in breast cancer patients treated with intravenous pamidronate: results from a multinational randomised controlled trial. *Journal of Clinical Oncology*, 14, 2552–9.

Delmas, P.D., Balena, R. & Confraveux, E. (1997). The bisphosphonate residronate prevents bone loss in women with artificial menopause due to chemotherapy of breast cancer: a double-blind, placebo-controlled study. *Journal of Clinical Oncology*, 15, 955–62.

Diel, I.J., Kaufmann, M., Costa, S.D. et al. (1996). Micrometastatic breast cancer cells in bone marrow at primary surgery: prognostic value in comparison with nodal status. *Journal of the National Cancer Institute*, 88, 1652–8.

Diel, I.J., Solomayer, E.F., Costa, S.D. et al. (1998). Reduction in new metastases in breast cancer with adjuvant clodronate treatment. *New England Journal of Medicine*, 339(6), 357–63.

Elomaa, I., Blomqvist, C., Porrka, L. et al. (1987). Treatment of skeletal disease in breast cancer: a controlled clinical trial. *Bone*, 8 (Suppl. 1), S53–S56.

Ernst, D.S. (1997). Role of bisphosphonates and other bone resorption inhibitors in metastatic bone pain. *Topics in Palliative Care*, 3, 117–37.

Ernst, D.S., Brasher, P., Hagen, N.A. et al. (1997). A randomised, controlled trial of intravenous clodronate in patients with metastatic bone disease and pain. *Journal of Pain and Symptom Management*, 13, 319–26.

Ernst, D.S., MacDonald, N., Paterson, A.H.G. et al. (1992). A double-blind cross-over trial of intravenous clodronate in metastatic bone pain. *Journal of Pain and Symptom Management*, 7, 4–11.

Ferreira, S.H. (1983). Prostaglandins: peripheral and central analgesia. *Advances in Pain Research and Therapy*, 5, 627–34.

Fisher, B., Constantino, J., Redmond, C. et al. (1989). A randomised clinical trial evaluating tamoxifen in the treatment of patients with node-negative breast cancer who have oestrogen receptor-positive tumours. *New England Journal of Medicine*, 320, 479–84.

Fleisch, H. (2000). *Bisphosphonates in bone disease – from the laboratory to the patient.* 4th edn. San Diego and London: Academic Press.

Goldhirsch, A., Gelber, R.D., Price, K.N. et al. (1994). Effect of systemic adjuvant treatment on first sites of breast cancer relapse. *Lancet*, 343, 377–81.

Grill, V., Ho, P., Body, J.J. et al. (1991). Parathyroid hormone-related protein: elevated levels in both humoral hypercalcemia of malignancy and hypercalcemia complicating metastatic breast cancer. *Journal of Clinical Endocrinology and Metabolism*, 73, 1309–15.

Hortobagyi, G.N., Theriault, R.L., Porter, L. et al. (1996). Efficacy of pamidronate in reducing skeletal complications in patients with breast cancer and lytic bone metastases. *New England Journal of Medicine*, 335, 1785–91.

Hughes, D.E., Wright, K.R., Uy, H.L. et al. (1995). Bisphosphonates promote apoptosis in murine osteoclasts in vitro and in vivo. *Journal of Bone and Mineral Research*, 10, 1478–87.

Kamenor, B., Kieran, M.W., Barrington-Leigh, J. et al. (1984). Homing receptors as functional markers for classification, prognosis, and therapy of leukemia and lymphomas. *Proceedings of the Society of Experimental Biology and Medicine*, 177, 211–19.

Kanis, J.A. & McCloskey, E.V. (1997). Bone turnover and biochemical markers in malignancy. *Cancer*, 80 (Suppl. 8), 1538–45.

Kanis, J.A., McCloskey, E.V., Powles, T. et al. (1999). A high incidence of vertebral fractures in women with breast cancer. *British Journal of Cancer*, 79 (7–8), 1179–81.

Kanis, J.A., Percival, R.C., Yates, A.J.P. et al. (1986). Effects of diphosphonates in hypercalcemia due to neoplasia. *Lancet*, i, 615–16.

Kanis, J.A., Powles, T., Paterson, A.H.G. et al. (1996). Clodronate and skeletal metastases. *Bone*, 19, 663–7.

Kanis, J.A., Urwin, G.H., Gray, R.E.S. et al. (1984). Effects of intravenous etidronate disodium on skeletal and calcium metabolism. *American Journal of Medicine*, 82 (Suppl. 2A), 55.

Kaplan, F.S. (1987). Osteoporosis: Pathophysiology and Prevention. In: *Clinical Symposia No 4.* Ciba-Geigy.

Krempien, B. (1994). Morphological findings in bone metastasis, tumourosteopathy and anti-osteolytic therapy. In *Metastatic Bone Disease. Fundamental and Clinical Aspects* (I.J. Diel, M. Kauffmann & G. Bastert, G., eds), Springer.

Macro, M., Bouvard, G., LeGangneux, E. et al. (1995). Intravenous aminohydroxy-propylidine bisphosphonate does not modify 99m Tc-hydroxy-methylene bisphosphonate bone scintigraphy: a prospective study. *Revue Du Rheumatisme*. English edition, 62, 99–104.

Major, P., Lortholary, A., Hon, J. et al. (2000). Zoledronic acid is superior to pamidronate in the treatment of tumor-induced hypercalcemia: a pooled analysis. *Proceedings of the American Society of Clinical Oncology*, 19, Abstract 2382.

McCloskey, E.V., Spector, T.D., Eyres, K.S. et al. (1993). The assessment of vertebral deformity: a method for use in population studies and clinical trials. *Osteoporosis International*, 3, 138–47.

Monkkonen, H., Moilanen, P., Monkkonen, J. et al. (2000). Analysis of adenine nucleotide-containing metabolite of clodronate using ion pair high-performance liquid chromatography-electrospray ionisation mass spectrometry. *Journal of Chromatography B Biomedical Sciences and Applications*, 11, 738(2), 395–403.

Mundy, G.R. (1987). Bone resorption and turnover in health and disease. *Bone*, 8 (Suppl. 1), S9–16.

Mundy, G.R. (1988). Hypercalcemia of malignancy revisited. *Journal of Clinical Investigation*, 82, 1–6.

Mundy, G.R. (1997). Mechanisms of bone metastasis. *Cancer*, 80 (Suppl. 8), 1546–56.

Mundy, G.R., Ibbotson, K.J., DeSouza, S.M. et al. (1984). The hypercalcemia of cancer: clinical implication and pathogenic mechanisms. *New England Journal of Medicine*, 310, 1718.

Nishikawa, M., Akatsu, T., Katayama, Y. et al. (1996). Bisphosphonates act on osteoblastic cells and inhibit osteoclast formation in mouse marrow cultures. *Bone*, 18, 9–14.

Paget, J. (1889). The distribution of secondary growths in cancer of the breast. *Lancet*, i, 571–3.

Paterson, A.H.G. (1987). Natural history of skeletal complications of breast cancer, prostate cancer and myeloma. *Bone*, 8 (Suppl. 1), S17–S22.

Paterson, A.H.G., Powles, T.J., Kanis, J.A. et al. (1993). Double-blind controlled trail of oral clodronate in patients with bone metastases from breast cancer. *Journal of Clinical Oncology*, 11, 59–65.

Pecherstorfer, M., Schilling, T., Janisch, S. et al. (1993). Effect of clodronate treatment on bone scintigraphy in metastatic breast cancer. *Journal of Nuclear Medicine*, 34, 1039–44.

Powles, T.J., McCloskey, E., Paterson, A.H.G. et al. (1997). Oral clodronate will reduce the loss of bone mineral density in women with primary breast cancer. *American Society of Clinical Oncology*, 16, 460, Abstract.

Powles, T.J., Muindi, J. & Coombes, C. (1982). Mechanisms for development of bone metastases and effects of anti-inflammatory drugs. In: *Prostaglandins and Cancer: First International Conference* (T.J. Powles, ed.). Alan R. Liss, 541–3.

Powles, T.J., Paterson, A.H.G., Navantaus, A. et al. (1998). Adjuvant clodronate reduces the incidence of bone metastases in patients with operable primary breast cancer. *Proceedings of ASCO*, 17, 468, Abstract.

Purohit, O.P., Radstone, C.R., Anthony, C. et al. (1995). A randomised double-blind comparison of intravenous pamidronate and clodronate in the hypercalcemia of malignancy. *British*

Journal of Cancer, 72, 1289–93.

Ralston, S.H., Thiebaud, D., Hermann, Z. et al. (1997). Dose response study of ibandronate in the treatment of cancer associated hypercalcemia. *British Journal of Cancer*, 75(2), 295–300.

Rogers, M.J., Chilton, K.M., Coxon, F.P. et al. (1996). Bisphosphonates induce apoptosis in mouse macrophage-like cells in vitro by a nitric oxide independent mechanism. *Journal of Bone and Mineral Research*, 11, 1482–91.

Rogers, M.J., Gordon, S., Benford, H.L. et al. (2000). Cellular and molecular mechanisms of action of bisphosphonates. *Cancer*, 88 (S12), 2961–78.

Ryzon, B., Martodam, R.R., Troxell, M. et al. (1985). Intravenous etidronate in the management of malignant hypercalcemia. *Archives of Internal Medicine*, 145, 449–52.

Saarto, T., Blomqvist, C., Valimaki, M. et al. (1997). Chemical castration induced by adjuvant cyclophosphamide, methotrexate and fluorouracil chemotherapy causes rapid bone loss that is reduced by clodronate: a randomised study in premenopausal breast cancer patients. *Journal of Clinical Oncology*, 15, 1341–7.

Saarto, T., Blomqvist, C., Virkkunen, P. et al. (1999). No reduction of bone metastases with adjuvant clodronate treatment in node-positive breast cancer patients. *Proceedings of the American Society of Clinical Oncology*, 18, Abstract 489.

Sahni, M., Guenther, H.L., Fleisch, H. et al. (1993). Bisphosphonates act on rat bone resorption through the mediation of osteoblasts. *Journal of Clinical Investigation*, 91, 2004–11.

Selander, K.S., Monkkonen, J., Karhukorpi, E.K. et al. (1996). Characteristics of clodronate-induced apoptosis in osteoclasts and macrophages. *Molecular Pharmacology*, 50, 1127–38.

Shipman, C.M., Rogers, M.J., Apperley, J.F. et al. (1997). Bisphosphonates induce apoptosis in human myeloma cell lines: a novel anti-tumour activity. *British Journal of Haematology*, 98, 665–72.

Singer, F.R., Ritch, P.S., Lad, T.E. et al. for the Hypercalcemia Study Group (1991). Treatment of hypercalcemia of malignancy with intravenous etidronate. A controlled, multicenter study. *Archives of Internal Medicine*, 151, 471–6.

Siwek, B., Lacroix, M., DePollak, C. et al. (1997). Secretory products of breast cancer cells specifically affect human osteoblastic cells: partial characterization of active factors. *Journal of Bone and Mineral Research*, 12, 552–60.

Smith, R., Jiping, W., Bryant, J. et al. (1999). Primary Breast Cancer (PBC) as a risk factor for bone recurrence (BR): NSABP experience. *Proceedings of the American Society of Clinical Oncology*, 18, Abstract 457.

Taube, T., Elomaa, I., Blomqvist, C. et al. (1993). Comparative effects of clodronate and calcitonin in metastatic breast cancer. *European Journal of Clinical Oncology*, 29, 1677–81.

Taube, T., Elomaa, I., Blomqvist, C. et al. (1994). Histomorphometric evidence for osteoclast medicated bone resorption in metastatic breast cancer. *Bone*, 15(2), 1616.

Turken, S., Siris, E., Seldin, D. et al. (1989). Effects of tamoxifen on spinal bone density in women with breast cancer. *Journal of the National Cancer Institute*, 81, 1086–8.

van der Pluijm, G., Vloedgraven, H., van Beek, E. et al. (1996). Bisphosphonates inhibit the adhesion of breast cancer cells to bone matrices in vitro. *Journal of Clinical Investigation*, 98, 698–705.

van Holten-Verzanvoort, A.T., Bijvoet, O.L., Cleton, F.J. et al. (1987). Reduced morbidity from skeletal metastases in breast cancer patients during long-term bisphosphonates (APD) treatment. *Lancet*, 11, 983–5.

van Holten-Verzanvoort, A.T., Hermans, J., Beex, L.F. et al. (1996). Does supportive pamidronate treatment prevent or delay the first manifestations of bone metastases in breast cancer patients? *European Journal of Cancer*, 32a, 450–4.

van Holten-Verzanvoort, A.T., Zwinderman, A.H., Aaranson, N.K. et al. (1991). The effect of supportive pamidronate treatment on aspects of quality of life of patients with advanced breast cancer. *European Journal of Cancer*, 27, 544–9.

Wronski, T.J., Dann, L.M., Qi, H. et al. (1993). Skeletal effects of withdrawal of oestrogen and diphosphonate treatment in ovariectomised rats. *Calcified Tissue International*, 53, 210–16.

Yoneda, T., Sasaki, A. & Mundy, G. (1994). Osteolytic bone metastasis in breast cancer. *Breast Cancer Research and Treatment*, 32, 72–84.

14

Palliative care in breast cancer

Janet Hardy

The Royal Marsden Hospital, Downs Road, Sutton, Surrey

Introduction

Chemotherapy and radiotherapy are probably the most effective means of palliation in metastatic breast cancer, but inevitably there will come a time when these modalities are no longer appropriate or possible to deliver. The emphasis must then be on pain and symptom control with the aim of maximizing quality of life.

Metastatic breast cancer is a chronic disease of relapse and recurrence, almost invariably ending in death. Although symptom care or palliative care tends to be positioned at the end of any schema documenting the management of advanced breast disease, this input should be available from the start, throughout the disease course and not just in the terminal phase. It is important that the transition from active anticancer treatment to palliative care is seamless for both the patient and her family (Royal College of Radiologists Clinical Information Network, 1999) (Figure 14.1). Moreover, the ideal palliative care model is interdisciplinary whereby the identity of the team is more important than the individuals in it. This is in contrast to the more traditional medical multidisciplinary team where the individuals are known more by their personal expertise and secondarily by their team affiliation (Cummings, 1998).

This chapter deals with the management of the common symptoms in women with metastatic breast cancer. These symptoms can often be directly related to the characteristic patterns of disease spread. Wherever possible, data has been taken from recent reviews or controlled studies. There is a paucity of evidence in palliative care however (Higginson, 1999), and much of the practice is based on personal experience and anecdotal evidence.

Pain

Uncontrolled pain is no longer something that needs to be feared as an inevitable consequence of cancer. It is still the most common symptom of advanced disease,

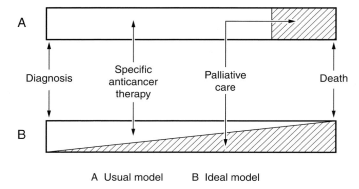

A Usual model   B Ideal model

Figure 41.1 Models for the place of palliative care in cancer care

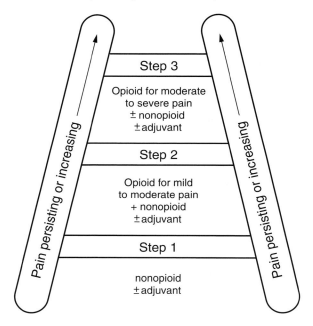

Figure 14.2 WHO analgesic ladder
Source: WHO 1996

however, and there is evidence that it is still poorly managed in many cases (NHS Executive, 1997). This is due not only to a reluctance on the part of many doctors to use strong analgesics but often because of a reluctance on the part of patients to accept them.

Pain control in cancer has been addressed as a major issue by the World Health Organization (WHO) and an international schema for pain control has been widely publicized in the form of the WHO analgesic ladder (Figure 14.2) (WHO,

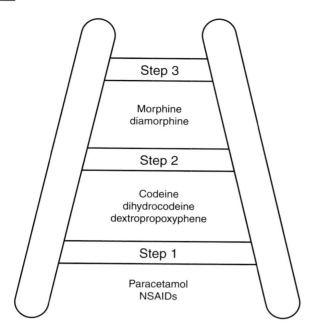

Figure 14.3   Drugs commonly used at each step of the WHO analgesic ladder

1996). It has been said that nothing would contribute more to pain relief world-wide than the dissemination of current knowledge. Although there has been some controversy in recent times regarding the WHO analgesic ladder and concern that its effectiveness in controlling pain has not been definitively proven (Jadad & Browman, 1995), it remains the 'gold standard' for the treatment of chronic cancer pain. In everyday practice, this schema provides a simple, easy-to-use, straightforward plan for pain management and requires an in-depth knowledge of relatively few drugs. The ladder has been revised (WHO, 1996) but the basic principles still apply, i.e. that analgesia should be given 'by mouth', 'by the clock', 'by the ladder', 'for the individual' and with 'attention to detail'.

The ladder defines different steps for mild, moderate and severe pain as shown in Figure 14.2. The drugs commonly used at each step are shown in Figure 14.3. At each step on the ladder, if complete pain control has not been achieved, coanal-gesics can be used according to the aetiology of the pain (Table 14.1).

Paracetamol and aspirin have until recently been the drugs of choice at step 1. Paracetamol is an effective drug, without significant side-effects and is quite safe when used at the recommended doses. Aspirin is usually avoided in cancer patients because of its gut toxicity and antithrombotic platelet effects. Non-steroidal anti-inflammatory drugs (NSAIDs) are now also classed as step 1 analgesics. They have proven efficacy in cancer pain (Eisenberg et al., 1994).

Table 14.1. Coanalgesics commonly used in cancer pain

Indication	Appropriate agents	Comments
(1) Neuropathic pain	Antidepressants e.g. amitriptyline, dothiepin	Analgesic effect via increased levels of serotonin in spinal cord. Recommended for dysaesthetic, aching neuropathic pain
	Anticonvulsants e.g. sodium valproate, carbamazepine, gabapentin	Analgesic effect via stabilization of neuronal membrane. Recommended for shooting, lancinating pain
	Anti-arrhythmics e.g. flecainide, mexiletine	Membrane stabilizers, usually used '3rd line'
	Corticosteroids	Reduce perineuronal oedema
	NMDA receptor antagonists e.g. methadone, ketamine	Specialist advice re use should be sought
(2) Bone pain	NSAIDs[a]	Anti-inflammatory action via inhibition of prostaglandin synthesis
	Bisphosphonates	Potent inhibitors of oesteoclast-mediated bone resorption
(3) Soft tissue inflammation	NSAIDs[a] Corticosteroids Antibiotics	Useful for inflammatory breast tumours
(4) Muscle spasm	Benzodiazepines	Added anxiolytic effect
	Baclofen	Can be sedative
(5) Intestinal colic	Hyoscine butylbromide	Antimuscarinic, antispasmodic and antisecretary

[a]WHO step 1 analgesic.

Anecdotally, they are particularly useful in bone pain although there is a lack of comparative studies demonstrating this. The evidence to support the use of NSAIDs is shown in Table 14.2. No single-dose study has shown an advantage of one NSAID over another. NSAID-induced analgesia has a trend to be dose dependent up to a ceiling. The side-effects (predominately gastric and renal toxicity) also have a dose-response relationship but with no ceiling. The incidence of side-effects increases with chronic use (Eisenberg et al., 1994). Meta-analysis has shown NSAIDs to be as effective if not better than paracetamol on a 'number needed to treat to get an effect' basis (NNT) and appear to be more effective than several of the weak opioids traditionally used either alone or in combination at

Table 14.2. NSAIDs – the evidence

- NSAIDs alone produce as good analgesia as single or multiple doses of weak opioids alone or in combination with nonopioid analgesics
- no single dose trial has shown any efficacy advantage of one NSAID over another
- the risk of NSAID-induced gastric bleeding is lowest with ibuprofen and increases with increasing age
- prophylactic misoprostol should be considered for preventing GI complications for high-risk patients (age > 75 years, history of peptic ulceration or GI bleeding)
- increasing doses above those recommended are more likely to increase adverse effects than to improve analgesia

McQuay & Moore, 1998.

step 2 of the analgesic ladder (Eisenberg et al., 1994; McQuay & Moore, 1998). Their mechanism of action is by the inhibition of prostaglandin synthesis via inhibition of the cyclo-oxygenase enzymes COX1 and COX2. Activation of COX1 forms prostaglandins that are protective to the gut and kidneys; COX2 is activated by inflammatory stimuli and produces prostaglandins that contribute to the pain and swelling of inflammation. The development of selective COX2 inhibitors may well be a major advance if the therapeutic effectiveness of these drugs can be maintained in the absence of COX1 type side-effects (Hawkey, 1999).

Step 2 opioids are those used for mild to moderate pain (previously known as 'weak' opioids). Those used most commonly at this step include codeine, dihydrocodeine and dextropropoxyphene. All are available as compound preparations (e.g. coproxamol and co-codamol 30/500) that contain adequate doses of the component drugs. Some combination preparations contain subtherapeutic doses of opioids (e.g. co-codamol 8/500) and should be avoided.

Step 3 opioids ('strong' opioids) are those used for severe pain. Morphine remains the opioid of choice at this level. When used correctly, it is a particularly useful, generally well-tolerated analgesic. Morphine is now available in a wide range of different formulations and dose sizes (Table 14.3). Advice on the correct use of morphine is given in Table 14.4 (European Association of Palliative Care, 1996). The correct use of morphine depends on the active and anticipatory treatment of its side-effects (Table 14.5). The initial drowsiness and light-headedness seen in many patients for the first few days is usually transitory, as is the associated nausea and vomiting. Patients never become tolerant to the constipating effects of opioids (Sykes, 1998). They must always be informed of this and provided with appropriate aperients.

There is no upper dose limit for morphine. The correct dose is that which controls the pain. Therefore, there is no logic in leaving morphine until 'the pain

Table 14.3. Commonly used morphine formulations

Immediate release oral preparations:

Duration of action 4 hours

• Morphine sulphate oral solution	• 10 mg/5 ml (taste mask)
• Concentrated oral morphine sulphate solution	• 100 mg/5 ml (no taste mask)
• Morphine sulphate unit dose vials	• 10 mg/5 ml, 30 mg/5 ml, 100 mg/5 ml
• Morphine tablets (Sevredol[R])	• 10 mg, 20 mg and 50 mg tablets
• Morphine suppositories	• 10, 15, 20, 30, 50, 100 mg

Delayed release oral preparations:

a. Duration of action 12 hours

• Morphine sulphate controlled release tablets	• 5, 10, 30, 60, 100 & 200 mg strength
e.g. MST Continus[R]	• 5, 10, 30, 60, 100 & 200 mg
Oramorph SR[R]	• 10, 30, 60, 100 mg
• Morphine sulphate controlled release capsules	
Morcap SR[R]	• 20, 50, 100 mg
Zomorph[R]	• 10, 30, 60, 100 & 200 mg
• Morphine sulphate slow release suspension	• 20, 30, 60, 100 & 200 mg (sachet of granules to mix with water)

b. Duration of action 24 hours

• Morphine sulphate controlled release capsules	• 30, 60, 90, 120, 150 & 200 mg
e.g. MXL[R]	
Morcap SR[R]	
• *Morphine sulphate injection*	10, 15, 20 & 30 mg/ml

gets really bad'. Similarly, it is always important to reassure a patient that starting on morphine does not imply that death is near. Morphine may even prolong survival if improved pain control results in greater activity with a reduced likelihood of venous thrombosis and infection, for example. Unfounded fears about morphine abound (Table 14.6). Many patients will require reassurance that morphine is not addictive and that the side-effects can be controlled. Many doctors will need reassurance that morphine when used correctly for patients in pain does not cause respiratory depression (Borgbjerg et al., 1996) and that when on a stable dose of morphine, patients may lead a near normal, fully active life. Driving ability in cancer patients receiving long-term morphine analgesia is not impaired (Vainio et al., 1995).

Morphine toxicity, characterized by drowsiness, miosis, confusion, hallucinations and myoclonic jerks is seen when the dose is escalated too quickly, or to too high a dose. As the major active metabolite of morphine (morphine-6-glucuronide) is excreted via the kidneys, the sudden development of toxicity in a previously

Table 14.4. Recommendations for the use of morphine for cancer pain

(1) The optimal route of administration of morphine is by mouth, either using immediate release (IR) or controlled release (CR)

(2) Commence titration with low dose of immediate release morphine, given every 4 hours with the same dose available for breakthrough pain

(3) The regular 4 hourly dose can be adjusted according to how many breakthrough doses are given

(4) Once the pain is controlled, convert to once or twice daily slow release morphine preparations

(5) After conversion to delayed release preparations, continue to supply appropriate breakthrough doses equivalent to the 4 hourly dose in an immediate release preparation

(6) Always prescribe a laxative to be taken concurrently; ensure that outpatients have a supply of antiemetics in case of opioid induced nausea

(7) Reassure that most of the initial side-effects e.g. drowsiness, light-headedness and nausea will pass

(8) Ensure appropriate patient review

From Royal Marsden Hospital NHS Trust Symptom Control Guidelines, 2000.

well-controlled patient suggests the presence of renal impairment (Faura et al., 1998).

There is now a wide range of 'alternate opioids' available, not only for use in those truly intolerant to morphine, but also as a theoretical means of improving pain control. The practice of 'opioid rotation' (changing the drug or the route of administration) has become popular (McQuay, 1999). The aim is not only to improve pain control but to reduce side-effects. The most simplistic explanation for this is that by switching to a new opioid, the toxic metabolites of the previous opioid are dispersed before the metabolites of the second opioid accumulate (de Stoutz et al., 1995). If the adverse effect is mediated via opioid receptors, however, it is difficult to see how similar effects would not occur with equianalgesic doses of different opioids acting at the same receptor (McQuay, 1999). The true benefit of such opioid rotation awaits further study. Some of the alternative opioids available in the UK are shown in Table 14.7 along with their potential benefits and limitations.

Special pain situations in breast cancer

Bone metastases (Figure 14.4)

The presence of bone metastases has been found to be the most common cause of cancer related pain (Twycross & Fairfield, 1982) and up to 85% of patients dying from breast cancer have evidence of bone involvement at postmortem (Nielsen et

Table 14.5. Opioid side-effects

Side-effect	Frequency	Action
(1) Constipation	Almost inevitable and tolerance does not develop	Always prescribe laxative concurrently when prescribing opioids
(2) Nausea and vomiting	Occurs in about 50% of patients started on morphine, but resolves in most	Ensure the availability of antiemetics and if fails to resolve, consider opioid rotation
(3) Drowsiness and unsteadiness	Common initial side-effects	Reassurance unless persistent, generally resolves within 2–3 days
(4) Dry mouth	Occasional	Encourage fluids, give artifical saliva spray and salivary stimulants plus diligent mouth care
(5) Pruritis	Rare, associated with intradermal histamine release	Antihistamines, anecdotal reports of benefit from $5HT_3$ antagonists, consider opioid rotation
(6) Sweating	Occasional	Anecdotal reports of benefit from low-dose thioridazine
(7) Hallucinations	Rare	If not associated with toxic doses, consider opioid rotation
(8) Myoclonus	Occasional	Reassure as to cause, check dose
(9) Miosis, frequent myoclonus and respiratory depression	Rare, evidence of toxicity	Check renal function, decrease dose or omit a dose, give less frequently in cases of renal impairment

al., 1991). Bone is the most common metastatic site in breast cancer and bone metastases are usually widespread by the time of first presentation. Women with bone metastases as their sole metastatic site are likely to live for a number of years (4-year median survival) and will require active palliation of their symptoms throughout their disease course.

The relationship between bone invasion and bone pain is unclear. Patients may

Table 14.6. Morphine – unfounded fears

Effect/fear	Comment
(1) Respiratory depression	Strong opioids do not cause clinically important respiratory depression in patients with pain when used correctly (Borgbjerg et al., 1996)
(2) Excessive drowsiness, sedation	Unlikely, as patients will probably have been on weak opioids already, and take oral medication with slow titration upwards to effective dose
(3) Impaired performance	Unusual when on a stable dose. Driving ability not impaired (Vainio et al., 1995)
(4) Addiction	Encompasses physical and psychological dependence; this is not a problem in cancer patients both from extensive clinical experience and the success of complete withdrawal in patients who no longer have pain (e.g. following a nerve block)

have multiple sites of bone metastases without related bone pain or pain from some sites but not others. The main mechanism of bone pain from small metastases is probably stimulation of nerve endings in the endosteum by chemical agents released from the destroyed bone tissue. Stretching of the periosteum probably contributes to the pain when the metastases enlarge (Nielsen et al., 1991).

Radiotherapy provides a very effective local treatment for painful bone metastases, giving response rates approaching 80% (Nielsen et al., 1991). Several studies have shown that there is no advantage of multiple fractions over a single dose of 8 GY (Bone Pain Trial Working Party, 1999). There is no difference with respect to onset or duration of pain relief, incidence or degree of pain relief or acute or late toxicity. There is also the potential for retreatment.

Bisphosphonates are potent inhibitors of normal and pathological bone resorption with a complex mechanism of action that is not fully understood (Body et al., 1998). Current evidence does suggest that these agents, especially pamidronate, have an analgesic effect as well as a positive effect on the reduction in morbidity of skeletal events (e.g. pathological fractures, bone pain requiring radiotherapy and hypercalcaemia) (Fulfaro et al., 1998).

Pooled data of phase 2 studies of pamidronate infusions show relief of pain in more than one-half of patients. Placebo-controlled trials of both pamidronate and

Table 14.7. 'Alternative' strong opioids

Drug	Comments
Diamorphine	• greater solubility than morphine allows injection of smaller volumes • drug of choice for subcutaneous strong opioid infusion at one third oral dose
Phenazocine	• often better tolerated in the elderly, can be given sublingually; dose limited by number of tablets (5 mg tablets only available), given 6–8 hourly • 5 mg phenazocine is equivalent to about 20–50 mg morphine po
Fentanyl Transdermal Patch	• skin patch changed every 3 days • ?less constipating than morphine • not suitable for dose titration in unstable pain • useful for patients unable to take oral medications
Methadone	• long half life • unique dosing schedule • toxic metabolites can accumulate with prolonged use • can be useful for control of neuropathic pain
Oxycodone	• synthetic opioid available in both oral and pr formulations
Hydromorphone	• analogue of morphine with similar pharmacokinetic properties • widely used in the USA
Tramadol	• opioid and nonopioid analgesia by enhancement of serotoninergic and adrenergic pathways; therefore fewer opioid side-effects • usually classed as a 'step 2' opioid
Pethidine	• less intense action at smooth muscle compared with morphine plus additional anticholinergic effects, toxic metabolites accumulate with prolonged use • short duration of action, not recommended for chronic pain
Dextramoramide	• short half-life, duration of action 1–2 hours, unsuitable for regular analgesia in chronic pain but can be useful for breakthrough analgesia

clodronate infusions have confirmed the analgesic effect (Body et al., 1998). Responding patients also showed an improvement in quality of life. Optimal doses and schedules have still to be determined but 60–90 mg pamidronate 3–4 weekly or 1500 mg clodronate fortnightly can be recommended for the palliation of bone

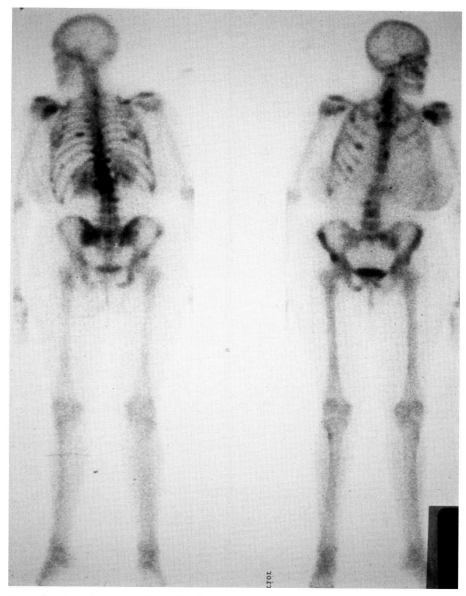

Figure 14.4   Bone showing widespreaad bone involvement

pain. Oral bisphosphonates are probably less effective but are much more con-
venient for many patients despite the low oral availability and the dietary restric-
tions (patients are advised to take the tablets on an empty stomach at least one
hour before eating). On the other hand, many women appreciate the close review

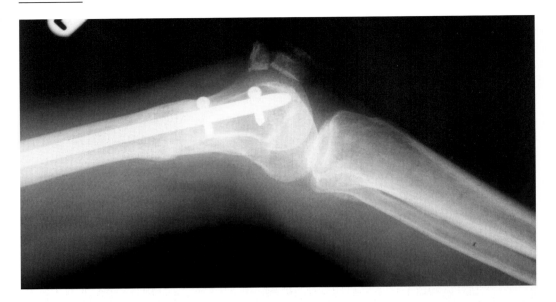

Figure 14.5 Fracture of the femur that has been pinned

inherent in attending monthly or fortnightly for intravenous therapy. It is also unclear when to start and when to stop bisphosphonate therapy. It is our practice to 'load' with intravenous therapy and to assess effectiveness before converting to oral medication. This practice is not based on any scientific evidence, however. The drugs are generally well tolerated, apart from occasional gastrointestinal effects and even cost-effective if their effect on the reduction in hospitalization secondary to reduced skeletal complications is taken into account (Bierman et al., 1991). This is also discussed in Chapters 11 and 13.

Pathological fractures (Figure 14.5)

Pathological fractures, most commonly involving the proximal femur and humeri, are not uncommon in breast cancer. Once 50% of bone cortex is destroyed by a lytic metastasis, fracture should be regarded as inevitable (British Association of Surgical Oncology (BASO), 1999) and prophylactic fixation should be undertaken. The aim of treatment is palliation, i.e. the relief of pain, and it is very difficult to achieve this without bone stabilization.

Incident pain (Figure 14.6)

This is a descriptive term for pain that occurs only on movement, e.g. pain from a lytic metastasis in the femur felt only when walking. This type of pain is difficult to control especially when pain control at rest is satisfactory. While a level of background analgesia will be necessary, short-acting opioids (e.g. immediate

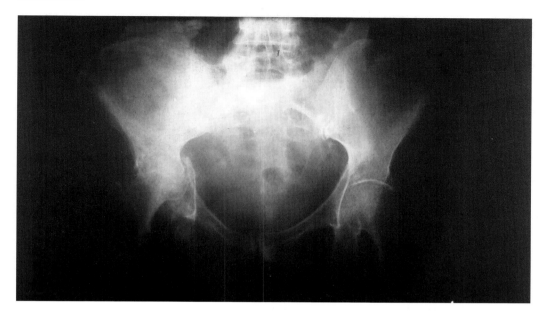

Figure 14.6 Pathological fracture of the acetabulum with upward displacement of the femoral head

release morphine or dextromoramide (Palfium)) given just prior to and/or post an anticipated activity will aid mobilization.

Liver capsular pain

Hepatomegaly or expanding intrahepatic metastases will produce pain in the right upper quadrant of the abdomen and occasionally in the back or mid-flank. The pain is generally described as dull and aching and is commonly associated with nausea and anorexia. The pain originates from stretching of the liver capsule or from compression or distension of vessels in the biliary tract. This pain generally responds to routine analgesia and there is evidence to support the use of NSAIDs in visceral pain such as this (Mercadente et al., 1999). A bleed into a hepatic metastases can result in sudden intense pain in the right subcostal area which does tend to resolve with time.

Neuropathic pain

Neuropathic pain from a brachial plexopathy secondary to either treatment or disease is unfortunately a not uncommon complication of breast cancer and one which can be very difficult to treat. This pain is often described as an aching burning unpleasant sensation which can occasionally be shooting or lancinating and associated with weakness and/or sensory changes (either hyper-aesthesia or sensory loss). It is seen not only with brachial plexopathies but is characteristic of any pain secondary to nerve damage, compression or infiltration.

Although standard analgesia according to the WHO guidelines provides the basis of pain control in this situation, there is some controversy surrounding the use of opioids for neuropathic pain. Some believe it to be completely opioid-insensitive (i.e. does not respond progressively to increasing opioid doses), where-as others believe it to be relatively insensitive (i.e. the dose-response curve is shifted to the right such that if high enough doses could be given, analgesia would be achieved) (McQuay, 1999). The problem with the latter is that the doses required are likely to be associated with unacceptable dose-related side-effects. The usual practice is therefore to use coanalgesics at a relatively early stage (Table 14.1). Coanalgesics or adjuvant analgesics are drugs which have relatively little analgesic activity in their own right but when used in conjunction with standard analgesics can add to the overall analgesic effect. The adjuvants used most commonly for neuropathic pain are the tricyclic antidepressants and/or anticon-vulsants. Despite widespread use, there is very little evidence to support the use of either class of drug in cancer-related neuropathic pain although anecdotal reports of their benefit abound.

Randomized studies against placebo have proven the analgesic effectiveness of anticonvulsants in *non-cancer* nerve pain but there are no trials comparing different anticonvulsants (McQuay & Moore, 1998). Sodium valproate is generally preferred over carbamazepine as it is perceived to have fewer side-effects. Gab-apentin is popular with some and has proven efficacy in diabetic neuropathy (Backonja et al., 1998) although its superiority over placebo has not been shown to be greater than that of other agents.

The tricyclic antidepressants have proven benefit in non-cancer-related nerve pain, with an efficacy similar to that of the anticonvulsants and little evidence of efficacy in cancer-related pain (McQuay et al., 1996). There is no evidence to date to support the use of the selective serotonin re-uptake inhibitors for the treatment of neuropathic pain.

All of these agents have significant side-effects and contraindications for use that must be taken into consideration when prescribing. Second-line management of neuropathic pain with agents such as the N-methyl-D-aspartic acid (NMDA) receptor antagonists (e.g. ketamine), antiarrhythmics (e.g. flecainide and mexilitene) and methadone is complex and potentially hazardous. The input of a pain or palliative care specialist is recommended. In the short term, steroids can have a dramatic effect on neuropathic pain, presumably by reducing the amount of tumour-associated oedema. Side-effects will generally preclude the chronic use of steroids in neuropathic pain unless they are used as a 'holding measure' until treatment of underlying disease causing the pain can be instigated (e.g. whilst awaiting radiotherapy for recurrent disease in the axilla). Acupuncture, TENS (transcutaneous electrical nerve stimulation), and various anaesthetic nerve blocks may all have additive roles in selected patients.

Headache

Headache in a woman with breast cancer, especially if associated with vomiting, should raise the possibility of brain metastases. Opioids are not contraindicated in this situation. Concerns about the possibility of opioid-induced respiratory depression and hypercapnia leading to reflex vasodilatation and exacerbation of headache are not justified. Opioid analgesia should be maximized to avoid the over use of steroids.

Spiritual pain

The concept of total body pain encompasses the anguish and grief inherent in the pain that a diagnosis of metastatic breast cancer can bring upon a woman. This pain is likely to be exacerbated by fear, anger, depression, misunderstanding and by the presence of other uncontrolled symptoms. Resolution of such issues can contribute greatly to pain relief.

Fatigue

Whereas pain is often quoted as being the most common symptom in cancer, fatigue is often underestimated, despite the fact that it probably is the most common unrelieved symptom of cancer (Stone et al., 1998). Fatigue is a subjective sensation of weakness, lack of energy or becoming easily tired. It is a symptom that cannot be easily measured as it is not always associated with demonstrable decrements in performance. The reported prevalence of fatigue in cancer patients receiving chemotherapy and radiotherapy ranges between 75–96%, and 75–100% respectively, and that in patients with advanced cancer is 33–89%. These reports generally come from uncontrolled studies, however, and do not take into account the high incidence of fatigue in the general population. In a controlled study of patients with locally advanced or metastatic breast cancer, Bruera and colleagues (Bruera et al., 1989) report an incidence of asthenia (defined as physical or mental fatigue/weakness) of 41% when measured against healthy controls. It is thought that fatigue in cancer patients is a result of a combination of physical (e.g. cachexia and weight loss, muscle abnormalities), biochemical, haematological and endocrine abnormalities and psychological causes (depression, personality, stress). When no obvious reversible cause (e.g. hypothyroidism) can be found for fatigue, treatment is difficult. Nondrug treatments include exercise, rest, information giving as well as psychological and behavioural interventions. Corticosteroids are often prescribed for their general beneficial effects in appetite and mood but there is little evidence that they improve fatigue. Other pharmacological treatments which have been evaluated include progestogens, anabolic steroids and psycho-stimulants but none of these agents has a proven role in this condition.

Depression

The incidence of nonorganic psychological morbidity is high in cancer patients and the prevalence increases in the terminal phases of disease (Breitbart et al., 1998). Moreover, depression and a hopelessness/helplessness personality type has recently been shown to be an indicator for poor survival in breast cancer (Watson et al., 1999). It is important, therefore, to identify these women at an early stage, and to have a low threshold for treatment not only to improve the quality of life of women with breast cancer but to optimize length of survival.

New agents for the treatment of depression, such as the selective serotonin re-uptake inhibitors, are less toxic than the tricyclic antidepressants, especially with respect to antimuscarinic and cardiotoxic effects. The sedative effect of drugs such as amitriptyline and dothiepin can be of great advantage in distressed women with insomnia (Kent, 2000).

Nausea

The most common causes of nausea in a woman with breast cancer are treatment (radiotherapy, chemotherapy), other drugs (especially analgesics), liver meta-stases, hypercalcaemia and brain metastases, but very often, no cause can be found. There are a large number of different antiemetics available (Table 14.8), some of which have specific indications (e.g. the 5-HT3 antagonists in radiotherapy or chemotherapy induced nausea and vomiting). Dexamethasone will almost always control the sickness associated with raised intracranial pressure, although side-effects generally preclude its use in the long term (see management of confusion). Similarly, low-dose steroids can provide effective palliation from the nausea and vomiting associated with liver metastases, sometimes for several months. Nausea and vomiting secondary to opioids is likely to settle after the first few days and patients should be informed of this. Haloperidol is the drug used most commonly to control chronic opioid nausea but there is no particular evidence to support this practice. The gastrokinetic agents (metoclopramide, domperidone) should theoretically be of benefit in cases of gastric stasis. Sickness associated with gastric irritation may best be controlled by stopping any nonsteroidal agents and prescribing lansoprazole or an H2 receptor antagonist. Levomepromazine is a phenothiazine closely related to chlor-promazine. It has a broad spectrum of cover as a dopamine antagonist, an anticholinergic, an antihistamine and a 5HT antagonist. It has proven efficacy in

Table 14.8. Nausea and vomiting in a woman with breast cancer

Possible cause	Treatment	Alternative(s)
Treatment (RT or chemotherapy)	5HT$_3$ antagonist e.g. granisetron 1 mg/po/od	Dexamethasone 4 mg/po/bd, Metoclopramide, Domperidone
Hypercalcaemia	i.v. bisphosphonates i.v. hydration	Metoclopramide, Cyclizine, Haloperidol, Levomepromazine
Brain metastases	Dexamethasone 4 mg/bd/po × 5 days (see text)	Cyclizine 50 mg/tds/po, Metoclopramide, Levomepromazine
Liver metastases	Dexamethasone 4 mg/bd/po, then reduce to lowest effective dose	Levomepromazine 6.25 mg/po/od → bd, Haloperidol, Metoclopramide
Drugs	Stop offending agent	Haloperidol 1.5 mg/po/od → bd, Levomepromazine
Gastric irritation	Stop NSAIDs	Lansoprazole 30 mg/od, Misoprostil
Gastric stasis	Metoclopramide 10–20 mg/po/tds → qds	Domperidone 10–20 mg/po/qds
Motion sickness, labyrinthine disorders	Prochlorperazine 5–20 mg/po/tds	Hyoscine e.g. Scopoderm TTS^R

the management of chemotherapy-induced nausea and vomiting and considerable anecdotal benefit in controlling nausea for which no specific cause can be determined, or which has been refractory to other antiemetics (Twycross et al., 1997). Because of its long plasma half-life, once or twice daily dosing is sufficient. The one major side-effect of levomepromazine is sedation; this can be used to advantage however in terminal care when a degree of sedation may be advisable. Most of the commonly used antiemetics can be given by the subcutaneous route for those unable to take food or fluid by mouth because of vomiting.

Dyspnoea

Shortness of breath in cancer patients is not always secondary to cancer. It is important to treat the treatable, e.g. anticoagulation for a pulmonary embolism, utilize bronchodilators for bronchospasm and antibiotics for chest infections. Similarly, cancer-related dyspnoea can often be palliated by such specific measures as draining a pleural effusion (with or without pleurodesis), irradiating a bronchial mass or stenting an obstructed bronchus. In the short term, corticosteroids can dramatically improve the respiratory distress of lymphangitis carcinomatosis. Dexamethasone is used most often in palliative care as it has little mineralocorticoid effect and is therefore less likely to cause fluid retention. Some physicians prefer prednisolone, claiming fewer side-effects in the way of proximal weakness, agitation and sleep disturbance. This needs further study.

The palliation of dyspnoea in patients with advanced disease with no reversible component is more difficult. Breathlessness or dyspnoea has been described as 'an uncomfortable awareness of breathing'. It is often difficult to correlate the sensation of breathlessness with measurable abnormalities. This is a subjective phenomena that encompasses an element of distress. Treatment options have not been as well defined as they have for the palliation of pain.

Standard practice in palliative care is to prescribe small doses of regular oramorph for the control of dyspnoea. There is some evidence to support this practice but the mechanism of action is unknown (Jennings & Broadley, 1999). Similarly, it is not known whether the beneficial effect is dose-related. Despite the recent enthusiasm for palliating dyspnoea with nebulized opioids, a recent systematic review has shown no evidence of effectiveness of opioids when given by this route (Jennings & Broadley, 1999).

Respiratory muscle fatigue is thought to be a contributing factor to dyspnoea (Le Grand & Walsh, 1999) suggesting that the methylxanthines (e.g. theophylline and aminophylline), which have a stimulatory effect on respiratory muscles and the diaphragm, may be of benefit. In practice, the narrow therapeutic range and the high incidence of side-effects, especially in frail patients, limits their potential usefulness.

Anxiety can play a major part in the exacerbation of dyspnoea. Buspirone is a non-benzodiazepam anxiolytic without respiratory depressant effects. Studies of its benefit in dyspnoea are contradictory (Le Grand & Walsh, 1999). Chlorpromazine has been shown to be effective in one study (Le Grand & Walsh, 1999). In practice, most practitioners in the field will use a small dose of diazepam, often in conjunction with opioids to palliate dyspnoea. The spiralling cycle of dyspnoea–anxiety–increased dyspnoea can sometimes be interrupted by the use of sublingual lorazepam. This route gives the patient a degree of control in that they can take out the tablet once a benefit is gained. Supportive care in the form of behavioural modification, relaxation therapy and acupuncture may all have a place in selected patients.

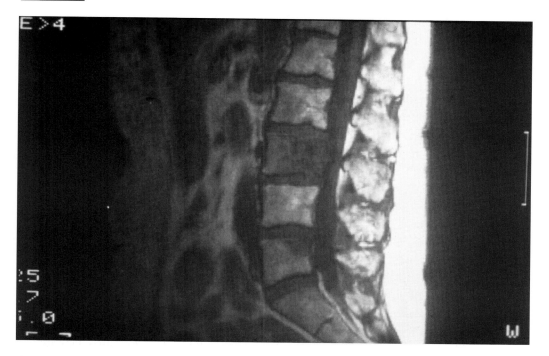

Figure 14.7 Spinal cord compression

Limb weakness/paraplegia

Limb weakness in association with personality change, confusion and/or seizures are common presenting features of brain metastases. Cerebral irradiation results in transitory amelioration of neurological defects in 60–85% of patients. Most patients will relapse after a median of 2–3 months (Lentzsch et al., 1999). Corticosteroids can result in a temporary improvement in symptoms by reducing peritumour oedema.

Spinal cord compression (SCC) (Figure 14.7) is an oncological emergency and must be considered in any woman with breast cancer who 'does not walk any more'. In most reported series of SCC, the three most common malignancies represented are lung, prostate and breast (Helweg-Larsen & Sorensen, 1994). Any of the symptoms of SCC may present in isolation but it is more common to find them in combination. Chronologically, back pain usually precedes motor weakness which in turn usually precedes sensory change and sphincter disturbance or dysfunction. It is generally accepted that the performance and neurological status of the patient at presentation is significant with respect to that patient's subsequent outcome. In a series of cancer patients found to have SCC on MRI scan, less than one-quarter of patients showed an improvement in functional ability. The majority showed either no change or a deterioration despite treatment (Cowap et al., 2000). This has major implications for the continuing care of these patients. Moreover, although this is often a manifestation of advanced disease, some women, especially those that present with SCC as the first metastatic event, will survive for a number of years and will require a high level of care for a prolonged period. SCC has the potential to change a woman's functional status dramatically. This has major implications for placement and for the palliative care services and resources that are frequently deployed in ongoing care and management.

Brachial plexopathy is a tragic consequence of both axillary recurrence and occasionally its treatment. In treatment-related disease, there is gradually progressive weakness associated with pain and sensory loss in the limb. The optimal management of this condition involves the multidisciplinary involvement of experts in pain control, lymphoedema, occupational therapy, physiotherapy and often psychological support. There are a number of support groups for patients including Radiotherapy Action Group Exposure (RAGE) and the British Association of Cancer United Patients (BACUP).

Confusion

Factors to consider in a previously asymtomatic woman with breast cancer who presents with confusion are hypercalcaemia, brain metastases, drug toxicity, electrolyte disturbance and infection.

In the past, tumour-induced hypercalcaemia (TIH) appeared to be an almost inevitable complication of metastatic bone disease. The impression is that it is becoming less common with the widespread use of bisphosphonates for bone pain and the prevention of skeletal morbidity, but there is no evidence to support such a premise. As well as confusion, the symptoms of TIH include thirst, polyuria, dehydration, nausea and vomiting, progressing to coma and death if left untreated. The prognosis of TIH is very poor unless the underlying disease can be successfully treated (Ling et al., 1995). Rehydration will reduce calcium levels by about 0.25 mmol/l but the effect is transient. Intravenous bisphosphonates are now firmly established as the treatment of choice for TIH (Body et al., 1998). Both clodronate 1500 mg and pamidronate 90 mg will result in normocalcaemia in the majority of patients within two to three days. The median duration of normocalcaemia following pamidronate is 28 days compared to 14 days for clodronate (Purohit et al., 1995). The TIH is likely to be recurrent and the success of treatment tends to decrease with repeated therapy. The wisdom of continued treatment in a woman with widespread metastatic disease in the absence of further anticancer treatment must be questioned if her symptoms can be controlled by alternative means.

Overt brain metastases occur in approximately 10–15% of women with breast cancer (di Stefano et al., 1979). As well as confusion, presenting features may include nausea and vomiting, headache and focal neurological signs. Treatment is aimed at relieving symptoms (see limb weakness/paraplegia). Cranial irradiation results in the transitory amelioration of neurological deficits in 60–85% of patients although most patients relapse after a median of 2–3 months (Lentzsch et al., 1999). The emphasis of palliative care at this stage must centre on the practical support of the patient and her family as well as the control of symptoms. Corticosteroids are often very effective at reducing the symptoms of brain metastases. Unfortunately, their long-term use is associated with distressing side-effects in the form of Cushingoid habitus, proximal weakness and skin changes, all resulting in profound effects on body image, as well as excessive hunger, hyperactivity and occasionally frank psychosis. Our policy is to avoid the use of steroids, if possible, by the aggressive treatment of pain and nausea as above. If steroid therapy is unavoidable, the use of high-dose steroid 'pulses' weaned as rapidly as possible to the lowest dose that will control symptoms will minimize steroid toxicity (Hardy, 1998). If steroids are no longer providing any benefit, they should be discontinued. Those patients remaining on steroids require close follow-up and guidance as to dose reduction.

Adverse drug effects amongst patients are not uncommon, especially in the elderly. For example, a recent systematic review has shown that 30% of patients with neuropathic pain treated with antidepressants will report adverse events, albeit minor. Similarly, the incidence of adverse events in controlled trials of anticonvulsants for the treatment of neuropathic pain varies between 25% and 50% (McQuay & Moore, 1998). The development of confusion, especially if associated with somnolence in a patient previously stable on opioids, should raise the suspicion of renal impairment. In turn, a common cause of renal impairment in the elderly is NSAID therapy.

Skin metastases and locally advanced disease

The most effective way of palliating local disease that can no longer be treated with specific anticancer therapy is by the use of appropriate wound dressings. The aim of all wound care in this situation is not to heal but to provide comfort. There are a large number of dressings available on the market with different indications for different types of wounds (Table 14.9). For advice on wound care management, readers are referred to the Royal Marsden nursing manual (Laverty, 2000).

Table 14.9. Wound management

---

(1) *Necrotic wounds*

Any brown-black hard eschar (dead tissue) must be removed to allow granulation of underlying skin; this requires debridment by surgery, hydrocolloid gels, hydrogels and/or enzymes

(2) *Sloughy wounds*

Any necrotic purulent or dead tissue must be removed to allow granulation of underlying skin; apply hydrogels, hydrocolloid gel sheets and pastes or alginate/hydrofibre dressings in cases of high exudate

(3) *Infected wounds*

These are likely to be painful and malodorous; there is likely to be surrounding swelling and erythema. Dressings need to be changed daily; systemic but not topical antibiotics may be appropriate, irrigate wounds with 0.9% NaCl and avoid topical antiseptic agents; hydrocolloid gel and hydrogel dressings are appropriate with the addition of alginate/hydrofibre or foam cavity dressings for high exudate wounds

(4) *Malodorous wounds*

This may be related to infections (see above); metronidazole gel can be used with primary and secondary dressings of choice; charcoal dressings can absorb odour

(5) *Granulating wounds*

These have a pink/red appearance and bleed easily; they therefore require protection; avoid frequent dressing changes but utilize hydrocolloid gels and sheets with hydrofibre/alginates or foam cavity dressings for high exudate

(6) *Bleeding wounds*

Initial management should be with pressure dressings and then consider adrenaline soaks, tranexamic acid (systemically and topically) and/or haemostatic swabs

(7) *Painful wounds*

Utilize breakthrough analgesia (using short-acting opioids) half an hour prior to dressing change and following dressing change as necessary; use of entonox during the procedure can be useful

---

Abdominal distension

Ascites can be classed as 'central' (where tumour involves hepatic parenchyma compressing portal venous and/or lymphatic systems resulting in elevated hydrostatic pressure and decreased oncotic pressure) or 'peripheral'. In the latter case, tumour cells on the surface of parietal or visceral peritoneum results in a mechanical block of venous and/or lymphatic drainage at the level of the peritoneal space. Patients with the central or a mixed form of malignant ascites often have increased renal sodium and water retention. In these cases, diuretic therapy with an aldosterone antagonist such as spironolactone, either alone or in combination with a loop diuretic such as frusemide, can be effective. Diuretics must be used with great caution, however, to avoid intravascular volume depletion, diminished renal perfusion and consequent prerenal failure. Studies have shown diuretic therapy to be of no benefit in the peripheral form of ascites (Pockros et al., 1992).

Abdominal paracentesis need not be a traumatic procedure if a fine bore tube such as a suprapubic catheter is used. Ultrasound can be used to identify the best site for insertion of the catheter. Some authors recommend the coadministration of intravenous albumin to reduce complications of hypovolaemia and renal underperfusion (Sharma & Walsh, 1995). It is important to inform the patient that the fluid is likely to reaccumulate but that the process can be repeated if necessary. Permanent drainage catheters left in situ have been used but are associated with a risk of sepsis (Sharma & Walsh, 1995). There are no studies which have compared the relative benefits and disadvantages of diuretic therapy and paracentesis.

Terminal care

Metastatic breast cancer is essentially an incurable disease and the overwhelming majority of women with metastatic disease will die from complications of breast cancer. It is important that women in the terminal phase of disease are cared for as actively as they are during the initial treatment phases, and that they and their families are fully supported.

Although many patients are said to want to die at home, the majority are still dying in hospital. This is not always by choice, although the proportion of patients wishing to die at home decreases as death approaches (Hinton, 1994; Higginson et al., 1998). In the UK, women with breast cancer who wish to die at home should be able to because of the widespread availability of community palliative care services, although the availability of these services does vary from region to region.

As the terminal phase approaches, all unnecessary investigations and medications should be discontinued. Some medications (e.g. antihypertensives) will no longer be appropriate whereas the continuation of others (e.g. analgesics) is essential. The requirement for food and fluids will decrease as death approaches. This must be explained to the family who need to be involved in all decisions such as the discontinuation of intravenous fluids.

The use of the subcutaneous route for the delivery of drugs to patients unable to swallow has revolutionized the care of the dying but has been criticized on the grounds of overmedicalization (O'Neil, 1994). The drugs commonly given by this route in the terminal phase are shown in Table 14.10. Diamorphine is used for pain control. It is much more soluble than morphine and is therefore more suitable for subcutaneous delivery.

Table 14.10. Drugs commonly used in the terminal phase by subcutaneous route

Indication	Drug	Usual dose range	Comments
Analgesia	Diamorphine	1/3 total/day morphine dose given	Preferred for s.c. use because of greater solubility
Terminal restlessness	Midazolam	10–60 mg/12 hr	Dose requirement may exceed 100 mg/12 hr
	Levomepromazine	12.5–100 mg/12 hr	Alternate agents should be sought if dose requirement exceeds 200 mg/12 hr, often used in conjunction with midazolam
	Haloperidol	3–15 mg/12 hr	
Antiemesis	Levomepromazine	6.25–25 mg/12 hr	Sedative effect can be used to advantage in the terminal phase as above
	Haloperidol	1.5–6 mg/12 hr	Sedative at higher dose range
Control of secretions	Glycopyrronium	400 mcg stat; 600–800 mcg/12 hr	No CNS effects, can be given to patients whilst they are awake and alert
	Hyoscine hydrobromide	600 mcg stat; 600–1200 mcg/12 hr	CNS side-effects can limit usefulness in alert patients
Miscellaneous	Dexamethasone	2–4 mg stat	Sudden cessation of long-term corticosteroids might exacerbate terminal agitation

It is important to recognize when death is imminent. The dying process is often but not always associated with the worsening of symptoms (Rees et al., 1998). The most common symptoms in a series of 200 consecutive hospice patients, in order of frequency, were noisy respirations, urinary dysfunction (incontinence or reten-

Table 14.11. Potential causes of terminal restlessness

(1) Drugs
    (a) withdrawal e.g. long-term benzodiazepines, antidepressants, barbiturates, corticosteroids
    (b) new drugs e.g. opioids, anticonvulsants
(2) Metabolic disturbance – hypercalcaemia, hepatic or renal failure
(3) Infection
(4) Fear, anxiety
(5) Pain/uncontrolled symptoms
    – distended bladder or rectum
    – painful joints resulting from immobility
    – pressure areas
(6) Confusion/delirium
    – directly related to disease e.g. brain metastases, metabolic disturbance, infection
    – related to treatment e.g. drugs
    – nonorganic disease e.g. psychological morbidity.

tion), pain, restlessness and agitation, dyspnoea, nausea and vomiting, sweating, jerking and twitching and confusion (Lichter & Hunt, 1990).

The term 'terminal restlessness' encompasses the agitation, anxiety, fear, mental anguish, general discontent and uneasiness of patients commonly seen as death approaches. As well as the obvious mental anguish, there are likely to be physical manifestations in the form of restlessness, inability to get comfortable, tossing and turning and fidgeting. This is a complex syndrome with multiple possible causes (Table 14.11), some of which can be relieved by simple measures, e.g. repositioning or toileting. On many occasions, however, it will develop because of progressive disease for which no further treatment is possible or appropriate (e.g. brain or liver metastases) or from metabolic causes that are inappropriate to correct (e.g. renal failure or TIH). In these circumstances, sedation is often used as the only means of achieving symptom control. The benzodiazepine midazolam, an anxiolytic sedative with amnesic and anticonvulsant properties, is the agent most frequently used in this context. It can be given subcutaneously either by 'stat' injections, or continuously via a syringe driver. The dose can be titrated upwards according to clinical need from a starting dose of 5–10 mg/12 hours. This drug is of particular use in patients at risk of seizure activity and those with myoclonus. Levomepromazine (a phenothiazine closely related to chlorpromazine) was originally developed as an antipsychotic. It is highly sedative and can be a useful alternative to midazolam for the control of terminal restlessness, especially in patients who are confused, anxious or agitated (O'Neill & Fountain, 1999). It is important to be aware that the dose necessary to control confusion or agitated delerium is likely to be much higher than that commonly used for the control of nausea and vomiting. Haloperidol is a phenothiazine-like drug which is less sedating than chlorpromazine, with fewer antimuscarinic effects but a tendency towards extrapyramidal side-effects. It is used 'first line' as a sedative in some units. Diazepam given rectally can avoid the need for setting up a pump in the community.

'Death rattle' is the rather unpleasant euphemism commonly used for the noise made by dying patients with retained bronchial and/or salivary secretions. It generally, but not always, occurs when patients are unconscious and heralds the dying process. It is often very distressing to attending relatives, carers and other patients in the ward. The drug most commonly used to control these 'noisy secretions' is hyoscine hydrobromide (hyoscine). This antimuscarinic agent re-laxes bronchial smooth muscle to reduce airway resistance and reduces salivary secretions. It can be given by either bolus injections or continuous infusion. Anecdotally, it needs to be given early, which can be difficult in conscious patients as the associated side-effects (i.e. confusion, hallucinations, behavioural abnor-malities) can be unpleasant, especially in the elderly. Hyoscine butylbromide (buscopan) is less lipophilic than hyoscine and therefore less likely to cause central nervous system toxicity when given early in the development of terminal secre-tions. Glycopyrrolate is the drug used 'first line' in some centres. It is more potent than hyoscine and does not cause sedation or agitation.

Continuous communication with relatives and carers is imperative. Palliative care is care of the whole family. This is particularly important for women with breast cancer who may well have young children whose continuing welfare need to be addressed. After the death of a wife, about one-third of surviving spouses will suffer a decline in physical or mental health of sufficient magnitude to justify them in seeking help (Pockros et al., 1992). Bereavement services should be offered in all cases and especially to those at risk.

Conclusion

There is little evidence on which to base practice in palliative care in breast cancer. One of the areas in which there is general agreement, however, is that palliative care should be seamless and built around the needs of the patient. This will require close cooperation between the general practitioner, the specialist breast team and the palliative care consultant.

REFERENCES

Backonja, M., Beydoun, A., Edwards, K.R. et al. (1998). Gabapentin for symptomatic treatment of painful neuropathy in patients with diabetes mellitus. *Journal of the American Medical Association*, 280(21), 1831–4.

Bierman, W.A., Cantor, R.I., Fellin, F.M. et al. (1991). An evaluation of the potential cost reductions resulting from the use of clodronate in the treatment of metastatic carcinoma of the breast to bone. *Bone*, 12 (Suppl. 1), S37–42.

Body, J.J., Bartl, R., Burckhardt, P.D. etal. (1998). Current use of bisphosphonates in oncology. International bone and cancer study group. *Journal of Clinical Oncolology*, 12, 3890–9.

Bone Pain Trial Working Party. (1999). 8 Gy single fraction radiotherapy for the treatment of metastatic skeletal pain randomized comparison with a multifraction schedule over 12 months of patient follow-up. *Radiotherapy and Oncology*, 52, 111–21.

Borgbjerg, F.M., Nielsen, K. & Franks, J. (1996). Experimental pain stimulates respiration and attenuates morphine-induced respiratory depression: a controlled study in human volunteers. *Pain*, 64, 123–8.

Breitbart, W., Chochinov, M. & Passik, S. (1998). Psychiatric aspects of palliative care. In: *Oxford Textbook of Palliative Medicine*, 2nd edn, Ed. D. Doyle, pp. 933–54.

British Association of Surgical Oncology (1999). The management of metastatic bone disease in the UK. *European Journal of Surgical Oncology*, 25, 3–23.

Bruera, E., Brenneis, C., Michaud, M. et al. (1989). Association between asthenia and nutritional status, lean body mass, anaemia, psychological status, and tumor mass in patients with advanced breast cancer. *Journal of Pain and Symptom Management*, 4(2), 59–63.

Cowap, J., Hardy, J. & A'Hern, R. (2000). Outcome of spinal cord compression at a cancer centre – implications for palliative care services. *Journal of Pain and Symptom Management*, 19(4), 257–64.

Cummings, I. (1998). The interdisciplinary team. In: *Oxford Textbook of Palliative Medicine*, 2nd edn, Ed. D. Doyle, pp. 19–30.

de Stoutz, N.D., Bruera, E. & Suarez-Almazor, M. (1995). Opioid rotation for toxicity reduction in terminal care patients. *Journal of Pain and Symptom Management*, 10, 378–84.

Di Stefano, A., Yong Yap, Y., Hortobagyi, G.N. et al. (1979). The natural history of breast cancer patients with brain metastases. *Cancer*, 44, 1913–18.

Eisenberg, E., Berkey, C.S., Carr, D.B. et al. (1994). Efficacy and safety of nonsteroidal anti-inflammatory drugs for cancer pain: a meta-analysis. *Journal of Clinical Oncology*, 12, 2756–65.

European Association of Palliative Care (1996). Morphine in cancer pain: modes of administration. *British Medical Journal*, 312, 823–6.

Faura, C.C., Collins, S.L., Moore, R.A. et al. (1998). Systematic review of factors affecting the ratios of morphine and its major metabolites. *Pain*, 74, 43–53.

Fulfaro, F., Casuccio, A., Ticozzi, C. et al. (1998). Role of bisphosphonates in treatment of painful metastatic bone disease: a review of phase III trials. *Pain*, 78, 157–69.

Hardy, J.R. (1998). The use of corticosteroids in palliative care. *European Journal of Palliative Care*, 5(2), 46–50.

Hardy, J.R. (2000). The Royal Marsden NHS Trust Symptom Control Guidelines.

Hawkey, C.J. (1999). COX-2 inhibitors. *Lancet*, 353, 307–14.

Helweg-Larsen, S. & Sorensen, P.S. (1994). Symptoms and signs in metastatic spinal cord compression: a study of progression from first symptom until diagnosis in 153 patients. *European Journal of Cancer*, 30(A)3, 396–8.

Higginson, I.J. (1999). Evidence based palliative care. *British Medical Journal*, 319, 462–3.

Higginson, I.J., Astin, P. & Dolan, S. (1998). Where do cancer patients die? Ten-year trends in the place of death of cancer patients in England. *Palliative Medicine*, 12, 353–63.

Hinton, J. (1994). Can home care maintain an acceptable quality of life for patients with terminal cancer and their relatives? *Palliative Medicine*, 8, 183–96.

Jadad, A.R. & Browman, G. (1995). The WHO analgesic ladder for cancer pain management. *Journal of the American Medical Association*, 274(23), 1870–3.

Jennings, A.-L. & Broadley, K.E. (1999). Systematic review of the palliative use of opioids in dyspnoea. 6th Congress of the European Association for Palliative Care, Geneva. Abstract No. S21/1514.

Kent, J.M. (2000). SnaRIs, NaSSAs, and NaRIs: new agents for the treatment of depression. *Lancet*, 355, 911–18.

Laverty, D. (2000). Wound management. In *The Royal Marsden NHS Trust Manual of Clinical Nursing Procedures*. In Press.

LeGrand, S.B. & Walsh, D. (1999). Palliative management of dyspnoea in advanced cancer. *Current Opinion in Oncology*, 11, 250–4.

Lentzsch, S., Reichardt, P., Weber, F. et al. (1999). Brain metastases in breast cancer: prognostic factors and management. *European Journal of Cancer*, 35(4), 580–5.

Lichter, I. & Hunt, E. (1990). The last 48 hours of life. *Journal of Palliative Care*, 6, 7–15.

Ling, P.J., A'Hern, R.P. & Hardy, J.R. (1995). Analysis of survival following treatment of tumour-induced hypercalcaemia with intravenous pamidronate. (APD). *British Journal of Cancer*, 72, 206–9.

McQuay, H. (1999). Opioids in pain management. *Lancet*, 353, 2229–32.

McQuay, H. & Moore, A. (1998). *An evidence-based resource for pain relief.* Oxford University Press.

McQuay, H.J., Tramer, M., Nye, B.A. et al. (1996). A systematic review of antidepressants in neuropathic pain. *Pain*, 68, 217–27.

Mercadante, S., Casuccio, A., Agnello, A. et al. (1999). Analgesic effects of nonsteroidal anti-inflammatory drugs in cancer pain due to somatic or visceral mechansims. *Journal of Pain and Symptom Management*, 17(5), 351–6.

NHS Executive (1997). Cancer Guidance Sub-Group of the Clinical Outcomes Group. *Guidance for purchasers – improving outcomes in breast cancer: the research evidence.* Crown Copyright. Department of Health.

Nielsen, O.S., Munro, A.J. & Tannock, I.F. (1991). Bone metastases: pathophysiology and management policy. *Journal of Clinical Oncology*, 9(3), 509–24.

O'Neil, W.M. (1994). Subcutaneous infusions – a medical last rite. *Palliative Medicine*, 8, 91–3.

O'Neill, J. & Fountain, A. (1999). Levomepromazine (methotrimeprazine) and the last 48 hours. *Hospital Medicine*, 60(8), 564–7.

Pockros, P.J., Esrason, K.T., Nguyen, C. et al. (1992). Mobilisation of malignant ascites with diuretics is dependent on ascitic fluid characteristics. *Gastroenterology*, 103, 1302–6.

Purohit, O.P., Radstone, C.R., Anthony, C. et al. (1995). A randomised double-blind comparison of intravenous pamidronate and clodronate in the hypercalcaemia of malignancy. *British Journal of Cancer*, 72, 1289–93.

Rees, E., Hardy, J., Ling, J. et al. (1998). The use of the Edmonton Symptom Assessment Scale (ESAS) within a palliative care unit in the United Kingdom. *Palliative Medicine*, 12, 75–82.

Royal College of Radiologists Clinical Information Network (COIN) (1999). Guidelines on the non-surgical management of breast cancer. *Clinical Oncology*, 11(3), Section 7, Palliative Care.

Sharma, S. & Walsh, D. (1995). Management of symptomatic malignant ascites with diuretics: two case reports and a review of the literature. *Journal of Pain and Symptom Management*, 10(3), 237–42.

Stone, P., Richards, M. & Hardy, J. (1998). Review article: fatigue in patients with cancer. *European Journal of Cancer*, 34, 1670–6.

Sykes, N. (1998). The treatment of morphine-induced constipation. *European Journal of Palliative Care*, 5(1), 12–15.

Twycross, R.G. & Fairfield, S. (1982). Pain in far-advanced cancer. *Pain*, 14, 303–10.

Twycross, R.G., Barkby, G.D. & Hallwood, P.M. (1997). The use of low dose levomepromazine (methotrimeprazine) in the management of nausea and vomiting. *Progress in Palliative Care*, 5(2), 49–53.

Vainio, A., Ollila, J., Matikainen, E. et al. (1995). Driving ability in cancer patients receiving long term morphine analgesia. *Lancet*, 346, 667–70.

Watson, M., Haviland, J.S., Greer, S. et al. (1999). Influence of psychological response on survival in breast cancer: a population based cohort study. *Lancet*, 354, 1331–6.

WHO (1996). *Cancer Pain Relief, with a guide to opioid availability*, 2nd edn, WHO.

Index